Fit & Well

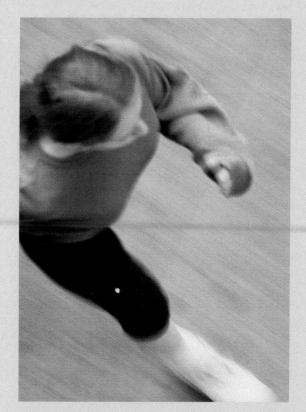

Fit&Well

Core Concepts and Labs in Physical Fitness and Wellness

FOURTH EDITION

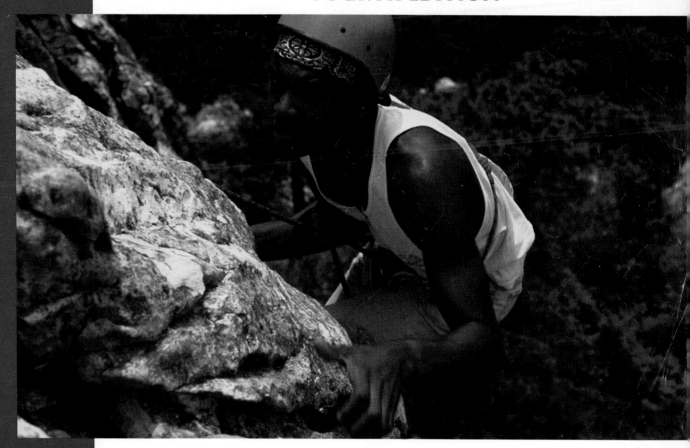

Thomas D. Fahey
California State University, Chico

Paul M. Insel
Stanford University

Walton T. Roth
Stanford University

Mayfield Publishing Company
Mountain View, California
London • Toronto

Library of Congress Cataloging-in-Publication Data
Fahey, Thomas D. (Thomas Davin)
    Fit & well : core concepts and labs in physical fitness and wellness / Thomas D. Fahey, Paul M. Insel, Walton T. Roth.—4th ed.
        p.   cm.
    Includes bibliographical references and index.
    ISBN 0-7674-1679-1
    1. Physical fitness.   2. Health.   I. Title: Fit and well.
II. Insel, Paul M.   III. Roth, Walton T.   IV. Title.
GV481.F26   2000
613.7'043—dc21   00-023785

Custom fitness edition with nutrition (Chapters 1–8)
ISBN: 0-7674-2067-5
Manufactured in the United States of America
10   9   8   7   6   5   4   3   2

Mayfield Publishing Company
1280 Villa Street
Mountain View, CA 94041

Sponsoring editor, Michele Sordi; *developmental editors,* Kathleen Engelberg, Kirstan Price, and Jeanne Woodward; *production editor,* Julianna Scott Fein; *manuscript editor,* Beverley J. DeWitt; *art director and text designer,* Jeanne M. Schreiber; *design manager,* Jean Mailander; *cover designer,* Scott Hammond; *cover photo,* © Leland Bobbe/Tony Stone Images; *art editor,* Robin Mouat; *illustrators,* John and Judy Waller; *photo researcher,* Brian Pecko; *manufacturing manager,* Randy Hurst. The text was set in 10.5/12 Berkeley Book by GTS Graphics, Inc., and printed on acid-free 45# Custom LG by Banta Book Group.

The Internet addresses listed in the text were accurate at the time of publication. The inclusion of a Web site does not indicate an endorsement by the authors or Mayfield Publishing Company, and Mayfield does not guarantee the accuracy of the information presented at these sites.

Photo Credits

Half-title page © Leland Bobbe/Tony Stone Images.
Title page © John Elk III/Stock Boston/Picture Quest.
Chapter 1   p. 1, © Index Stock Imagery; p. 4, © David Maung/ Impact Visuals.
Chapter 2   p. 19, © Ken Coleman/PhotoEdit; p. 22, © Patrick O'Lear/PhotoEdit; p. 24, © David Young-Wolff/PhotoEdit; p. 30, © Mark Burnett/Photo Researchers, Inc.
Chapter 3   p. 39, © Michael Newman/PhotoEdit; p. 45, © David Young-Wolff/PhotoEdit; p. 50, Courtesy Shirlee Stevens; p. 54, © David Young-Wolff/PhotoEdit; p. 64, Courtesy Shirlee Stevens.
Chapter 4   p. 69, © Karl Weatherly/AllStock/Picture Quest; pp. 73, 74, 80, Courtesy Neil A. Tanner; p. 88, Courtesy Shirlee Stevens; p. 89, Courtesy Neil A. Tanner; pp. 90T, 90B, 91, 92, 93T, Courtesy Shirlee Stevens; p. 94, Courtesy Neil A. Tanner; pp. 95, 96, Courtesy Shirlee Stevens; p. 97T, Courtesy Neil A. Tanner; pp. 97B, 98T, Courtesy Shirlee Stevens; p. 98B, Courtesy Neil A. Tanner; p. 99, Courtesy Shirlee Stevens; pp. 103, 104, Photos furnished by Universal Gym Equipment, Inc., Cedar Rapids, Iowa; pp. 105, 107, 108, 110, Courtesy Neil A. Tanner.
Chapter 5   p. 115, © Joel Gordon; pp. 120, 121, 122T, 122M, Courtesy Shirlee Stevens; pp. 122B, 123T, Courtesy Neil A. Tanner; pp. 123M, 123B, 124, Courtesy Shirlee Stevens; pp. 125, 129, Courtesy Neil A. Tanner; pp. 130, 131, Courtesy Shirlee Stevens; p. 132, Courtesy Neil A. Tanner; p. 137, Courtesy Shirlee Stevens; p. 138, Courtesy Neil A. Tanner.
Chapter 6   p. 145, © Index Stock Imagery; p. 152, Courtesy Shirlee Stevens; p. 153, © Frank Siteman/Stock Boston; p. 158, Courtesy Shirlee Stevens.
Chapter 7   p. 165, © Jonathan Nourok/PhotoEdit; p. 166, © Kate & David Davis/Photo Researchers, Inc.; p. 175, © Gary Conner/ PhotoEdit.
Chapter 8   p. 191, © Joyce Photographics/Photo Researchers, Inc.; p. 200, © Kathy Ferguson/PhotoEdit; p. 213, © Myrleen Ferguson Cate/PhotoEdit.
Chapter 9   p. 241, © Jonathan Nourok/PhotoEdit; p. 246, © Donna Binder/Impact Visuals; p. 253, © Spencer Grant/PhotoEdit; p. 258, © Alán Gallegos/AG Photograph.
Chapter 10   p. 269, © Brian Giza; p. 273, © Spencer Grant/ PhotoEdit; p. 276, © Joel Gordon; p. 280, © Vicki Silbert/ PhotoEdit.
Chapter 11   p. 291, © Blair Seitz/Photo Researchers, Inc.; p. 295, © Joel Gordon; p. 301, © Michael Newman/PhotoEdit; p. 303, © Amy C. Etra/PhotoEdit.
Chapter 12   p. 309, © David M. Phillips/Photo Researchers, Inc.; p. 311, © Richard Renaldi/Impact Visuals; p. 315, © Joel Gordon; p. 320, © Felicia Martinez/PhotoEdit.
Chapter 13   p. 329, © Michael Newman/PhotoEdit; p. 331, © Alán Gallegos/AG Photograph; p. 336, © David Young-Wolff/Photo Edit; p. 345, © Alán Gallegos/AG Photograph.
Chapter 14   p. 355, © Jonathan Nourok/PhotoEdit; p. 358, © Joel Gordon; p. 365, © Mary Kate Denny/PhotoEdit; p. 368, © Joel Gordon.
Chapter 15   p. 375, © David Young-Wolff/PhotoEdit; p. 378, © John Boykin/PhotoEdit; p. 382, © Robert Brenner/PhotoEdit; p. 387, © Will & Deni McIntyre/Photo Researchers, Inc.

Preface

For today's fitness-conscious student, *Fit and Well: Custom Fitness Edition with Nutrition* offers expert knowledge based on the latest findings in exercise physiology, sports medicine, and nutrition along with tools for self-assessment and guidelines for becoming fit. This Custom Fitness Edition with Nutrition contains the first 8 of the 15 chapters and two of the 4 appendixes that appear in the full version of *Fit and Well*. To create this book, we have drawn on our combined expertise and experience in exercise physiology, athletic training, personal health, scientific research, and teaching.

OUR AIMS

Our aims in writing this book can be stated simply:

- To show students that becoming fit and well greatly improves the quality of their lives
- To show students how they can become fit and well
- To motivate students to make healthy choices and to provide them with tools for change

The first of these aims means helping students see how their lives can be enhanced by a fit and well lifestyle. This book offers convincing evidence of a simple truth: To look and feel our best, to protect ourselves from degenerative diseases, and to enjoy the highest quality of life, we need to place fitness among our top priorities. *Fit and Well* makes clear both the imprudence of our modern, sedentary lifestyle and the benefits of a fitness lifestyle.

Our second aim is to give students the tools and information they need to become fit. This book provides students with everything they need to create their own personal fitness programs, including instructions for fitness tests, explanations of the components of fitness and guidelines for developing them, descriptions and illustrations of exercises, sample programs, and more. In addition, *Fit and Well* provides accurate, up-to-date, scientifically based information about key topics and issues in nutrition.

We have balanced the coverage of complex topics with student-friendly features designed to make the book accessible. Written in a straightforward, easy-to-read style and presented in a colorful, open format, *Fit and Well* invites the student to read, learn, and remember. Boxes, labs, tables, figures, artwork, photographs, and other features add interest to the text and highlight areas of special importance.

Our third aim is to involve students in taking responsibility for their fitness. *Fit and Well* makes use of interactive features to get students thinking about their own levels of physical fitness. We offer students assessment tools and laboratory activities to evaluate themselves in terms of each component of physical fitness and in the key area of nutrition.

We also show students how they can make difficult lifestyle changes by using the principles of behavior change. Chapter 1 contains a step-by-step description of this simple but powerful tool for change. The chapter not only explains the five-step process but also offers a wealth of tips for ensuring success. Behavior management aids, including personal contracts, behavior checklists, and self-tests, appear throughout the book. *Fit and Well*'s combined emphasis on self-assessment, self-development in each area of wellness, and behavior change ensures that students not only are inspired to become fit and well but also have the tools to do so.

CONTENT AND ORGANIZATION OF THE FOURTH EDITION

The basic content of *Fit and Well* remains unchanged in the fourth edition. Chapter 1 provides an introduction to fitness and wellness and explains the principles of behavior change. Chapters 2–7 focus on the various areas of physical fitness. Chapter 2 provides an overview, discussing the five components of fitness, the principles of physical training, and the factors involved in designing a well-rounded, personalized exercise program. Chapter 3 provides basic information on how the cardiorespiratory system functions, how the body produces energy for exercise, and how individuals can create successful cardiorespiratory fitness programs. Chapters 4, 5, and 6 look at muscular strength and endurance, flexibility, and body composition, respectively. Chapter 7 "puts it all together," describing the nature of a complete program that develops all the components of fitness. This chapter also includes sample exercise programs for developing overall fitness. Chapter 8 treats the important wellness area of nutrition.

For the fourth edition, each chapter was carefully reviewed, revised, and updated. The following list gives a sample of some of the new and updated material included in the fourth edition of *Fit and Well*:

- Dietary Guidelines for Americans, 2000
- New Dietary Supplements labeling requirements
- New American College of Sports Medicine (ACSM) guidelines for exercise
- "Performance aids": nutritional supplements and drugs
- The role of moderate daily physical activity in wellness
- The female athlete triad
- Benefits of exercise for older adults
- Genetically modified foods, functional foods, food irradiation, food additives, and foodborne illnesses

Taken together, the chapters of the book provide students with a complete, up-to-date guide to maximizing their fitness, now and through their entire lives.

FEATURES OF THE FOURTH EDITION

This edition of *Fit and Well* builds on the features that attracted and held our readers' interest in previous editions. These features are designed to help students increase their understanding of the key concepts of wellness and to make better use of the book.

Laboratory Activities

To help students apply the principles of fitness to their own lives, *Fit and Well* includes **laboratory activities** for classroom use. These hands-on activities give students the opportunity to assess their current level of fitness, to create plans for changing their lifestyle to improve fitness, and to monitor their progress. They can assess their daily physical activity, for example, or their level of cardiorespiratory endurance, or they can design a program to improve muscular strength or endurance.

Many of the laboratory activities in the text are also found on the *Fit and Well Interactive* Student CD-ROM, a supplement described later in the preface. Labs that appear on the CD are indicated with a CD icon. For a complete list of laboratory activities, see p. xvi in the table of contents.

Illustrated Exercise Sections

To ensure that students understand how to perform important exercises and stretches, *Fit and Well* includes three separate **illustrated exercise sections**, one in Chapter 4 and two in Chapter 5. The section in Chapter 4 covers a total of 23 exercises for developing muscular strength and endurance, as performed both with free weights and on weight machines. One section in Chapter 5 presents 12 stretches for flexibility, and the other presents 11 exercises to stretch and strengthen the lower back. Each exercise is illustrated with one or more full-color photographs showing proper technique.

Sample Programs

To help students get started, Chapter 7 offers seven complete **sample programs** designed to develop overall fitness. The programs are built around four popular cardiorespiratory endurance activities: walking/jogging/running, bicycling, swimming, and in-line skating. They also include weight training and stretching exercises. Each one includes detailed information and guidelines on equipment and technique; target intensity, duration, and frequency; calorie cost of the activity; record keeping; and adjustments to make as fitness improves. The chapter also includes general guidelines for putting together a personal fitness program—setting goals; selecting activities; setting targets for intensity, duration, and frequency; making and maintaining a commitment; and recording and assessing progress.

Boxes

Boxes are used in *Fit and Well* to explore a wide range of current topics in greater detail than is possible in the text itself. Boxes fall into five different categories, each marked with a special icon and label.

 Tactics and Tips boxes distill from the text the practical advice students need to apply information to their own lives. By referring to these boxes, students can easily find information about such topics as becoming more active, rehabilitating athletic injuries, exercising in hot weather, adding whole-grain foods to the diet, judging serving sizes, and many others.

Critical Consumer boxes are designed to help students develop and apply critical thinking skills, thereby enabling them to make sound choices in areas such as choosing a health club, exercise, and using food labels to make informed dietary choices.

Dimensions of Diversity boxes highlight fitness concerns for particular population groups. Topics include fitness for people with disabilities, gender differences in muscular strength, and ethnic foods.

Wellness Connection boxes explore the close connection between mind and body, looking at such topics as the effects of exercise on mood and mental functioning.

A Closer Look boxes highlight current topics and issues of particular interest to students. These boxes focus on such topics as benefits of physical activity, exercise machines versus free weights, diabetes, and risk factors for low-back pain.

Vital Statistics

Vital Statistics tables and figures highlight important facts and figures in an accessible format. From tables and figures marked with the Vital Statistics label, students learn about such matters as the leading causes of death for Americans and the factors that play a part in each one, the relationship between level of physical fitness and mortality, and the most popular fitness activities. For students who learn best when material is displayed graphically or numerically, Vital Statistics tables and figures offer a way to grasp information quickly and directly.

Common Questions Answered

Sections called **Common Questions Answered** appear at the ends of Chapters 2–8. In these student-friendly sections, the answers to frequently asked questions are presented in easy-to-understand terms. Included are such questions as, Are there any stretching exercises I shouldn't do? Do I need more protein in my diet when I train with weights? and Are kickboxing and Tae Bo effective forms of exercise?

Quick-Reference Appendixes

Included in the Custom Fitness Edition with Nutrition are two of the appendixes from the full version of *Fit and Well:*

Appendix B, Nutritional Content of Common Foods, allows students to assess their daily diet in terms of 11 nutrient categories, including protein, fat, saturated fat, fiber, added sugar, cholesterol, and sodium. Keyed to the software available with the text, this guide puts vital nutritional information at students' fingertips.

Appendix D, Monitoring Your Progress, is a log that enables students to record and summarize the results of the assessment tests they complete as part of the laboratory activities. With space for preprogram and postpro-

gram assessment results, the log provides an easy way to track the progress of a behavior change program.

Several specific learning aids have been incorporated in *Fit and Well*. At the beginning of each chapter, under the heading **Looking Ahead,** five or six questions preview the main points of the chapter for the student and serve as learning objectives. Within each chapter, important terms appear in boldface type and are defined on the same or facing page of text in a **running glossary,** helping students handle new vocabulary.

Chapter summaries offer students a concise review and a way to make sure they have grasped the most important concepts in the chapter. Also found at the end of chapters are **selected bibliographies** and sections called **For More Information.** These sections list books, journal articles, newsletters, organizations, hotlines, and Web sites that may be of interest to students, as well as campus and community resources.

TEACHING TOOLS

Available with the fourth edition of *Fit and Well* is a comprehensive package of supplementary materials designed to enhance teaching and learning. Included in the package are the following items:

- Instructor's Resource Binder
- Transparency acetates
- Instructor's CD-ROM
- Computerized test bank
- Nutritional analysis software
- Students on Health: Custom Video to Accompany *Fit and Well*
- *Fit and Well* Web site
- *Fit and Well Interactive* Student CD-ROM
- Nutrition and Weight Management Journal
- Daily Fitness Log
- Internet guide

The **Instructor's Resource Binder** contains a variety of helpful teaching materials in an easy-to-use form.

- The **Instructor's Resource Guide,** prepared for the fourth edition by Diane Lowry, Kennesaw State University, includes learning objectives; extended chapter outlines; lists of additional resources;

descriptions of the labs, transparencies, and handouts; and other teaching tools.

- The **Internet Handbook** provides a brief introduction to the Internet, a complete directory of all sites listed in the text and Instructor's Resource Guide, guidelines for evaluating Internet information, and worksheets with student Internet activities.

- The **Examination Questions,** completely revised and updated for the fourth edition by Rob Schurrer, Black Hills State University, include more than 1000 true/false, multiple-choice, and essay questions.

- 80 **Additional Laboratory Activities** supplement the labs that are included in the text.

- More than 120 **Transparency Masters and Handouts** are provided as additional lecture resources.

A set of 50 **transparency acetates,** half of which are in color, is also available as a lecture resource.

The **Instructor's CD-ROM** contains an **Image Bank** of more than 80 full-color images from the text, as well as images from the acetates, masters, and handouts. A complete set of **PowerPoint slides,** developed by Christopher M. Janelle, University of Florida, provides lecture outlines for each chapter of the book. The complete **Instructor's Resource Guide** can be downloaded from the CD and customized to fit any course organization. The CD can be used with both IBM-compatible and Macintosh computers.

The **computerized test bank** (Microtest III from Chariot Software Group) allows instructors to design tests using the provided test questions and/or their own questions. **Dine Healthy software** provides an easy way for students to evaluate the nutritional value of their current diet and to track their energy expenditure. Both programs are available for Windows and Macintosh.

Students on Health and Wellness: Custom Video to Accompany *Fit and Well* features students from college campuses across the country discussing how their daily lives are affected by their choices in such wellness areas as exercise, nutrition, and stress. The accompanying Instructor's Video Guide provides summaries of each segment and discussion questions. Other **videos, software,** and **multimedia,** on topics such as weight training, healthy diets, and heart disease, are also available.

Expanded for the forth edition, the *Fit and Well* Web site (http://www.mayfieldpub.com/fahey) contains fully interactive resources for both instructors and students. Password-protected instructor's resources include a **syllabus builder** that allows instructors to construct and edit their syllabus, which can then be printed or accessed online. Other downloadable instructor's materials include PowerPoint slides, the Image Bank, and the Instructor's Resource Guide; web-based testing options are also available. Student resources include the **Online Behavior Change Workbook,** Internet activities, interactive quizzes, chapter objectives and summaries, an extensive set of links, and guidelines for evaluating the credibility of online information.

New to the fourth edition, the *Fit and Well* **Interactive Student CD-ROM** is designed to help students learn and apply key concepts. From point-and-click activities featuring images from the text, students can see important concepts animated, hear pronunciations of key terms, and learn additional information. Interactive quizzes provide immediate feedback, and video segments highlight issues of special concern to students. Also included are a pronunciation guide to all key terms, all the images from the text, chapter objectives and summaries, and links to the *Fit and Well* Web site and the Online Behavior Change Workbook.

Fit and Well Interactive also includes **electronic versions of lab activities** and **the Daily Fitness Log.** The lab activities component calculates and prints the results of selected self-assessment and fitness tests; it also provides information about behavior change and a behavior change contract. The fitness log can be used to track a fitness program for up to 40 weeks; students can print out their logs and graph their progress. The CD can be used with both IBM-compatible and Macintosh computers and can be packaged with the text for students.

Other practical items for the student can also be shrinkwrapped with the text:

- **The Nutrition and Weight Management Journal** guides students in assessing their current diet and making appropriate changes.

- The **Daily Fitness Log** contains logs for students to plan and track the progress of their general fitness and weight training programs for up to 40 weeks.

- Available in a new edition is *Mayfield's Quick View Guide to the Internet for Students of Health, Physical Education, and Exercise Science, Version 2.0.* It provides step-by-step instructions on how to access the Internet; how to find, evaluate, and use online information about fitness and wellness; and many other topics.

If you have any questions concerning the book or teaching package, please call your local Mayfield sales representative or the Marketing and Sales Department at 800-433-1279. You may also e-mail Mayfield at calpoppy@mayfieldpub.com.

A NOTE OF THANKS

Fit and Well has benefited from the thoughtful commentary, expert knowledge, and helpful suggestions of many people. We are deeply grateful for their participation in the project.

Academic reviewers of the first three editions:

Mary Jo Adams, Illinois State University
Liz Applegate, University of California, Davis
Viviane L. Avant, University of North Carolina at Charlotte
E. Harold Blackwell, Lamar University
Elaine H. Blair, Indiana University of Pennsylvania
Laura L. Borsdorf, Ursinus College
Susan Brown, Johnson County Community College
Vicki Boye, Concordia College
William J. Considine, Springfield College
Arlene Crosman, Linn-Benton Community College
Robert Cross, Salisbury State University
Todd Crowder, U.S. Military Academy
Anita D'Angelo, Florida Atlantic University
Jean F. Dudney, San Antonio College
Michael A. Dupper, University of Mississippi
Robert Femat, El Paso Community College
Richard J. Fopeano, Rowan College of New Jersey
Carol A. Giroud, Monmouth University
Eunice Goldgrabe, Concordia College
Dorothy P. Haugen, Bethel College
Susan J. Hibbs, Bloomsburg University of Pennsylvania
William Hottinger, Wake Forest University
Joyce Huner, Macomb Community College
Mike Johnson, Berea College
Kenneth W. Kambis, College of William and Mary
Elizabeth Fell Kelly, Monroe Community College
Jeanne M. Mathias, Binghamton University
Patricia A. Miller, Anderson University
Christine M. Miskec, Mankato State University
Russell R. Pate, University of South Carolina
Charles J. Pelitera, Canisius College
Margaret A. Peterson, Central Oregon Community College
Jacalyn J. Robert, Texas Tech University
Steve Sansone, Chemeketa Community College
Susan T. Saylor, Shelton State Community College
Roland J. Schick, Tyler Junior College
Rob Schurrer, Black Hills State University
Eugenia S. Scott, Butler University
Charles R. Seager, Miami-Dade Community College
J. L. Sexton, Fort Hays State University
Lois M. Smith, University of Maryland, Eastern Shore
Jack Stovall, Salisbury State University
Karen Teresa Sullivan, Marymount University
Mark G. Urtel, Indiana University–Purdue University at Indianapolis
Ann Ward, University of Wisconsin–Madison
Glenn R. West, Transylvania University
Christopher J. Womack, Longwood College
Anthony Zaloga, Frostburg State University

Special fitness consultants for the third edition:

Warren D. Franke, Iowa State University
David C. Nieman, Appalachian State University
Michael Pollock, University of Florida

Technology focus group participants:

Ken Allen, University of Wisconsin–Oshkosh
Lisa Farley, Butler University
Barbara Greenburg, Butler University
Bill Johnson, Stephen F. Austin State University
Rita Nugent, University of Evansville
Patricia Dotson Pettit, Nebraska Wesleyan University
Carol Plugge, Lamar University
Steve Sedbrook, Fort Hays State University
Marilyn Strawbridge, Butler University

Academic reviewers of the fourth edition:

Joel R. Barton III, Lamar University
Phillip Bogle, Eastern Michigan University
Bill Brewer, Rochester Institute of Technology
Ronnie Carda, University of Wisconsin-Madison
Barbara Coleman, Northern Michigan University
Dale DeVoe, Colorado State University
Karen Avery Hixson, Salem College
Shahla Khan, Kennesaw State University
Alan M. Kramer, Abraham Baldwin College
Michelle Miller, Indiana University
Dennis M. Mishko, Keystone College
Deb Power, Iowa State University
Gary Preston, Gainesville College
Jerry J. Swope, Millersville University

Special fitness consultants for the fourth edition:

Patty Freedson, University of Massachusetts–Amherst
Lawrence A. Golding, University of Nevada at Las Vegas

We are also grateful to the staff of Mayfield Publishing Company and the *Fit and Well* book team, without whose efforts the book could not have been published. Special thanks to Michele Sordi, sponsoring editor; Kirstan Price, Susan Shook Malloy, Jeanne Woodward, and Kate Engelberg, developmental editors; Julianna Scott Fein, production editor; Jeanne M. Schreiber, art director; Robin Mouat, art manager; Marty Granahan, permissions editor; Brian Pecko, photo researcher; Randy Hurst, manufacturing manager; Reid Hester, marketing manager; and Jay Bauer, marketing communications specialist.

Thomas D. Fahey
Paul M. Insel
Walton T. Roth

Brief Contents

Contents

BOXES

TACTICS AND TIPS

CRITICAL CONSUMER

DIMENSIONS OF DIVERSITY

WELLNESS CONNECTION

A CLOSER LOOK

LABORATORY ACTIVITIES

◎ Indicates a laboratory activity that is also found on the Lab Activities and Fitness Log Software.

Introduction to Wellness, Fitness, and Lifestyle Management

1

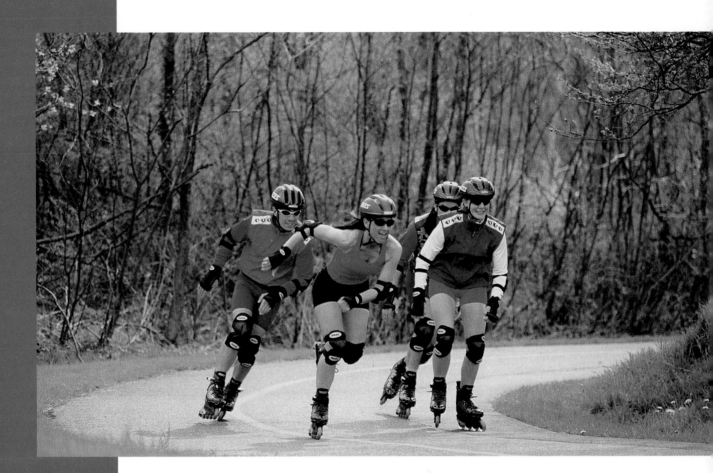

LOOKING AHEAD

After reading this chapter, you should be able to answer these questions about wellness, fitness, and behavior change:

- What is wellness?

- What are the major health problems in the United States today, and what are their principal causes?

- What behaviors are part of a fit and well lifestyle?

- What is physical fitness, and why is it important to wellness?

- What are the components of a behavior change program?

1

A first-year college student resolves to meet the challenge of making new friends. A long-sedentary senior starts riding her bike to school every day instead of taking the bus. A busy graduate student volunteers to plant trees in a blighted inner-city neighborhood. What do these people have in common? Each is striving for optimal health and well-being. Not satisfied to be merely free of major illness, these individuals want more. They want to live life actively, energetically, and fully, in a state of optimal personal, interpersonal, and environmental well-being. They have taken charge of their health and are on the path to wellness.

WELLNESS: THE NEW HEALTH GOAL

Wellness is an expanded idea of health. Many people think of health as being just the absence of physical disease. But wellness transcends this concept of health, as when individuals with serious illnesses or disabilities rise above their physical or mental limitations to live rich, meaningful, vital lives. Some aspects of health are determined by your genes, your age, and other factors that may be beyond your control. But true wellness is largely determined by the decisions you make about how to live your life. In this book, we will use the terms "health" and "wellness" interchangeably to mean the ability to live life fully—with vitality and meaning.

The Dimensions of Wellness

No matter what your age or health status, you can optimize your health in each of the following six interrelated dimensions. Wellness in any dimension is not a static goal but a dynamic process of change and growth (Figure 1-1).

Physical Wellness Optimal physical health requires eating well, exercising, avoiding harmful habits, making responsible decisions about sex, learning about and recognizing the symptoms of disease, getting regular medical and dental checkups, and taking steps to prevent injuries at home, on the road, and on the job. The habits you develop and the decisions you make today will largely de-

termine not only how many years you will live, but the quality of your life during those years.

Emotional Wellness Optimism, trust, self-esteem, self-acceptance, self-confidence, self-control, satisfying relationships, and an ability to share feelings are just some of the qualities and aspects of emotional wellness. Maintaining emotional wellness requires monitoring and exploring your thoughts and feelings, identifying obstacles to emotional well-being, and finding solutions to emotional problems, with the help of a therapist if necessary.

Intellectual Wellness The hallmarks of intellectual health include an openness to new ideas, a capacity to question and think critically, and the motivation to master new skills, as well as a sense of humor, creativity, and curiosity. An active mind is essential to overall wellness; it detects problems, finds solutions, and directs behavior. People who enjoy intellectual wellness never stop learning. They seek out and relish new experiences and challenges.

Spiritual Wellness To enjoy spiritual health is to possess a set of guiding beliefs, principles, or values that give meaning and purpose to your life, especially during difficult times. Spiritual wellness involves the capacity for love, compassion, forgiveness, altruism, joy, and fulfillment. It is an antidote to cynicism, anger, fear, anxiety, self-absorption, and pessimism. Spirituality transcends the individual and can be a common bond among people. Organized religions help many people develop spiritual health. Many others find meaning and purpose in their lives on their own—through nature, art, meditation, political action, or good works.

Interpersonal and Social Wellness Satisfying relationships are basic to both physical and emotional health. We need to have mutually loving, supportive people in our lives. Developing interpersonal wellness means learning good communication skills, developing the capacity for intimacy, and cultivating a support network of caring friends and/or family members. Social wellness requires participating in and contributing to your community, country, and world.

Environmental, or Planetary, Wellness Increasingly, personal health depends on the health of the planet— from the safety of the food supply to the degree of violence in a society. Other examples of environmental threats to health are ultraviolet radiation in sunlight, air and water pollution, lead in old house paint, and second-hand tobacco smoke in indoor air. Wellness requires learning about and protecting yourself against such hazards—and doing what you can to reduce or eliminate them, either on your own or with others.

TERMS **wellness** Optimal health and vitality, encompassing physical, emotional, intellectual, spiritual, interpersonal and social, and environmental well-being.

infectious disease A disease that is communicable from one person to another.

chronic disease A disease that develops and continues over a long period of time; usually caused by a variety of factors, including lifestyle factors.

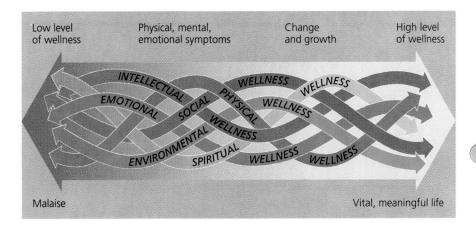

| Low level of wellness | Physical, mental, emotional symptoms | Change and growth | High level of wellness |

INTELLECTUAL WELLNESS
EMOTIONAL WELLNESS
SOCIAL WELLNESS
PHYSICAL WELLNESS
ENVIRONMENTAL WELLNESS
SPIRITUAL WELLNESS

Malaise

Vital, meaningful life

Figure 1-1 The wellness continuum. Wellness is composed of six interrelated dimensions, all of which must be developed in order to achieve overall wellness.

The six dimensions of wellness interact continuously, influencing and being influenced by one another. Making a change in one dimension often affects some or all of the others. For example, regular exercise (developing the physical dimension of wellness) can increase feelings of well-being and self-esteem (emotional wellness), which in turn can increase feelings of confidence in social interactions and achievements at work or school (interpersonal and social wellness). Maintaining good health is a dynamic process, and increasing your level of wellness in one area of life often influences many others. Some of the key links among different dimensions of wellness are highlighted in this text in boxes labeled Wellness Connection.

New Opportunities, New Responsibilities

Wellness is a relatively recent concept. A century ago, people considered themselves lucky just to survive to adulthood. A child born in 1890, for example, could expect to live only about 40 years. Many people died as a result of common **infectious diseases** and poor environmental conditions (unrefrigerated food, poor sanitation, air and water pollution). However, over the past 100 years, the average life expectancy has nearly doubled, thanks largely to the development of vaccines and antibiotics to prevent and fight infectious diseases and to public health campaigns to improve environmental conditions.

But a different set of diseases has emerged as our major health threat—**chronic diseases** such as cardiovascular disease (CVD), cancer, hypertension (high blood pressure), diabetes, osteoporosis, kidney disease, and cirrhosis of the liver. Even though people are living longer, many suffer a declining quality of life in their later years as a result of these diseases. For example, although life expectancy in the United States was 76.7 years in 1998, the average American could expect only about 64 years of healthy life. Of the chronic diseases, the most widespread and devastating are heart disease, cancer, and stroke, the three leading causes of death for Americans today (Table 1-1). Treating these and other chronic, degenerative dis-

eases is enormously expensive and extremely difficult. The best treatment for these diseases is prevention—people having a greater awareness about health and about taking care of their bodies.

The good news is that people do have some control over whether they develop CVD, cancer, and other chronic diseases. People make choices every day that either increase or decrease their risks for these diseases—lifestyle choices involving such behaviors as exercise, diet, smoking, and drinking. When researchers look at the lifestyle factors that contribute to death in the United States (see the last column in Table 1-1), it becomes clear that individuals can profoundly influence their own health risks. This knowledge has led to the realization that wellness cannot be prescribed; physicians and other health care professionals can do little more than provide information, advice, and encouragement—the rest is up to each of us.

This chapter provides an overview of a lifestyle that promotes wellness and describes a method that can help you make lasting changes in your life to promote good health. The chapters that follow provide more detailed information about fitness, nutrition, and other components of a wellness lifestyle. The book as a whole is designed to be used in a very real way, to help you take charge of your behavior and improve the quality of your life—to become fit and well.

Behaviors That Contribute to Wellness

A lifestyle based on good choices and healthy behaviors maximizes the quality of life. It helps people avoid disease, remain strong and fit, and maintain their physical and mental health as long as they live. The most important behaviors and habits are described in the following sections.

Be Physically Active Perhaps the single most important choice individuals can make to promote wellness is to be physically active. Unfortunately, a sedentary lifestyle

| TABLE 1-1 | Ten Leading Causes of Death in the United States | | | | |

Rank	Cause of Death	Number of Deaths	Percent of Total Deaths	Female/Male Ratio*	Lifestyle Factors
1	Heart disease	724,269	31.0	51/49	D I S A
2	Cancer	538,947	23.0	48/52	D I S A
3	Stroke	158,060	6.7	61/39	D I S A
4	Chronic obstructive lung diseases	114,381	4.9	49/51	S
5	Pneumonia and influenza	94,828	4.1	55/45	S
6	Unintentional injuries	93,207	4.0	35/65	S A
	Motor vehicle–related	(41,826)	(1.8)	(34/66)	
	All others	(51,382)	(2.2)	(36/64)	
7	Diabetes mellitus	64,574	2.8	55/45	D I S
8	Suicide	29,264	1.3	20/80	A
9	Kidney disease	26,295	1.1	52/48	D
10	Chronic liver disease and cirrhosis	24,936	1.1	35/65	A
	All causes	2,338,075			

Key D Cause of death in which diet plays a part
I Cause of death in which an inactive lifestyle plays a part
S Cause of death in which smoking plays a part
A Cause of death in which excessive alcohol consumption plays a part

*Ratio of females to males who died of each cause. For example, about the same number of women and men died of heart disease, but only about half as many women as men died of motor vehicle–related injuries and four times as many men as women committed suicide.

SOURCES: Martin, J. A., et al. 1999. Births and deaths: Preliminary data for 1998. *National Vital Statistics Reports* 47(25). Hyattsville, Md.: National Center for Health Statistics. Hoyert, D. L., K. D. Kochanek, and S. L. Murphy. 1999. Deaths: Final data for 1997. *National Vital Statistics Reports* 47(19). Hyattsville, Md.: National Center for Health Statistics. Pamuk, E., et al. 1998. Socioeconomic status and health chartbook. In *Health, United States, 1998.* Hyattsville, Md.: National Center for Health Statistics, pp.108–118. Doyle, R. 1996. Deaths due to alcohol. *Scientific America*, December.

is common among Americans today: More than 60% of Americans are not regularly physically active, and 25% are not active at all. The human body is designed to work best when it is active. It readily adapts to nearly any level of activity and exertion; in fact, **physical fitness** is defined as a set of physical attributes that allow the body to respond or adapt to the demands and stress of physical effort. The more we ask of our bodies—our muscles, bones, heart, lungs—the stronger and more fit they become. However, the reverse is also true: The less we ask of them, the less they can do. When our bodies are not kept active, they begin to deteriorate. Bones lose their density, joints stiffen, muscles become weak, and cellular energy systems begin to degenerate. To be truly well, human beings must be active.

The benefits of physical activity are both physical and mental, immediate and long term (see the box "Benefits of Regular Physical Activity"). In the short term, being physically fit makes it easier to do everyday tasks, such as lifting; it provides reserve strength for emergencies; and it

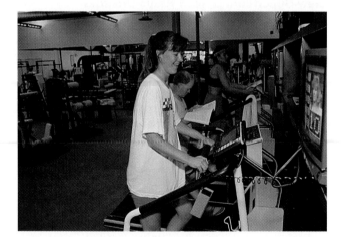

Healthy choices will help this young woman to live life actively, energetically, and fully. To enjoy health and vigor later in life, people have to cultivate wellness while they are young.

helps people look and feel good. In the long term, being physically fit confers protection against chronic diseases and lowers the risk of dying prematurely (Figure 1-2). Physically active individuals are less likely to develop or die from heart disease, respiratory disease, high blood pressure, cancer, diabetes, and osteoporosis. Their cardiorespiratory systems tend to resemble those of people

TERMS **physical fitness** A set of physical attributes that allows the body to respond or adapt to the demands and stress of physical effort.

Regular physical activity improves physical and mental health in the following ways:

- Reduces the risk of dying prematurely from all causes
- Reduces the risk of dying from heart disease
- Reduces the risk of developing diabetes
- Reduces the risk of developing high blood pressure
- Helps reduce blood pressure in people who already have high blood pressure
- Reduces the risk of developing colon cancer
- Reduces feelings of depression and anxiety
- Helps control weight, develop lean muscle, and reduce body fat

- Helps build and maintain healthy bones, muscles, and joints
- Helps older adults become stronger and better able to move about without falling
- Promotes psychological well-being

(The changes and benefits that occur in response to physical activity are discussed in Chapters 2–6.)

SOURCE: National Center for Chronic Disease Prevention and Health Promotion. 1996. *Physical Activity and Health: A Report of the Surgeon General.* Superintendent of Documents, P.O. Box 371954, Pittsburgh, PA 15250-7954.

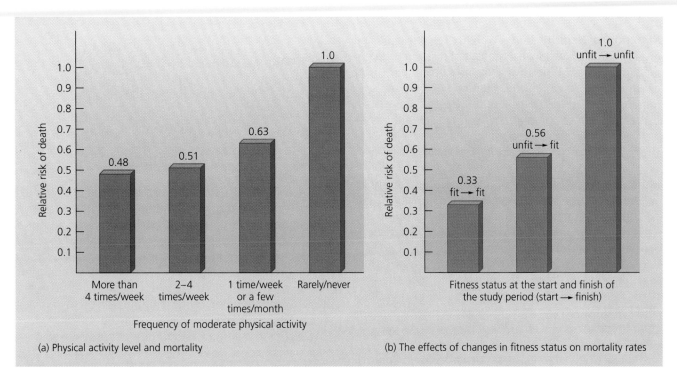

(a) Physical activity level and mortality

(b) The effects of changes in fitness status on mortality rates

VITAL STATISTICS

Figure 1-2   Physical activity, physical fitness, and mortality.   Many long-term research studies have demonstrated the benefits of regular physical activity. These benefits can be expressed in terms of risk of death—a statistic representing, in the studies shown here, the risk of death for those in each activity or fitness category compared with the risk of death for those in the least-active or least-fit category (represented by 1.0). **(a)** A 7-year study of 40,000 postmenopausal women found that the more frequently women engaged in physical activity, the lower their relative risk of death was. **(b)** An 18-year study of 9700 men that tracked changes in fitness level over a period of years found that the more physically fit the men were, the lower their relative risk of death was. Men who improved from unfit to fit during the study saw their risk of death decline by 44% compared with men who remained unfit.   SOURCES: Kushi, L. H., et al. 1997. Physical activity and mortality in postmenopausal women. *Journal of the American Medical Association* 277(16): 1287–1292. Blair, S. N., et al. 1995. Changes in physical fitness and all-cause mortality: A prospective study of healthy and un-healthy men. *Journal of the American Medical Association* 273(14): 1093–1098.

10 or more years younger than themselves. As they get older, they may be able to avoid weight gain, muscle and bone loss, fatigue, and other problems associated with aging. With healthy hearts, strong muscles, lean bodies, and a repertoire of physical skills they can call on for recreation and enjoyment, fit people can maintain their physical and mental well-being throughout their lives.

Choose a Healthy Diet   In addition to being sedentary, many Americans have a diet that is too high in calories, fat, and added sugars and too low in fiber and complex carbohydrates. This diet is linked to a number of chronic diseases, including heart disease, stroke, and certain kinds of cancer. It has been estimated that 15% of deaths in the United States can be attributed to poor diet combined with lack of exercise. A healthy diet promotes wellness in both the short and long term. It provides necessary nutrients and sufficient energy without also providing too much of the dietary substances linked to diseases.

Maintain a Healthy Body Weight   Overweight and obesity are associated with a number of disabling and potentially fatal conditions and diseases, including heart disease, cancer, and diabetes. Healthy body weight is an important part of wellness—but short-term dieting is not part of a fit and well lifestyle. Maintaining a healthy body weight requires a lifelong commitment to regular exercise, a healthy diet, and effective stress management.

Manage Stress Effectively   Many people cope with stress by eating, drinking, or smoking too much. Others don't deal with it at all. In the short term, inappropriate stress management can lead to fatigue, sleep disturbances, and other unpleasant symptoms. Over longer periods of time, poor management of stress can lead to less efficient functioning of the immune system and increased susceptibility to disease. There *are* effective ways to handle stress, and learning to incorporate them into daily life is an important part of a fit and well lifestyle.

Avoid Use of Tobacco and Use Alcohol Wisely, If at All
Tobacco use is associated with 7 of the top 10 causes of death in the United States; it kills more Americans each year than any other behavioral or environmental factor (Figure 1-3). A hundred years ago, before cigarette smoking was widespread, lung cancer was considered a rare disease. Today, with nearly 25% of the American population smoking, lung cancer is the most common cause of cancer death among both men and women and one of the leading causes of death overall.

Excessive alcohol consumption is linked to 6 of the top 10 causes of death and results in more than 100,000 deaths a year in the United States. It is an especially notable factor in the death and disability of young people,

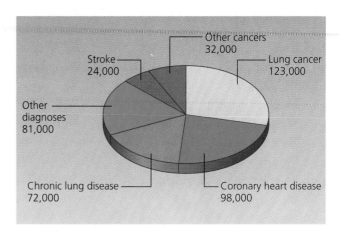

VITAL STATISTICS

Figure 1-3   The cost of smoking.   Each year, tobacco use in the United States kills 430,000 people; 1 out of every 5 deaths is smoking related. Besides the health consequences, there are financial ones, too. Smoking-related illnesses cost the nation more than $100 billion each year.   SOURCES: Shalala, D. E. 1999. *Targeting Tobacco Use: The Nation's Leading Cause of Death.* National Center for Chronic Disease Prevention and Health Promotion (http://www.cdc.gov/tobacco; retrieved August 15, 1999). Centers for Disease Control and Prevention. 1997. *Morbidity and Mortality Weekly Report 1997* 46(20): 448–451.

particularly through **unintentional injuries** (such as drownings and car crashes caused by drunken driving) and violence.

Protect Yourself from Disease and Injury   The most effective way of dealing with disease and injury is to prevent them. Many of the lifestyle strategies discussed here—being physically active, managing body weight, and so on—help protect you against chronic illnesses. In addition, you can take specific steps to avoid infectious diseases, particularly those that are sexually transmitted. These diseases are preventable through responsible sexual behavior, another component of a fit and well lifestyle.

Unintentional injuries are the leading cause of death for people age 45 and under, but they, too, can be prevented. Learning and adopting safe, responsible behaviors is also part of a fit and well lifestyle.

Other important behaviors in a fit and well lifestyle include developing meaningful relationships, planning ahead for successful aging, becoming knowledgeable about the health care system, and acting responsibly in relation to the environment. Lab 1-1 will help you evaluate your behaviors as they relate to wellness.

The Role of Other Factors in Wellness

Of course, behavior isn't the only factor involved in good health. Heredity, the environment, and access to adequate

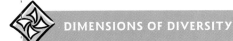
When it comes to striving for wellness, most differences among people are insignificant. We all need to exercise, eat well, and manage stress. We need to know how to protect ourselves from heart disease, cancer, sexually transmitted diseases, and injuries.

But some of our differences—differences among us both as individuals and as members of groups—do have implications for wellness. Some of us, for example, have grown up eating foods that increase our risk of obesity or heart disease. Some of us have inherited predispositions for certain health problems, such as osteoporosis or high cholesterol levels. These health-related differences among individuals and groups can be biological—determined genetically—or cultural—acquired as patterns of behavior through daily interactions with our family, community, and society. Many health conditions are a function of biology and culture combined.

When we talk about wellness issues as they relate to diverse populations, we face two related dangers. The first is the danger of stereotyping, of talking about people as groups rather than as individuals. The second is that of overgeneralizing, of ignoring the extensive biological and cultural diversity that exists among people who may be grouped together because of their gender, socioeconomic status, or ethnicity. Every person is an individual with her or his own unique genetic endowment as well as unique experiences in life. However, many of these influences are shared with others of similar genetic and cultural backgrounds. Information about group similarities relating to wellness issues can be useful; for example, it can alert people to areas that may be of special concern for them and their families.

Wellness-related differences among groups can be identified and described along several different dimensions, including the following:

- *Gender.* Men and women have different life expectancies and different incidences of many diseases, including heart disease, cancer, and osteoporosis. They also differ in body composition and certain aspects of physical performance.

- *Socioeconomic status.* People with low income levels have higher rates of many conditions and diseases, including overweight, alcohol and drug abuse, heart disease, and HIV infection.

- *Ethnicity.* A genetic predisposition for a particular health problem can be linked to ethnicity as a result of each ethnic group's relatively distinct history. Diabetes is more prevalent among individuals of Native American or Latino heritage, for example, and African Americans have higher rates of hypertension. Ethnic groups may also vary in other ways that relate to wellness: traditional diets; patterns of family and interpersonal relationships; and attitudes toward using tobacco, alcohol, and other drugs, to name just a few.

These are just some of the "dimensions of diversity"—differences among people and groups that are associated with different wellness concerns. Other factors, too, such as age, educational attainment, and disability, can present challenges as an individual strives for wellness. In this book, topics and issues relating to wellness that affect different American populations are given special consideration in boxes labeled Dimensions of Diversity. All of these discussions are designed to deepen our understanding of the concepts of wellness and vitality in the context of ever-growing diversity.

---

health care are other important influences. These factors can interact in ways that raise or lower the quality of a person's life and the risk of developing particular diseases. For example, a sedentary lifestyle combined with a genetic predisposition for diabetes can greatly increase a person's risk for developing the disease. If this person also lacks adequate health care, he or she is much more likely to suffer dangerous complications from diabetes and to have a lower quality of life. (For a discussion of how different factors affect people as members of groups, see the box "Wellness Issues for Diverse Populations.")

But in many cases, behavior can tip the balance toward health even if heredity or environment is a negative factor. Breast cancer, for example, can run in families, but it also may be associated with overweight and a sedentary lifestyle. A woman with a family history of breast cancer is less likely to die from the disease if she controls her weight, exercises, performs regular breast self-exams, and consults with her physician about mammograms. By tak-

ing appropriate action, this woman can influence the effects of heredity on her health.

National Wellness Goals

You may think of health and wellness as personal concerns, goals that you strive for on your own for your own benefit. But the U.S. government also has a vital interest in the health of all Americans. A healthy population is the nation's greatest resource, the source of its vigor and wealth. Poor health, in contrast, drains the nation's resources and raises national health care costs. As the embodiment of our society's values, the federal government also has a humane interest in people's health.

---

unintentional injury   An injury that occurs without harm being intended.   **TERMS**

TABLE 1-2   *Selected* Healthy People 2010 *Objectives*

Objective	Estimate of Current Status	Goal
Increase the proportion of adults who engage regularly, preferably daily, in moderate physical activity for at least 30 minutes per day.	15%	30%
Increase the proportion of persons age 2 and older who consume at least three daily servings of vegetables, with at least one-third being dark-green or deep-yellow vegetables.	3%	50%
Increase the proportion of adults who are at a healthy weight.	42%	60%
Reduce the proportion of adolescents who use tobacco products.	43%	21%
Reduce the proportion of college students engaging in binge drinking.	39%	20%
Increase the proportion of adolescents who abstain from sexual intercourse or who use condoms if currently sexually active.	85%	95%
Increase the proportion of people who take protective measures when exposed to sunlight.	49%	75%
Increase the use of safety belts by motor vehicle occupants.	69%	92%
Reduce the proportion of persons living in homes with firearms that are loaded and unlocked.	19%	16%
Increase the proportion of persons with health insurance.	86%	100%

SOURCE: Department of Health and Human Services. 2000. *Healthy People 2010.* Conference Edition. Washington, D.C.: DHHS.

The U.S. government's national Healthy People initiative seeks to prevent unnecessary disease and disability and to achieve a better quality of life for all Americans. Healthy People reports, published first in 1980 and revised every decade, set national health goals based on 10-year agendas. Each report includes both broad goals—such as increasing the quality and years of healthy life for all Americans and eliminating health disparities among special populations within our society—and specific, measurable targets in many different priority areas of wellness (fitness, nutrition, and so on). Healthy People targets serve as the basis for national monitoring and tracking of health status, health risks, and use of preventive services. They encompass individual actions as well as larger-scale changes in environmental and medical services.

Examples of individual health promotion objectives from *Healthy People 2010,* as well as estimates of how we are tracking toward the goals, appear in Table 1-2. (For information on the Healthy People initiative and the development of *Healthy People 2010* objectives, contact the Healthy People office or Web sites listed in the For More Information section at the end of the chapter.) As you can see, the objectives are tied closely to the wellness lifestyle described in this chapter. The principal topics covered in this book parallel the priority concerns of the Healthy

People initiative, and the approach of *Fit and Well* is based on the initiative's premise that personal responsibility is a key to achieving wellness.

REACHING WELLNESS THROUGH LIFESTYLE MANAGEMENT

The picture drawn here of a fit and well lifestyle may seem complex and out of reach to you right now. Many people fall into a lifestyle that puts them at risk. Some aren't aware of the damage they're doing, others don't want to or know how to change, and still others want to change but can't get started. These are all real problems, but they aren't insurmountable. If they were, there would be no ex-smokers, recovering alcoholics, or people who have successfully lost excess body weight. People can and do make difficult changes in their lives.

Taking big steps toward wellness may at first seem like too much work, but as you make progress, it gets easier. At first you'll be rewarded with a greater sense of control over your life, a feeling of empowerment, higher self-esteem, and more joy. These benefits will encourage you to make further improvements. Over time, you'll come to know what wellness feels like—more energy; greater vitality; deeper feelings of curiosity, interest, and enjoyment; and a higher quality of life.

How do people go about actually making changes in their health-related behaviors? One theory that has become popular in recent years is the Stages of Change model developed by psychologist James O. Prochaska. Studying thousands of people trying to make changes like quitting smoking or starting an exercise program, Prochaska found that we move through six stages as we work to change our behavior: precontemplation, contemplation, preparation, action, maintenance, and termination. In the precontemplation stage, people either deny that a problem exists or believe they have no control over it. Contemplaters recognize the problem and try to understand it but have only vague thoughts about how to solve it. The preparation stage involves making a specific plan of action, such as setting a date to quit smoking or joining a health club and buying exercise clothes. The action stage requires the most discipline and commitment; this is the phase in which change happens. The maintenance stage begins when a behavior change goal has been reached. A period of struggling against lapses and relapses can last from months to a lifetime. The final stage is reached when the problem and the temptation to relapse no longer exist and the cycle of change is complete. However, people with certain problems, such as drug addiction, may never reach this stage; avoiding relapse may be a lifelong effort.

This section introduces the general process of behavior change and highlights the decisions and challenges you'll face at each stage. For additional help and advice, work through the activities in the Behavior Change Workbook at the end of the text.

Getting Serious About Your Health

Before you can start changing a wellness-related behavior, you have to know that the behavior is problematic and that you *can* change it. To make good decisions, you need information about relevant topics and issues. You also need knowledge about yourself—how you relate to the wellness lifestyle described in this chapter and what strengths you can draw on to change your behavior and improve your health. Although knowledge is a necessary ingredient, it isn't usually enough to make you act. Millions of smokers stick to their habit, for example, even though they know it's bad for their health.

Many people start to consider changing a behavior when they get help from others. An observation from a friend, family member, or physician can help you see yourself as others do and may get you thinking about your behavior in a new way. For example, Jason has been getting a lot of stomachaches lately. His girlfriend, Anna, notices other changes as well and suggests that the stress of classes plus a part-time job and serving as president of the school radio station might be causing some of Jason's problems. Jason never thought much about trying to control the stressors in his life, but with encouragement from Anna he starts noticing what events trigger stress for him.

Landmark events can also get you thinking about behavior change. A birthday, the birth of a child, or the death of someone close to you can be a powerful motivator for thinking seriously about behaviors that affect wellness. New information can also help you get started. As you read this text, you may find yourself reevaluating some of your wellness-related behaviors. This could be a great opportunity to make healthful changes that will stay with you for the rest of your life.

What Does It Take to Change?

As we all know, change doesn't happen just because we want it to. Some people are able to change and grow fairly easily, whereas others get stuck in problem behaviors for years. What are the secrets of moving toward wellness?

Motivation   Once you recognize that you have an unhealthy behavior, you may consider changing it. But before you can change, you need strong motivation to do so. Although some people are motivated by long-term goals, such as avoiding a disease that may hit them in 20 or 30 years, most are more likely to be moved to action by shorter-term, more personal goals. Looking better, being more popular, doing better in school, getting a good job, improving at a sport, and increasing self-esteem are common sources of motivation.

You can strengthen your motivation by raising your consciousness about your problem behavior. This will enable you to focus on the negatives of the behavior and imagine the consequences if you don't make a change. At the same time, you can visualize the positive results of changing your behavior. Ask yourself: What do I want for myself, now and in the future?

For example, Ruby has never worried much about her smoking because the problems associated with it seem so far away. But lately she's noticed her performance on the volleyball team isn't as good as it used to be. Over the summer she visited her aunt, who has chronic emphysema from smoking and can barely leave her bed. Ruby knows she wants to have children and a career as a teacher someday, and seeing her aunt makes her wonder if her smoking habit could make it difficult for her to reach these goals. She starts to wonder whether her smoking habit is worth the short- and long-term sacrifices.

Social pressures can also increase the motivation to make changes. In Ruby's case, anti-smoking ordinances make it impossible for her to smoke in her dorm and in many public places. The inconvenience of finding a place to smoke—and pressure from her roommate, who doesn't like the smoky smell of Ruby's clothes in their room—add to Ruby's motivation to quit.

Locus of Control When you start thinking about changing a health behavior, a big factor in your eventual success is whether you believe you can change. Who do you believe is controlling your life? Is it your parents, friends, or school? Is it "fate"? Or is it you?

Locus of control refers to the figurative "place" a person designates as the source of responsibility for the events in his or her life. People who believe they are in control of their own lives are said to have an internal locus of control. Those who believe that factors beyond their control—heredity, friends and family, the environment, fate, luck, or other outside forces—are more important in determining the events of their lives are said to have an external locus of control. Most people are not purely "internalizers" or "externalizers"; their locus of control changes in response to the situation.

For lifestyle management, an internal locus of control is an advantage because it reinforces motivation and commitment. An external locus of control can sabotage efforts to change behavior. For example, if you believe you are destined to die of breast cancer because your mother died from the disease, you may view monthly breast self-exams and regular checkups as a waste of time. In contrast, an internal locus of control is an advantage. If you believe you can take action to reduce your hereditary risk of breast cancer, you will be motivated to follow guidelines for early detection of the disease.

People who tend to have an external locus of control can learn to view the events in their lives differently. Examine your attitudes carefully. If you find yourself attributing too much influence to outside forces, gather more information about your wellness-related behaviors. List all the ways that making lifestyle changes will improve your health. If you believe you'll succeed, and if you recognize and accept that you are in charge of your life, you're on your way to wellness.

Choosing a Target Behavior

The worst thing you can do is try to change everything at once—quit smoking, give up high-fat foods, eat a good breakfast, start jogging, plan your study time better, avoid drugs, get enough sleep. Overdoing it leads to burnout. Concentrate on one behavior that you want to change, your **target behavior,** and work on it systematically. Start with something simple, like substituting olive oil for butter in your diet or low-fat milk for whole milk. Or concentrate on getting to sleep by 10:00 P.M. Working on even one behavior change will make high demands on your energy.

Developing a Behavior Change Plan

Once you are committed to making a change, it's time to put together a plan of action. Your key to success is a well-thought-out plan that sets goals, anticipates problems, and includes rewards.

1. Monitor Your Behavior and Gather Data Begin by keeping careful records of the behavior you wish to change (your target behavior) and the circumstances surrounding it. Keep these records in a health journal, a notebook in which you write the details of your behavior along with observations and comments. Note exactly what the activity was, when and where it happened, what you were doing, and what your feelings were at the time. In a journal for a weight-loss plan, for example, you would typically record how much food you ate, the time of day, the situation, the location, your feelings, and how hungry you were (Figure 1-4). If your goal is to start an exercise program, use your journal to track your daily activities to determine how best to make time for your workouts. Keep your journal for a week or two to get some solid information about the behavior you want to change.

2. Analyze the Data and Identify Patterns After you have collected data on the behavior, analyze the data to identify patterns. When are you most likely to overeat? What events trigger your appetite? Perhaps you are especially hungry at midmorning or when you put off eating dinner until 9:00. Perhaps you overindulge in food and drink when you go to a particular restaurant or when you're with certain friends. Note the connections between your feelings and such external cues as time of day, location, situation, and the actions of others around you. Do you always think of having a cigarette when you read the newspaper? Do you always bite your fingernails when you're studying?

3. Set Specific Goals It's a good idea to break your ultimate goal down into a few small steps. Your plan will seem less overwhelming and more manageable, increasing the chances that you'll stick to it. You'll also build in more opportunities to reward yourself (discussed in step 4), as well as milestones you can use to measure your progress.

If you plan to lose 30 pounds, for example, you'll find it easier to take off 10 pounds at a time. If you want to start an exercise program, begin by taking 10- to 15-minute walks a few times a week. Then gradually increase the amount of exercise you do. Take easier steps first and work up to harder steps.

TERMS **locus of control** The figurative "place" where a person locates the source of responsibility for the events in his or her life.

target behavior An isolated behavior selected as the basis for a behavior change program.

Date ___November 5___   Day   M (TU) W TH F SA SU

Time of day	M/S	Food eaten	Cals.	H	Where did you eat?	What else were you doing?	How did someone else influence you?	What made you want to eat what you did?	Emotions and feelings?	Thoughts and concerns?
7:30	M	1 C Crispix cereal 1/2 C skim milk coffee, black 1 C orange juice	110 40 — 120	3	dorm cafeteria	reading newspaper	eating w/ friends, but I ate what I usually eat	I always eat cereal in the morning	a little keyed up & worried	thinking about quiz in class today
10:30	S	1 apple	90	1	library	studying	alone	felt tired & wanted to wake up	tired	worried about next class
12:30	M	1 C chili 1 roll 1 pat butter 1 orange 2 oatmeal cookies 1 soda	290 120 35 60 120 150	2	cafeteria terrace	talking	eating w/ friends; we decided to eat at the cafeteria	wanted to be part of group	excited and happy	interested in hearing everyone's plans for the weekend

M/S = Meal or snack   H = Hunger rating (0–3)

Figure 1-4 Sample health journal entries.

4. Devise a Strategy or Plan of Action

As you write in your health journal, you gather a lot of information about your target behavior—the times it typically occurs; the situations in which it usually happens; the ways sight, smell, mood, situation, and accessibility trigger it. You can probably trace the chain of events that leads to the behavior and perhaps also identify points along the way where making a different choice would mean changing the behavior.

MODIFY YOUR ENVIRONMENT   You can be more effective in changing behavior if you control the environmental cues that provoke it. This might mean not having cigarettes or certain foods or drinks in the house, not going to parties where you're tempted to overindulge, or not spending time with particular people, at least for a while. If you always get a candy bar at a certain vending machine, change your route so you don't pass by it. If you always end up taking a coffee break and chatting with friends when you go to the library to study, choose a different place to study, such as your room.

It's also helpful to control other behaviors or habits that are linked to the target behavior. You may give in to an urge to eat when you have a beer (alcohol increases the appetite) or watch TV. Try substituting other activities for habits that are linked with your target behavior, such as exercising to music instead of plopping down in front of the TV. Or, if possible, put an exercise bicycle in front of the set and burn calories while watching your favorite show.

You can change the cues in your environment so they trigger the new behavior you want instead of the old one. Tape a picture of a cyclist speeding down a hill on your TV screen. Leave your exercise shoes in plain view. Put a chart of your progress in a special place at home to make your goals highly visible and inspire you to keep going. When you're trying to change a strong habit, small cues can play an important part in keeping you on track.

REWARD YOURSELF   A second powerful way to affect your target behavior is to set up a reward system that will reinforce your efforts. Most people find it difficult to change longstanding habits for rewards they can't see right away. Giving yourself instant, real rewards for good behavior will help you stick with a plan to change your behavior.

Carefully plan your reward payoffs and what they will be. In most cases, rewards should be collected when you reach specific objectives or subgoals in your plan. For example, you might treat yourself to a movie after a week of avoiding extra snacks. Don't forget to reward yourself for good behavior that is consistent and persistent—if you simply stick with your program week after week. Decide on a reward after you reach a certain goal or mark off the sixth week or month of a valiant effort. Write it down in your health journal and remember it as you follow your plan—especially when the going gets rough.

Make a list of your activities and favorite events to use as rewards. They should be special, inexpensive, and preferably unrelated to food or alcohol. You might treat yourself to a concert, a ball game, a new CD, a long-distance phone call to a friend, a day off from studying for a long hike in the woods—whatever is rewarding to you.

INVOLVE THE PEOPLE AROUND YOU   Rewards and support can also come from family and friends. Tell them about your plan, and ask for their help. Encourage them to be active, interested participants. Ask them to support you when you set aside time to go running or avoid second helpings at Thanksgiving dinner. You may have to remind them not to do things that make you "break training" and not to be hurt if you have to refuse something when they forget. Getting encouragement, support, and praise from important people in your life can powerfully reinforce the new behavior you're trying to adopt.

5. Make a Personal Contract
Once you have set your goals and developed a plan of action, make your plan into a personal contract. A serious personal contract—one that commits your word—can result in a higher chance of follow-through than a casual, offhand promise. Your contract can help prevent procrastination by specifying the important dates and can also serve as a reminder of your personal commitment to change.

Your contract should include a statement of your goal and your commitment to reaching it. Include details of your plan: the date you'll begin, the steps you'll use to measure your progress, the concrete strategies you've developed for promoting change, and the date you expect to reach your final goal. Have someone—preferably someone who will be actively helping you with your program—sign your contract as a witness.

A Sample Behavior Change Plan
Let's take the example of Michael, who wants to break a longstanding habit of eating candy and chips every afternoon and evening. Michael begins by keeping track of his snacking in a journal. He discovers that he always buys candy or a bag of chips at the snack bar on campus between two of his afternoon classes. In the evenings, he eats several candy bars or a large bag of chips while he studies at home.

Next, Michael sets specific goals. He sets a start date and decides to break his plan into two parts. He will begin by cutting out his afternoon snack of candy or chips. Once he successfully reaches this goal, he'll concentrate on his evening snacking. He decides to allow 3 weeks for each half of his behavior change plan.

Michael decides to make several changes in his behavior to help control his urges to buy and eat candy and chips. He plans to bring a healthy snack, such as an apple or orange, to eat between his afternoon classes. He decides to avoid going near the snack bar; instead, he'll spend his between-classes break taking a walk around campus or reading in the student union. To help break his evening habit, he decides to study at the library instead of at home; when he's at home, he'll try studying in a different room. He also plans to stock the refrigerator with healthy snacks. Finally, Michael decides on some rewards he'll give himself when he meets his goals, choosing things he likes that aren't too expensive.

After Michael has thought through his plan to stop snacking on candy and chips, he's ready to create and sign a behavior change contract. He decides to enlist one of his housemates as a witness to his contract; he also asks his housemate to check on his progress and offer encouragement (Figure 1-5). Once Michael has signed his contract, he's ready to take action.

Putting Your Plan into Action

The starting date has arrived, and you are ready to put your plan into action. This stage requires commitment, the resolve to stick with the plan no matter what temptations you encounter. Remember all the reasons you have to make the change—and remember that *you* are the boss.

Use all your strategies to make your plan work. Substitute behaviors are often very important—go for a walk after class instead of eating a bag of chips. Make sure your environment is change-friendly by keeping cues that trigger the problem behavior to a minimum.

Social support can make a big difference as you take action. Try to find a buddy who wants to make the same changes you do. You can support and encourage each other, as well as exchange information and motivation. For example, an exercise buddy can provide companionship and encouragement for times when you might be tempted to skip that morning jog. Or you and a friend can watch to be sure that you both have only one alcoholic beverage at a party.

Let the people around you know about your plan, and enlist their support in specific ways. Perhaps you know people who have reached the goal you are striving for; they could be role models or mentors for you. Talk to them about what strategies worked for them.

Use your health journal to keep track of how well you are doing in achieving your ultimate goal. Record your daily activities and any relevant details, such as how far you walked or how many calories you ate. Each week, chart your progress on a graph and see how it compares with the subgoals on your contract. You may want to track more than one behavior, such as the time you spend exercising each week and your weight.

If you aren't making progress, analyze your plan to see what might be causing the problem. Possible barriers to success are listed in the section "Staying with It," along

- *Make your efforts cost-effective and time-effective.* Be sure your new behavior has a real and lasting value for you personally. Be realistic about the amount of time and energy you can put into it. Choose a strategy or approach that works for you. For example, many activities—from walking to bicycle racing—lead to physical fitness; for long-term success, choose one that you enjoy and that fits smoothly into your schedule.

- *Find a buddy.* A buddy can provide support, encouragement, and motivation. The fear of letting your buddy down makes it less likely that you'll take a day off, and, in a crisis, your buddy can help overcome an urge to slip (and vice versa). If you can't find a buddy who shares your goal from among your friends, family members, and classmates, try joining a group such as Weight Watchers for a ready-made set of buddies.

- *Prepare for problem situations.* If you know in advance that you're going to be in a situation that will trigger your target behavior, rehearse what you'll do. If you don't want to drink too much at a party, decide on your drink limit ahead of time, and switch to a soft drink when you reach your limit.

- *Expect success.* Change your ideas about yourself as you change your behavior. Drop your old self-image and start thinking of yourself in a new way—as a jogger, a nonsmoker, a person in control.

- *Realize that lasting change takes time.* Major life changes involve giving up a familiar and comfortable part of your life in exchange for something new and unknown. They happen one day at a time, with lots of ups and downs.

- *Forgive and forget.* If you slip—miss a workout or eat a bag of candy—focus on discovering what triggered the slip and how to deal with it next time. Don't waste time blaming yourself. Keeping up your self-esteem will help you stay with your plan; negative feelings will get in your way.

My Personal Contract for Giving Up Snacking on Candy and Chips

I agree to stop snacking on candy and chips twice every day. I will begin my program on __10/4__ and plan to reach my final goal by __11/15__. I have divided my program into two parts, with two separate goals. For each step in my program, I will give myself the reward listed.

1. I will stop having candy or chips for an afternoon snack on __10/4__ .
(Reward: __new CD__)

2. I will stop having candy or chips for an evening snack on __10/25__ .
(Reward: __Concert__)

My plan for stopping my snacking includes the following strategies:

1. _Avoiding snack bar by taking a walk or reading at student union._
2. _Eating healthy snacks instead of candy and chips._
3. _Studying at the library instead of at home._

I understand that it is important for me to make a strong personal effort to make this change in my behavior. I sign this contract as an indication of my personal commitment to reach my goal.

Michael Cook   9/28

Witness: _Katie Lim_   9/28

Figure 1-5 A sample behavior change contract.

with suggestions for addressing them. Once you've identified the problem, revise your plan. Refer to the box "Maximizing Your Chances of Success" for additional suggestions.

Be sure to reward yourself for your successes by treating yourself as specified in your contract. And don't forget to give yourself a pat on the back—congratulate yourself, notice how much better you look or feel, and feel good about how far you've come and how you've gained control of your behavior.

Staying with It

As you continue with your program, don't be surprised when you run up against obstacles; they're inevitable. In fact, it's a good idea to expect problems and give yourself time to step back, see how you're doing, and make some changes before going on. If your program is grinding to a halt, identify what is blocking your progress. It may come from one of these sources.

Social Influences   Take a hard look at the reactions of the people you're counting on, and see if they're really supporting you. If they come up short, connect and network with others who will be more supportive.

A related trap is trying to get your friends or family members to change *their* behaviors. The decision to make a major behavior change is something people come to only after intensive self-examination. You may be able to influence someone by tactfully providing facts or support, but that's all. Focus on yourself. If you succeed, you may become a role model for others.

Levels of Motivation and Commitment   You won't make real progress until an inner drive leads you to the stage of change at which you are ready to make a personal commitment to the goal. If commitment is your problem, you may need to wait until the behavior you're dealing with makes your life more unhappy or unhealthy; then your desire to change it will be stronger. Or you may find that changing your goal will inspire you to keep going. If you really want to change but your motivation comes and goes, look at your support system and at your own level of confidence. Building these up may be the key to pushing past a barrier. For more ideas, refer to Activity 9 in the Behavior Change Workbook at the end of the text.

Choice of Techniques and Level of Effort   If your plan is not working as well as you thought it would, make changes where you're having the most trouble. If you've lagged on your running schedule, for example, maybe it's because you don't like running. An aerobics class might suit you better. There are many ways to move toward your goal. Or you may not be trying hard enough. You do have to push toward your goal. If it were easy, you wouldn't need to have a plan.

Stress Barrier   If you've hit a wall in your program, look at the sources of stress in your life. If the stress is temporary, such as catching a cold or having a term paper due, you may want to wait until it passes before strengthening your efforts. If the stress is ongoing, find healthy ways to manage it, such as taking a half-hour walk after lunch. You may even want to make stress management your highest priority for behavior change (see Chapter 10).

Procrastinating, Rationalizing, and Blaming   Try to detect the games you might be playing with yourself so that you can stop them. If you're procrastinating ("It's Friday already; I might as well wait until Monday to begin"), break your plan down into still smaller steps that you can accomplish one day at a time. If you're rationalizing or making excuses ("I wanted to go swimming today, but I wouldn't have had time to wash my hair afterward"), remember that when you "win" by deceiving yourself, it's not much of a victory. If you're wasting time blaming yourself or others ("Everyone in that class talks so much that I don't get a chance to speak"), recognize that blaming is a way of taking your focus off the real problem and denying responsibility for your actions. Try refocusing by taking a positive attitude and renewing your determination to succeed.

Getting Outside Help

Outside help is often needed for changing behavior that may be too deeply rooted for a self-management approach. Alcohol and other drug addictions, excessive overeating, and other conditions or behaviors that put you at a serious health risk fall into this category; so do behaviors that interfere with your ability to function. Many communities have programs to help with these problems—Weight Watchers, Alcoholics Anonymous, Smoke Enders, and Coke Enders, for example.

On campus, you may find courses in physical fitness, stress management, and weight control. The student health center or campus counseling center may also be a source of assistance. Many communities offer a wide variety of low-cost services through adult education, school programs, health departments, and private agencies. Consult the yellow pages, your local health department, or the United Way (which often sponsors local referral services). Whatever you do, don't be stopped by a problem when you can tap into resources to help you solve it.

Being Fit and Well for Life

Your first attempts at making behavior changes may never go beyond the project stage. Those that do may not all succeed. But as you experience some success, you'll start to have more positive feelings about yourself. You may discover physical activities you enjoy; you may encounter new situations and meet new people. Perhaps you'll surprise yourself by accomplishing things you didn't think were possible—breaking a nicotine habit, competing in a race, climbing a mountain, developing a lean, muscular body. Most of all, you'll discover the feeling of empowerment that comes from taking charge of your health (see the box "Ten Warning Signs of Wellness").

Once you've started, don't stop. Assume that health improvement is forever. Take on the easier problems first, and then use what you learn to tackle more difficult problems later. Periodically review what you've accomplished to make sure you don't fall into old habits. And keep informed about the latest health news and trends. Research is constantly providing new information that directly affects daily choices and habits.

This book will introduce you to the main components of a fit and well lifestyle, show you how to assess your

1. The persistent presence of a support network.

2. Chronic positive expectations; the tendency to frame events in a constructive light.

3. Episodic outbreaks of joyful, happy experiences.

4. A sense of spiritual involvement.

5. A tendency to adapt to changing conditions.

6. Rapid response and recovery of stress response systems to repeated challenges.

7. An increased appetite for physical activity.

8. A tendency to identify and communicate feelings.

9. Repeated episodes of gratitude and generosity.

10. A persistent sense of humor.

SOURCE: Ten warning signs of good health. 1996. *Mind/Body Health Newsletter* 5(1). Reprinted by permission.

current health status, and help you put together a program that will lead to wellness. You can't control every aspect of your health—there are too many unknowns in life for that to be possible. But you can create a lifestyle that minimizes your health risks and maximizes your enjoyment of life and well-being. You can take charge of your health in a dramatic and meaningful way. *Fit and Well* will show you how.

SUMMARY

- Wellness is the ability to live life fully, with vitality and meaning. Wellness is dynamic and multidimensional; it incorporates physical, emotional, intellectual, spiritual, interpersonal and social, and environmental dimensions.

- People today have greater control over, and greater responsibility for, their health than ever before.

- Behaviors that promote wellness include being physically active; choosing a healthy diet; maintaining a healthy body weight; managing stress effectively; avoiding use of tobacco and using alcohol wisely, if at all; and protecting oneself from disease and injury.

- Although heredity, environment, and health care all play roles in wellness and disease, behavior can mitigate their effects.

- Knowledge about topics in wellness and about yourself is necessary to begin making changes in behavior. Observations by others and landmark events can help get people started on change.

- Strong motivation to change and an internal locus of control are keys to successful behavior change. It is best to concentrate on one target behavior at a time.

- A specific plan for change can be developed by (1) monitoring behavior by keeping a journal; (2) analyzing the recorded data; (3) setting specific goals; (4) devising strategies for modifying the environment, rewarding yourself, and involving others; and (5) making a personal contract.

- To start and maintain a behavior change program you need commitment, a well-developed and manageable plan, social support, and a system of rewards. It is also important to monitor the progress of your program, revising it as necessary.

- Obstacles sometimes come in the form of unsupportive people; a low level of motivation or commitment; inappropriate techniques; too much stress; and procrastinating, rationalizing, and blaming. Taking advantage of outside resources can help.

FOR MORE INFORMATION

Books

Columbia University's Health Education Program. 1998. *The "Go Ask Alice" Book of Answers.* New York: Henry Holt. *Presents answers to a variety of student-oriented health questions from the popular "Go Ask Alice" Web site.*

Prochaska, J. O., J. C. Norcross, and C. C. DiClemente. 1994. *Changing for Good: The Revolutionary Program That Explains the Six Stages of Change and Teaches You How to Free Yourself from Bad Habits.* New York: Morrow. *Outlines the authors' model of behavior change and offers suggestions and advice for each stage of change.*

Swartzberg, J. E., and S. Margen. 1998. *The UC Berkeley Wellness Self-Care Handbook.* New York: Rebus. *Provides information and strategies for promoting lifelong health.*

Newsletters

Consumer Reports on Health, P.O. Box 56356, Boulder, CO 80323.

Harvard Health Letter, P.O. Box 420300, Palm Coast, FL 32142 (http://www.health.harvard.edu/newsletters/hltext.html).

Harvard Men's Health Watch, P.O. Box 420099, Palm Coast, FL 32142.

Harvard Women's Health Watch, P.O. Box 420068, Palm Coast, FL 32142.

HealthNews, P.O. Box 52924, Boulder, CO 80322 (http://www.onhealth.com).

Mayo Clinic Health Letter, P.O. Box 53889, Boulder, CO 80322.

Mind/Body Health, P.O. Box 381069, Boston, MA 02238.

SickbayToday, 510 Broadhollow Road, Suite 300, Melville, NY 11747 (http://sickbay.com).

University of California, Berkeley Wellness Letter, P.O. Box 420148, Palm Coast, FL 32142 (http://www.berkeleywellness.com).

Organizations, Hotlines, and Web Sites

The Internet addresses (also called uniform resource locators, or URLs) listed here were accurate at the time of publication. If a site has moved and there is no link to the new URL, you can use a search engine to locate the new site.

Centers for Disease Control and Prevention. The CDC provides materials on HIV infection, national health statistics, governmental nutrition recommendations, and much more.

> 404-332-4555 (CDC Infoline); 888-CDC-FAXX (CDC fax)
> http://www.cdc.gov

Go Ask Alice. Provides answers to student questions about stress, sexuality, fitness, and many other wellness topics.

> http://www.goaskalice.columbia.edu

Healthfinder. A gateway to online publications, Web sites, support and self-help groups, and agencies and organizations that produce reliable health information.

> http://www.healthfinder.gov

Healthy People 2000/Healthy People 2010. Provide information on Healthy People objectives and priority areas.

> 800-367-4725
> http://odphp.osophs.dhhs.gov/pubs/hp2000
> http://web.health.gov/healthypeople

National Health Information Center (NHIC). Provides information on more than 100 health-related organizations and an extensive list of toll-free numbers.

> 800-336-4797
> http://nhic-nt.health.org

National Women's Health Information Center. Provides information and answers to frequently asked questions.

> 800-994-WOMAN
> http://www.4woman.org

NOAH: New York Online Access to Health. Provides consumer health information in both English and Spanish.

> http://www.noah.cuny.edu

The following are just a few of the many sites that provide consumer-orientated information on a variety of health issues:

American Medical Association Health Insight:
> http://www.ama-assn.org/consumer.htm

Dr. Koop's Community: http://www.drkoop.com

HealthIndex Health Information Directory:
> http://www.healthindex.org

InteliHealth: Johns Hopkins Health Information:
> http://www.intelihealth.com

Mayo Health Oasis: http://www.mayohealth.org

OnHealth: http://www.onhealth.com

Sickbay: http://www.sickbay.com

The following sites provide daily health news updates:

CNN/Health: http://www.cnn.com/Health

HealthScout: http://www.healthscout.com

New York Times Your Health Daily:
> http://www.yourhealthdaily.com

Yahoo Health News: http://dailynews.yahoo.com/headlines/hl

SELECTED BIBLIOGRAPHY

American Cancer Society. 2000. *Cancer Facts and Figures 2000.* Atlanta: American Cancer Society.

American Heart Association. 2000. *2000 Heart and Stroke Statistical Update.* Dallas, Tex.: American Heart Association.

Blair, S. N., et al. 1996. Influences of cardiorespiratory fitness and other precursors on cardiovascular disease and all-cause mortality in men and women. *Journal of the American Medical Association* 276(3): 205–210.

Bureau of the Census. 1999. *Resident Population of the United States: Estimates by Sex, Race, and Hispanic Origin* (http://www.census.gov/population/estimates/nation/intfile3–1.txt; retrieved July 27, 1999).

Curl, W. W. 2000. Aging and exercise: Are they compatible in women? *Clinical Orthopedics and Related Research* 372: 151–158.

Department of Health and Human Services. 2000. *Healthy People 2010.* Conference Edition. Washington, D.C.: DHHS.

Department of Health and Human Services. 1996. *Physical Activity and Health: A Report of the Surgeon General.* Atlanta, Ga.: DHHS.

Douglas, K. A., et al. 1997. Results from the 1995 National College Health Risk Behavior Survey. *Journal of American College Health* 46(2): 55–56.

Fuller, P. R., et al. 1998. Effects of a personalized system of skill acquisition and an educational program in the treatment of obesity. *Addictive Behavior* 23(1): 97–100.

Grace, T. W. 1997. Health problems of college students. *Journal of American College Health* 45(6): 243–250.

Hunink, M. G. M., et al. 1997. The recent decline in mortality from coronary heart disease, 1980–1990. *Journal of the American Medical Association* 277(7): 535–542.

King, A. C., et al. 2000. Comparative effects of two physical activity programs on measured and perceived physical functioning and other health-related quality of life outcomes in older adults. *Journals of Gerontology. Series A, Biological Sciences and Medical Sciences* 55(2): M74–83.

Lee, I. M., C. C. Hsieh, and R. S. Paffenbarger. 1995. Exercise intensity and longevity in men. The Harvard Alumni Health Study. *Journal of the American Medical Association* 273(15): 1179–1184.

National Center for Health Statistics. 1998. *Health, United States, 1998.* Hyattsville, Md.: Public Health Service.

Ni, M. C., B. M. Margetts, and V. M. Speller. 1997. Applying the stages-of-change model to dietary change. *Nutrition Reviews* 55(1 Pt. 1): 10–16.

Nieman, D. C. 1999. *Exercise Testing and Prescription: A Health-Related Approach,* 4th ed. Mountain View, Calif.: Mayfield.

Reif, C. J., and A. B. Elster. 1998. Adolescent preventive services. *Primary Care* 25(1): 1–21.

Wei, M. et al., 2000. Low cardiorespiratory fitness and physical inactivity as predictors of mortality in men with type 2 diabetes. *Annals of Internal Medicine* 132(8): 605–611.

LAB 1-1 *Lifestyle Evaluation*

The following brief test will give you some idea about how your current lifestyle compares with the lifestyle recommended for wellness. For each question, choose the answer that best describes your behavior; then add up your score for each section.

Exercise/Fitness

	Almost Always	Sometimes	Never
1. I engage in moderate exercise, such as brisk walking or swimming, for 20–60 minutes, three to five times a week.	4	1	0
2. I do exercises to develop muscular strength and endurance at least twice a week.	2	1	0
3. I spend some of my leisure time participating in individual, family, or team activities, such as gardening, bowling, or softball.	2	1	0
4. I maintain a healthy body weight, avoiding overweight and underweight.	2	1	0

Exercise/Fitness Score: _____

Nutrition

	Almost Always	Sometimes	Never
1. I eat a variety of foods each day, including five or more servings of fruits and/or vegetables.	3	1	0
2. I limit the amount of fat and saturated fat in my diet.	3	1	0
3. I avoid skipping meals.	2	1	0
4. I limit the amount of salt and sugar I eat.	2	1	0

Nutrition Score: _____

Tobacco Use

If you never use tobacco, enter a score of 10 for this section and go to the next section.

	Almost Always	Sometimes	Never
1. I avoid using tobacco.	2	1	0
2. I smoke only low-tar-and-nicotine cigarettes, or I smoke a pipe or cigars, or I use smokeless tobacco.	2	1	0

Tobacco Use Score: _____

Alcohol and Drugs

	Almost Always	Sometimes	Never
1. I avoid alcohol, or I drink no more than 1 (women) or 2 (men) drinks a day.	4	1	0
2. I avoid using alcohol or other drugs as a way of handling stressful situations or the problems in my life.	2	1	0
3. I am careful not to drink alcohol when taking medications (such as cold or allergy medications) or when pregnant.	2	1	0
4. I read and follow the label directions when using prescribed and over-the-counter drugs.	2	1	0

Alcohol and Drugs Score: _____

Emotional Health

1. I enjoy being a student, and I have a job or do other work that I enjoy. 2 1 0
2. I find it easy to relax and express my feelings freely. 2 1 0
3. I manage stress well. 2 1 0
4. I have close friends, relatives, or others whom I can talk to about personal matters and call on for help when needed. 2 1 0
5. I participate in group activities (such as community or church organizations) or hobbies that I enjoy. 2 1 0

Emotional Health Score: _____

Safety

1. I wear a safety belt while riding in a car. 2 1 0
2. I avoid driving while under the influence of alcohol or other drugs. 2 1 0
3. I obey traffic rules and the speed limit when driving. 2 1 0
4. I read and follow instructions on the labels of potentially harmful products or substances, such as household cleaners, poisons, and electrical appliances. 2 1 0
5. I avoid smoking in bed. 2 1 0

Safety Score: _____

Disease Prevention

1. I know the warning signs of cancer, heart attack, and stroke. 2 1 0
2. I avoid overexposure to the sun and use sunscreen. 2 1 0
3. I get recommended medical screening tests (such as blood pressure checks and Pap tests), immunizations, and booster shots. 2 1 0
4. I practice monthly breast/testicle self-exams. 2 1 0
5. I am not sexually active *or* I have sex with only one mutually faithful, uninfected partner *or* I always engage in "safer sex" (using condoms), *and* I do not share needles to inject drugs. 2 1 0

Disease Prevention Score: _____

What Your Scores Mean

Scores of 9 and 10   Excellent! Your answers show that you are aware of the importance of this area to your health. More important, you are putting your knowledge to work for you by practicing good health habits. As long as you continue to do so, this area should not pose a serious health risk. It's likely that you are setting an example for your family and friends to follow. Because you got a very high test score on this part of the test, you may want to consider other areas where your scores indicate room for improvement.

Scores of 6 to 8   Your health practices in this area are good, but there is room for improvement. Look again at the items you answered with a "Sometimes" or "Never." What changes can you make to improve your score? Even a small change can often help you achieve better health.

Scores of 3 to 5   Your health risks are showing! Would you like more information about the risks you're facing and about why it's important for you to change these behaviors? Perhaps you need help in deciding how to successfully make the changes you desire. In either case, help is available.

Scores of 0 to 2   Obviously, you were concerned enough about your health to take the test, but your answers show that you may be taking serious and unnecessary risks with your health. Perhaps you are not aware of the risks and what to do about them. You can easily get the information and help you need to improve, if you wish. The next step is up to you.

The behaviors covered in this test are recommended for most Americans, but some may not apply to people with certain chronic diseases or disabilities or to pregnant women, who may require special advice from their physician.

SOURCE: Adapted from *Healthstyle: A Self-Test*, developed by the U.S. Public Health Service.

Basic Principles of Physical Fitness

2

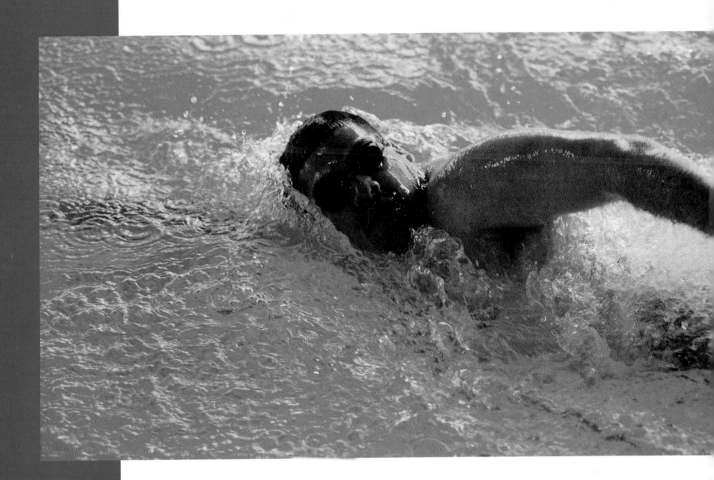

LOOKING AHEAD

After reading this chapter, you should be able to answer these questions about physical fitness:

- How much exercise is recommended for developing health and fitness?

- What are the components of physical fitness, and how does each one affect wellness?

- What is the goal of physical training, and what are the basic principles of training?

- What principles are involved in designing a well-rounded exercise program? What kinds of activities should be included?

- What steps can be taken to make an exercise program safe, effective, and successful?

Any list of the benefits of physical activity is impressive. A physically active lifestyle helps you generate more energy, control your weight, manage stress, and boost your immune system. It provides psychological and emotional benefits, contributing to your sense of competence and well-being. It offers protection against heart disease, diabetes, high blood pressure, osteoporosis, some types of cancer, and even premature death. Exercise increases your physical capacity so that you are better able to meet the challenges of daily life with energy and vigor. Although people vary greatly in the levels of physical fitness and performance they can ultimately achieve, the benefits of regular physical activity are available to everyone. (For more on the benefits of exercise, see the box "A Runner's Rationale.")

This chapter provides an overview of physical fitness. It explains how lifestyle physical activity and more formal exercise programs contribute to wellness. It describes the components of fitness, the basic principles of physical training, and the essential elements of a well-rounded exercise program. Chapters 3–6 provide an in-depth look at each of the elements of a fitness program; Chapter 7 will help you put all these elements together into a complete, personalized program.

PHYSICAL ACTIVITY AND EXERCISE FOR HEALTH AND FITNESS

Despite the many benefits of an active lifestyle, levels of physical activity have declined in recent years and remain low for all populations of Americans (Table 2-1). More than 60% of U.S. adults do not engage in recommended amounts of physical activity; 25% are not active at all. In the summer of 1996, the U.S. Surgeon General published *Physical Activity and Health,* a landmark report designed to reverse these trends and get Americans moving. Here is a summary of its findings:

- People of all ages benefit from regular physical activity.

- People can obtain significant health benefits by including a moderate amount of physical activity on most, if not all, days of the week. Through a modest increase in daily activity, most Americans can improve their health and quality of life.

- Additional health benefits can be gained through greater amounts of physical activity. People who can

VITAL STATISTICS

TABLE 2-1	*Adults Who Regularly Engage in Physical Activity*	
	Moderate Intensity[a]	High Intensity[b]
Overall	20.1%	14.4%
Sex		
Men	21.5	12.9
Women	18.9	15.8
Ethnicity		
White	20.8	15.3
Black	15.2	9.4
Hispanic (Latino)	20.1	11.9
Education		
Less than 12 years	15.6	8.2
12 years	17.8	11.5
13–15 years	22.7	14.9
16 or more years	23.5	21.9
Income		
Less than $10,000	17.6	9.0
$10,000–$19,999	18.7	10.8
$20,000–$34,999	20.3	14.2
$35,000–$49,999	20.9	16.3
$50,000 or more	23.5	20.5
Geographic region		
Northeast	20.2	13.8
North Central	18.2	13.7
South	19.0	13.8
West	24.0	16.8

[a]Adults who engage in moderate-intensity physical activity five or more times per week for at least 30 minutes per session.
[b]Adults who engage in high-intensity physical activity three or more times per week for at least 20 minutes per session.

SOURCE: Department of Health and Human Services. 1996. *Physical Activity and Health: A Report of the Surgeon General.* Atlanta, Ga.: DHHS.

maintain a regular regimen of more vigorous or longer-duration activity are likely to obtain even greater benefits.

Evidence is growing that simply becoming more physically active may be the single most important lifestyle change for promoting health and well-being.

Physical Activity on a Continuum

Physical activity can be defined as any body movement carried out by the skeletal muscles and requiring energy. Different types of physical activity can be arranged on a continuum based on the amount of energy they require. Quick, easy movements such as standing up or walking down a hallway require little energy or effort; more intense, sustained activities such as cycling 5 miles or running in a race require considerably more.

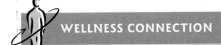
Much of the attention surrounding exercise focuses on its benefits for physical health. But for many exercisers, improved health and longevity are only part of the reason they begin and continue to train. In this selection, long-time Runner's World *columnist George Sheehan highlights the diverse and interconnected nature of the wellness benefits of exercise.*

When I lecture, I often begin with a short film on running. The opening scene is the start of the Boston Marathon. Thousands of runners stream toward the camera, while the narrator remarks that these marathoners are only the visible elite of millions of runners now surging along the world's roads and filling its parks. "The nonrunner watches," he says, "and wonders—*why?*"

The audience almost always laughs at that question. To the people in the film, running is normal; to those in my audience, running—especially marathon running—is a mystery. When the film ends and the lights go on, I ascend the stage and address the question, Why do people run?

My answer is direct: Their lives depend upon it. People begin running for any number of motives, but we stick to it for one basic reason—to find out who we really are. Running or some other form of exercise is essential in the drive to become and perpetuate the ultimate self, because finding out who we are means finding out what our limits are—and we have to *test* ourselves to do that.

I run because my life in all its aspects depends upon it. The length of my life, certainly; the hours in my day, just as surely. The person I am, my productivity, my creativity, my pursuit of happiness—all are conditioned and determined by my hours on the road.

Most non-exercisers are unaware of this global, whole-life effect of athletic training. The experts—physicians, psychologists, sociologists, teachers, even philosophers—carve out discrete territories in which they operate. They focus on certain parts of our lives, but not life in its totality—not Life with a capital *L.*

The physician tells me that my life span is related to my lifestyle. When I began running, my coronary risk factors practically disappeared. I stopped smoking, my weight returned to what it had been in college, and my blood pressure didn't rise as I got older. Running also added hours to my day. My physical

work capacity is far greater than it was when I was 38 years old and (presumably) in my prime. Clearly, my body benefits from fitness.

But my mind does, too. The psychologist tells me that. The negative feelings—anxiety and depression, anger and hostility—are all reduced by training. While these destructive feelings diminish, constructive ones such as self-esteem and self-confidence rise.

And the public me benefits also: The sociologist argues that my professional success is linked to the fitness I earn from running. It is no longer simply survival of the fittest, it is also success to the fittest. Fit people occupy the upper echelons in education, position, and salary.

The educator views my running and racing as a laboratory where I learn about such things as sacrifice and solitude, courage and cooperation, victory and defeat. And the philosopher reminds me that creative thinking requires the inner and outer solitude that running confers.

So it goes: Each specialist sees the role of exercise through the prism of that particular specialty. I explain this fragmentation to the audience, and then I tell them that no one piece of the puzzle is enough. Each of these experts sees only a bit of me. But I am not a cholesterol level, I am not a Rorshach profile. I am not an ergometer reading or an IQ. I am a physician, a student, a problem solver. I am also a parent, a sibling, a lover, a friend.

But none of these entirely defines me. "I absolutely deny," wrote D. H. Lawrence, "that I am a soul, or a body or an intelligence, or a nervous system or a bunch of glands, or any of the rest of the bits of me. The whole is greater than the sum of my parts. . . . I am a total living human being."

I look out over the audience and ask them, "Are you content with this total living person you are now?" American writer Lewis Mumford once remarked that today might be a fair sample of eternity. If so, who you are today would be the eternal you, the final product of your years on earth. If this were your last day, would you be satisfied?

There it is—my *why* of running, my reason for exercise—no less than the creation of the human being I become. [1986]

Runner's World, January 1995. Reprinted with the permission of the estate of George Sheehan.

Exercise refers to a subset of physical activity—planned, structured, repetitive movement of the body designed specifically to improve or maintain physical fitness. As discussed in Chapter 1, physical fitness is a set of physical attributes that allows the body to respond or adapt to the demands and stress of physical effort—to perform moderate-to-vigorous levels of physical activity without becoming overly tired. Levels of fitness depend on such physiological factors as the heart's ability to pump blood and the size of muscle fibers. To develop fitness, a person must perform enough physical activity to stress the body and cause

long-term physiological changes. Only exercise will develop fitness. Knowing this is important for setting goals and developing a program.

Lifestyle Physical Activity for Health Promotion

The Surgeon General's report recommends that all Americans include a moderate amount of physical activity on most, preferably all, days of the week. The report suggests a goal of expending 150 calories a day, or about 1000 calories a week, in physical activity. The same amount of activity can be obtained in longer

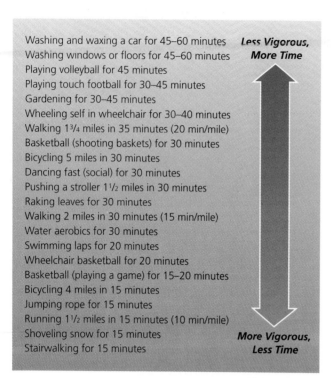

Washing and waxing a car for 45–60 minutes — **Less Vigorous, More Time**
Washing windows or floors for 45–60 minutes
Playing volleyball for 45 minutes
Playing touch football for 30–45 minutes
Gardening for 30–45 minutes
Wheeling self in wheelchair for 30–40 minutes
Walking 1¾ miles in 35 minutes (20 min/mile)
Basketball (shooting baskets) for 30 minutes
Bicycling 5 miles in 30 minutes
Dancing fast (social) for 30 minutes
Pushing a stroller 1½ miles in 30 minutes
Raking leaves for 30 minutes
Walking 2 miles in 30 minutes (15 min/mile)
Water aerobics for 30 minutes
Swimming laps for 20 minutes
Wheelchair basketball for 20 minutes
Basketball (playing a game) for 15–20 minutes
Bicycling 4 miles in 15 minutes
Jumping rope for 15 minutes
Running 1½ miles in 15 minutes (10 min/mile)
Shoveling snow for 15 minutes
Stairwalking for 15 minutes — **More Vigorous, Less Time**

Figure 2-1 Examples of moderate amounts of physical activity.
A moderate amount of physical activity is roughly equivalent to physical activity that uses approximately 150 calories of energy a day, or 1000 calories a week. Some activities can be performed at various intensities; the suggested durations correspond to expected intensity of effort.   SOURCE: Department of Health and Human Services. 1996. *Physical Activity and Health: A Report of the Surgeon General.* Atlanta, Ga.: DHHS.

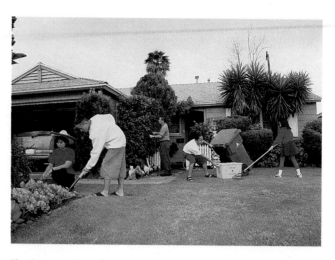

The Surgeon General recommends that all Americans accumulate at least 30 minutes of moderate-intensity activity on most days of the week. Yard work is one of many household chores that can contribute to your daily total of physical activity.

sessions of moderately intense activities as in shorter sessions of more strenuous activities. Thus, 30 minutes of brisk walking or leaf raking is equivalent to 15 minutes of running or snow shoveling. Examples of moderate physical activities are given in Figure 2-1.

In this lifestyle approach to physical activity, the daily total of activity can be accumulated in multiple short bouts—for example, two 10-minute bicycle rides to and from class and a brisk 15-minute walk to the post office. People can choose activities that they find enjoyable and that fit into their daily routine; everyday tasks at school, work, and home can be structured to contribute to the daily activity total. (See the box "Becoming More Active" for suggestions.) In addition to recommending moderate-intensity physical activity, the Surgeon General's report recommends that people perform resistance training (exercising against an opposing force such as a weight) at least twice a week to build and maintain muscular strength.

By increasing lifestyle physical activity in accordance with the guidelines given in the Surgeon General's report, people can expect to significantly improve their health and well-being. If all the Americans who are now completely sedentary were to adopt a more active lifestyle, there would be enormous benefit to the public's health and to individual well-being. Such a program may not, however, increase physical fitness.

Exercise Programs to Develop Physical Fitness   The Surgeon General's report also summarizes the benefits of more formal exercise programs. It concludes that people can obtain even greater health benefits by increasing the duration and intensity of activity. Thus, a person who engages in a structured, formal exercise program designed to measurably improve physical fitness will obtain even greater improvements in quality of life and greater reductions in disease and mortality risk.

How Much Physical Activity Is Enough?

Some experts feel that people get most of the health benefits of an exercise program simply by becoming more active over the course of the day. Others feel that the activity goal set by the lifestyle approach is too low; they argue that people should exercise long enough and intensely enough to improve their body's capacity for exercise—that is, to improve physical fitness. More research is needed to clarify the health effects of moderate-intensity vs. high-intensity exercise and continuous vs. intermittent exercise. However, there is probably truth in both of these positions.

Regular physical activity, regardless of intensity, makes you healthier and can help protect you from many chronic diseases. However, exercising at low intensities does little to improve physical fitness. Although you get many of the health benefits of exercise by simply being more active, you obtain even more benefits when you are

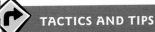
- Take the stairs instead of the elevator or escalator.
- Walk to the mailbox, post office, store, bank, or library whenever possible.
- Park your car a mile or even just a few blocks from your destination, and walk briskly.
- Do at least one chore every day that requires physical activity: wash the windows or your car, clean your room or house, mow the lawn, rake the leaves.
- Take study or work breaks to avoid sitting for more than 30 minutes at a time. Get up and walk around the library, your office, or your home or dorm; go up and down a flight of stairs.

- Stretch when you stand in line or watch TV.
- When you take public transportation, get off one stop down the line and walk to your destination.
- Go dancing instead of to a movie.
- Walk to visit a neighbor or friend rather than calling him or her on the phone. Go for a walk while you chat.
- Put your remote controls in storage; when you want to change TV or radio stations, get up and do it by hand.
- Seize every opportunity to get up and walk around. Move more and sit less.

physically fit. In addition to long-term health benefits, fitness also significantly contributes to quality of life. Fitness can give you freedom—freedom to move your body the way you want. Fit people have more energy and better body control. They can enjoy a more active lifestyle—cycling, hiking, skiing, and so on—than their more sedentary counterparts. Even if you don't like sports, you need physical energy and stamina in your daily life and for many nonsport leisure activities—visiting museums, playing with children, gardening, and so on.

Where does this leave you? Most experts agree that some physical activity is better than none, but that more—as long as it does not result in injury—is probably better than some. At the very least, strive to become more active and meet the goal set by the Surgeon General's report of using about 150 calories a day in physical activity. Choose to be active whenever you can. For even better health and well-being, participate in a structured exercise program that develops physical fitness. Any increase in physical activity will contribute to your health and well-being, now and in the future.

Next, let's take a closer look at the components of physical fitness and the basic principles of fitness training.

HEALTH-RELATED COMPONENTS OF PHYSICAL FITNESS

Physical fitness has many components, some related to general health and others related more specifically to particular sports or activities. The five components of fitness most important for health are cardiorespiratory endurance, muscular strength, muscular endurance, flexibility, and body composition. Health-related fitness contributes to your capacity to enjoy life, helps your body withstand physical and psychological challenges, and protects you from chronic disease.

Cardiorespiratory Endurance

Cardiorespiratory endurance is the ability to perform prolonged, large-muscle, dynamic exercise at moderate-to-high levels of intensity. It depends on such factors as the ability of the lungs to deliver oxygen from the environment to the bloodstream, the heart's capacity to pump blood, the ability of the nervous system and blood vessels to regulate blood flow, and the capability of the body's chemical systems to use oxygen and process fuels for exercise.

When levels of cardiorespiratory fitness are low, the heart has to work very hard during normal daily activities and may not be able to work hard enough to sustain high-intensity physical activity in an emergency. As cardiorespiratory fitness improves, the heart begins to function more efficiently. It doesn't have to work as hard at rest or during low levels of exercise. The heart pumps more blood per heartbeat, resting heart rate slows, blood volume increases, blood supply to the tissues improves, the body is better able to cool itself, and resting blood pressure decreases. A healthy heart can better withstand the strains of everyday life, the stress of occasional emergencies, and the wear and tear of time. Endurance training also improves the functioning of the chemical systems, particularly in the muscles and liver, thereby enhancing the body's ability to use energy supplied by food.

Cardiorespiratory endurance is a central component of health-related fitness because the functioning of the heart

cardiorespiratory endurance   The ability of the body to perform prolonged, large-muscle, dynamic exercise at moderate-to-high levels of intensity.   **TERMS**

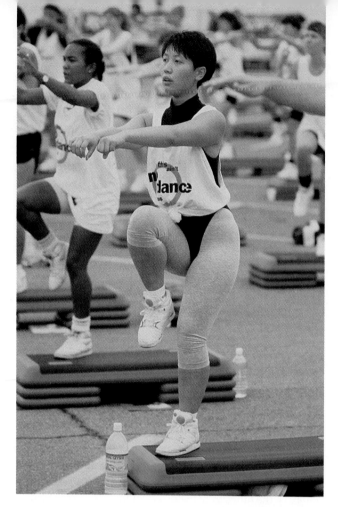

Cardiorespiratory endurance is a key component of health-related fitness. These participants in a step aerobics class are conditioning their hearts and lungs as well as gaining many other health benefits.

and lungs is so essential to overall good health. A person can't live very long or very well without a healthy heart. Low levels of cardiorespiratory fitness are linked with heart disease, the leading cause of death in the United States.

Muscular Strength

Muscular strength is the amount of force a muscle can produce with a single maximum effort. Strong muscles are important for the smooth and easy performance of everyday activities, such as carrying groceries, lifting boxes, and climbing stairs, as well as for emergency situations. They help keep the skeleton in proper alignment, preventing back and leg pain and providing the support necessary for good posture. Muscular strength has obvious importance in recreational activities. Strong people can hit a tennis ball harder, kick a soccer ball farther, and ride a bicycle uphill more easily. Muscle tissue is an important element of overall body composition. Greater muscle mass means a higher rate of **metabolism** and faster energy use. Maintaining strength and muscle mass

is vital for healthy aging. Older people tend to lose both number and size of muscle cells. Many of the muscle cells that remain become slower, and some become nonfunctional because they lose their attachment to the nervous system. Strength training helps maintain muscle mass and function and possibly helps decrease the risk of osteoporosis in older people, which greatly enhances their quality of life and prevents life-threatening injuries.

Muscular Endurance

Muscular endurance is the ability to sustain a given level of muscle tension—that is, to hold a muscle contraction for a long period of time or to contract a muscle over and over again. Muscular endurance is important for good posture and for injury prevention. For example, if abdominal and back muscles can't hold the spine correctly, the chances of low-back pain and back injury are increased. Muscular endurance helps people cope with the physical demands of everyday life and enhances performance in sports and work. It is also important for most leisure and fitness activities.

Flexibility

Flexibility is the ability to move the joints through their full range of motion. Although range of motion isn't a significant factor in everyday activities for most people, inactivity causes the joints to become stiffer with age. Stiffness often causes older people to assume unnatural body postures that can stress joints and muscles. Stretching exercises can help ensure a healthy range of motion for all major joints.

Body Composition

Body composition refers to the proportion of fat and **fat-free mass** (muscle, bone, and water) in the body. Healthy body composition involves a high proportion of fat-free mass and an acceptably low level of body fat, adjusted for age and gender. A person with excessive body fat is more likely to experience a variety of health problems, including heart disease, high blood pressure, stroke, joint problems, diabetes, gallbladder disease, some types of cancer, and back pain. The best way to lose fat is through a lifestyle that includes a sensible diet and exercise. The best way to add muscle mass is through resistance training, also known as strength training or, when weights are used, weight training.

In addition to these five health-related components of physical fitness, physical fitness for a particular sport or activity might include any or all of the following: coordination, speed, reaction time, agility, balance, and skill. Sport-specific skills are best developed through practice. The skill and coordination needed to play basketball, for example, are developed by playing basketball.

Exercise and physical activity are just as important for people with disabilities as for those who are able-bodied. The benefits are the same. They include improved overall physical functioning, stronger emotional and mental state of mind, intellectual alertness, muscular and strength development, healthier blood and glucose readings, greater stamina, new friends, self confidence, and a sense of accomplishment.

Thanks to the Americans with Disabilities Act, many public places, such as health clubs, have become accessible to people with disabilities. These facilities may offer activities and events at several levels. There are also many recreational activities for people of all ages and types of disabilities. Popular activities include adaptive horseback riding, golf, swimming, fishing, and skiing. Competitive sports are also available. For example, there are wheelchair versions of billiards, tennis, hockey, and basketball, as well as sports for people with hearing or visual impairments or mental retardation. Sporting events may be held at regional, state, and national levels.

The most famous sporting competition is the Paralympics, an event for elite athletes with disabilities that is held at about the same time and place as the Olympic Games. Participants in the Paralympics include people with cerebral palsy, those who are blind, paraplegics, quadriplegics, and amputees. They train year-round, and their performance makes it clear that people with disabilities can be active, healthy—and extraordinarily fit.

One example of just how fit people with disabilities can be is Jamie Goldman, who in 1988 lost both legs below the knee from frostbite. After being fitted with carbon fiber artificial legs, Jamie now runs competitively. You may have seen her in an advertisement promoting the year 2000 Olympic and Paralympic Games. "In life, you have a choice," says Goldman. "You can be stuck where you are or you can try to do something."

Currently some 54 million Americans are estimated to have chronic, significant disabilities—the result of injury, illness, chronic pain such as that caused by arthritis, or birth defects. If you have a disability and are considering starting an exercise, sport, or recreational program, call your local community center, YMCA/YWCA, independent living center, or health club. You can also create a workout or exercise corner right in your own home. Be sure to check with your doctor to make sure that the activity you've chosen is right for you, and don't substitute it for any physical therapy you may now be doing. Remember that no matter what your level of ability or disability, it's possible to make exercise an integral part of your life.

SOURCES: Richards, P. 1999. Once a skier, she lost her legs to discover the joy of running. *Indianapolis Star*, 13 July, B-1. *Fit for Life*. 1997. New York State Department of Health brochure. McNeil, J. A. 1997. Americans with disabilities: 1994–95. *Current Population Reports*, August, 5–6 (Table 1).

PRINCIPLES OF PHYSICAL TRAINING: ADAPTATION TO STRESS

The human body is very adaptable. The greater the demands made on it, the more it adjusts to meet those demands. Over time, immediate, short-term adjustments translate into long-term changes and improvements. When breathing and heart rate increase during exercise, for example, the heart gradually develops the ability to pump more blood with each beat. Then, during exercise, it doesn't have to beat as fast to meet the cells' demands for oxygen. The goal of **physical training** is to bring about these long-term changes and improvements in the body's functioning. Although people differ in the maximum levels of physical fitness and performance they can achieve through training, the wellness benefits of exercise are available to everyone (see the box "Fitness and Disability").

Particular types and amounts of exercise are most effective in developing the various components of fitness. To put together an effective exercise program, a person should first understand the basic principles of physical training. Important principles are specificity, progressive overload, reversibility, and individual differences. All of these rest on the larger principle of adaptation.

Specificity—Adapting to Type of Training

To develop a particular fitness component, exercises must be performed that are specifically designed for that component. This is the principle of **specificity**. Weight training,

TERMS

muscular strength The amount of force a muscle can produce with a single maximum effort.

metabolism The sum of all the vital processes by which food energy and nutrients are made available to and used by the body.

muscular endurance The ability of a muscle or group of muscles to remain contracted or to contract repeatedly for a long period of time.

flexibility The range of motion in a joint or group of joints; flexibility is related to muscle length.

body composition The proportion of fat and fat-free mass (muscle, bone, and water) in the body.

fat-free mass The nonfat component of the human body, consisting of skeletal muscle, bone, and water.

physical training The performance of different types of activities that cause the body to adapt and improve its level of fitness.

specificity The training principle that the body adapts to the particular type and amount of stress placed on it.

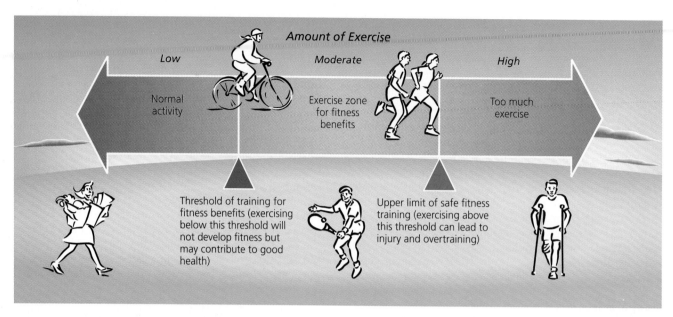

Figure 2-2 Amount of exercise for improving physical fitness. Your current level of fitness determines the amount and intensity of exercise that will increase fitness or cause injury. Olympic athletes must exercise harder than sedentary people to improve fitness. They can also tolerate more exercise than most people can without getting injured.

for example, develops muscular strength, not cardiorespiratory endurance or flexibility. Specificity also applies to the skill-related fitness components—to improve at tennis, you must practice tennis—and to the different parts of the body—to develop stronger arms, you must exercise your arms. A well-rounded exercise program includes exercises geared to each component of fitness, to different parts of the body, and to specific activities or sports.

Progressive Overload—Adapting to Amount of Training

The body adapts to the demands of exercise by improving its functioning. When the amount of exercise (also called overload or stress) is progressively increased, fitness continues to improve. This is the principle of **progressive overload.**

The amount of overload is very important. Too little exercise will have no effect on fitness (although it may improve health); too much may cause injury. The point at which exercise becomes excessive is highly individual—it occurs at a much higher level in an Olympic athlete than in a sedentary person. For every type of exercise, there is a training threshold at which fitness benefits begin to oc-

cur, a zone within which maximum fitness benefits occur, and an upper limit of safe training (Figure 2-2). The amount of exercise needed depends on the individual's current level of fitness, his or her fitness goals, and the component being developed. A novice, for example, might experience fitness benefits from jogging a mile in 10 minutes, but this level of exercise would cause no physical adaptations in a trained distance runner. Beginners should start at the lower end of the fitness benefit zone; fitter individuals will make more rapid gains by exercising at the higher end of the fitness benefit zone.

The amount of overload needed to maintain or improve a particular level of fitness is determined in terms of three dimensions: exercise frequency (how often), intensity (how hard), and duration (how long).

Frequency Developing fitness requires regular exercise. Optimum exercise frequency, expressed in number of days per week, varies with the component being developed and the individual's fitness goals. For most people, a frequency of 3–5 days per week for cardiorespiratory endurance exercise and 2–3 days per week for resistance and flexibility training is appropriate for a general fitness program.

Intensity Fitness benefits occur when a person exercises harder than his or her normal level of activity. The appropriate exercise intensity varies with each fitness component. To develop cardiorespiratory endurance, for example, a person must raise his or her heart rate above normal; to develop muscular strength, a person must lift

TERMS **progressive overload** The training principle that placing increasing amounts of stress on the body causes adaptations that improve fitness.

reversibility The training principle that fitness improvements are lost when demands on the body are lowered.

a heavier weight than normal; to develop flexibility, a person must stretch muscles beyond their normal length.

Duration Fitness benefits occur when you exercise for an extended period of time. For cardiorespiratory endurance exercise, 20–60 minutes is recommended; exercise can take place in a single session or in several sessions of 10 or more minutes. The greater the intensity of exercise, the less time needed to obtain fitness benefits. For high-intensity exercise, such as running, for example, 20–30 minutes is appropriate. For more-moderate-intensity exercise, such as walking, 45–60 minutes may be needed. High-intensity exercise poses a greater risk of injury than lower-intensity exercise, so if you are a nonathletic adult, it's probably best to emphasize lower-to-moderate-intensity activity of longer duration.

For muscular strength, muscular endurance, and flexibility, similar amounts of time are advisable, but these exercises are more commonly organized in terms of a specific number of repetitions of particular exercises. For resistance training, for example, a recommended program includes 1 or more sets of 8–12 repetitions of 8–10 different exercises that work the major muscle groups.

Reversibility—Adapting to a Reduction in Training

Fitness is a reversible adaptation. The body adjusts to lower levels of physical activity the same way it adjusts to higher levels. This is the principle of **reversibility**. When a person stops exercising, up to 50% of fitness improvements are lost within 2 months. If a training schedule must be curtailed temporarily, fitness improvements are best maintained if exercise intensity is kept constant and frequency and/or duration is reduced.

Individual Differences—Limits on Adaptability

Anyone watching the Olympics, a professional football game, or a tennis championship match can readily see that, from a physical standpoint, we are not all created equal. There are large individual differences in our ability to improve fitness and perform and learn sports skills. Some people are able to run longer distances, or lift more weight, or kick a soccer ball more skillfully than others will ever be able to, no matter how much they train. There are limits on the adaptability—the potential for improvement—of any human body. The body's ability to transport and use oxygen, for example, can be improved by only about 15–30% through training. An endurance athlete must therefore inherit a large metabolic capacity in order to reach competitive performance levels. In the past few years, scientists have identified specific genes that control body fat, strength, and endurance.

However, an individual doesn't have to be an Olympic sprinter to experience health benefits from running. Physical training improves fitness regardless of heredity. For the average person, the body's adaptability is enough to achieve all fitness goals.

Physical training works best when you have a plan. A plan helps you make gradual but steady progress toward your goals. Planning for physical fitness consists of assessing how fit you are now, determining where you want to be, and choosing the right activities to help you get there. These activities are discussed next, along with some general guidelines for training.

Assessment

The first step in creating a successful fitness program is to assess your current level of physical activity and fitness for each of the five health-related fitness components. The results of the assessment tests will help you set specific fitness goals and plan your fitness program. Lab 2-1 gives you the opportunity to assess your current overall level of activity and determine if it is appropriate. Assessment tests in Chapters 3, 4, 5, and 6 will help you evaluate your cardiorespiratory endurance, muscular strength, muscular endurance, flexibility, and body composition.

Setting Goals

The ultimate goal of every health-related fitness program is the same—wellness that lasts a lifetime. Whatever your goals, they must be important enough to you to keep you motivated. Studies have shown that exercising for yourself, rather than for the impression you think you'll make on others, is more likely to lead to long-lasting commitment. After you complete the assessment tests in Chapters 3–6, you will be able to set goals directly related to each fitness component, such as working toward a 3-mile jog or doing 20 push-ups. First, though, think carefully about your overall goals, and be clear about why you are starting a program.

Choosing Activities for a Balanced Program

An ideal fitness program combines a physically active lifestyle with a systematic exercise program to develop and maintain physical fitness. This overall program is shown in the physical activity pyramid in Figure 2-3. If you are currently sedentary, your goal is to start at the bottom of the pyramid and gradually increase the amount of moderate-intensity physical activity in your daily life. Appropriate activities include brisk walking, climbing stairs, yard work, and washing your car. You don't have to exercise vigorously, but you should experience a moderate increase in your heart and breathing rates. As described earlier, your activity time can be broken up into small blocks over the course of a day.

The next two levels of the pyramid illustrate parts of a formal exercise program. The principles of this program are consistent with those of the American College of Sports Medicine (ACSM), the professional organization for people involved in sports medicine and exercise

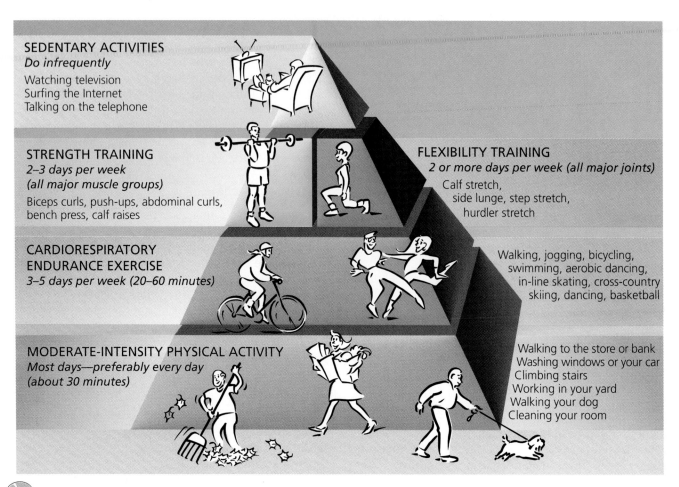

SEDENTARY ACTIVITIES
Do infrequently
Watching television
Surfing the Internet
Talking on the telephone

STRENGTH TRAINING
2–3 days per week
(all major muscle groups)
Biceps curls, push-ups, abdominal curls,
bench press, calf raises

FLEXIBILITY TRAINING
2 or more days per week (all major joints)
Calf stretch,
   side lunge, step stretch,
      hurdler stretch

CARDIORESPIRATORY
ENDURANCE EXERCISE
3–5 days per week (20–60 minutes)

Walking, jogging, bicycling,
   swimming, aerobic dancing,
      in-line skating, cross-country
         skiing, dancing, basketball

MODERATE-INTENSITY PHYSICAL ACTIVITY
Most days—preferably every day
(about 30 minutes)

Walking to the store or bank
Washing windows or your car
Climbing stairs
Working in your yard
Walking your dog
Cleaning your room

Figure 2-3 Physical activity pyramid. Similar to the Food Guide Pyramid, this physical
activity pyramid is designed to help people become more active. If you are currently sedentary,
begin at the bottom of the pyramid and gradually increase the amount of moderate-intensity
physical activity in your life. If you are already moderately active, begin a formal exercise program
that includes cardiorespiratory endurance exercise, flexibility training, and strength training to help
you develop all the health-related components of fitness.

science. The ACSM has established guidelines for creating
an exercise program that will develop physical fitness
(Table 2-2). A balanced program includes activities to develop all the health-related components of fitness.

- *Cardiorespiratory endurance* is developed by continuous rhythmic movements of large-muscle groups
  in activities such as walking, jogging, cycling, swimming, and aerobic dance and other forms of group
  exercise. Choose activities that you enjoy and that
  are convenient. Other popular choices are in-line
  skating, dancing, and backpacking. Start-and-stop
  activities such as tennis, racquetball, and soccer
  can also develop endurance if one's skill level is
  sufficient to enable periods of continuous play.
  Training for cardiorespiratory endurance is discussed in Chapter 3.

- *Muscular strength and endurance* can be developed
  through resistance training—training with weights
  or performing calisthenic exercises such as push-ups

and sit-ups. Training for muscular strength and endurance is discussed in Chapter 4.

- *Flexibility* is developed by stretching the major muscle groups, regularly and with proper technique.
  Flexibility is discussed in Chapter 5.

- *Healthy body composition* can be developed through a
  sensible diet and a program of regular exercise. Endurance exercise is best for reducing body fat; resistance training builds muscle mass, which, to a small
  extent, helps increase metabolism. Body composition is discussed in Chapter 6.

There are as many different fitness programs as there
are individuals. Consider the following examples:

- Maggie is a person whose life revolves around
  sports. She's been on softball teams and swim teams, and
  now she's on her college varsity soccer team. She follows
  a rigorous exercise regimen established by her soccer
  coach. Soccer practice is from four to six afternoons a

TABLE 2-2 *Exercise Recommendations for Healthy Adults*

Exercise to Develop and Maintain Cardiorespiratory Endurance and Body Composition

Mode of activity	Any activity that uses large-muscle groups, can be maintained continuously, and is rhythmic and aerobic in nature; for example, walking-hiking, running-jogging, cycling-bicycling, cross-country skiing, aerobic dance and other forms of group exercise, rope skipping, rowing, stair climbing, swimming, skating, and endurance game activities.
Frequency of training	3–5 days per week.
Intensity of training	55/65–90% of maximum heart rate or 40/50–85% of maximum oxygen uptake reserve.* The lower intensity values (55–64% of maximum heart rate and 40–49% of maximum oxygen uptake reserve) are most applicable to individuals who are quite unfit. For average individuals, intensities of 70–85% of maximum heart rate are appropriate.
Duration of training	20–60 total minutes of continuous or intermittent (in sessions lasting 10 or more minutes) aerobic activity. Duration is dependent on the intensity of activity; thus, lower-intensity activity should be conducted over a longer period of time (30 minutes or more). Lower-to-moderate-intensity activity of longer duration is recommended for the nonathletic adult.

Exercise to Develop and Maintain Muscular Strength and Endurance, Flexibility, and Body Composition

Resistance training	One set of 8–10 exercises that condition the major muscle groups should be performed 2–3 days per week. Most people should complete 8–12 repetitions of each exercise; for older and more frail people (approximately 50–60 years of age and above), 10–15 repetitions with a lighter weight may be more appropriate. Multiple-set regimens may provide greater benefits if time allows.
Flexibility training	Stretches for the major muscle groups should be performed a minimum of 2–3 days per week; at least 4 repetitions, held for 10–30 seconds, should be completed.

*Instructions for calculating target heart rate intensity for cardiorespiratory endurance exercise are presented in Chapter 3.

SOURCE: American College of Sports Medicine. 1998. Position stand: The recommended quantity and quality of exercise for developing and maintaining cardiorespiratory and muscular fitness, and flexibility in healthy adults. *Medicine and Science in Sports and Exercise* 30(6): 975–991.

week. It begins with warm-ups, drills, and practice in specific skills, and it ends with a scrimmage and then a jog around the soccer field. Games are every Saturday. Maggie likes team sports, but she also enjoys exercising alone, so she goes on long bicycle rides whenever she can fit them in. She can't imagine what it would be like not to be physically active every day.

• Maria is a busy young mother of twins. To keep in shape, she joined a health club with a weight room, exercise classes, and child care. Every Monday, Wednesday, and Friday morning, she takes the twins to the club and attends the 7:00 "wake-up" low-impact aerobics class. The instructor leads the class through warm-ups; a 20-minute aerobic workout; exercises for the arms, abdomen, buttocks, and legs; stretches; and a relaxation exercise. Maria is exhilarated and ready for the rest of the day before 9:00 A.M.

• Tom is an engineering student with a lot of studying to do and an active social life as well. For exercise, he plays tennis three times a week. He likes to head for the courts around 6:00 P.M., when most people are eating dinner. He warms up for 10 minutes by practicing his forehand and backhand against a backboard and then plays a hard, fast game with his regular partner for 45 minutes to an hour. Afterwards, he does some stretching exercises while his muscles are still warm. Then he showers and gets ready for dinner. Twice a week he works out at the gym, with particular attention to keeping his arms strong and his shoulders limber. On Saturday nights, he goes dancing with friends.

Each of these people has worked an adequate or more-than-adequate fitness program into their busy daily routine. Chapter 7 contains guidelines to help you choose activities and put together a complete exercise program that suits your goals and preferences.

What about the tip of the activity pyramid? Although sedentary activities are often unavoidable—attending class, studying, working in an office, and so on—many people choose inactivity over activity during their leisure time. Change sedentary patterns by becoming more active whenever you can. Move more and sit less.

Guidelines for Training

The following guidelines will make your exercise program more effective and successful.

• *Train the way you want your body to change.* Stress your body such that it adapts in the desired direction.

To have a more muscular build, lift weights. To be more flexible, do stretching exercises. To improve performance in a particular sport, practice that sport or the movements used in it.

• *Train regularly.* Consistency is the key to improving fitness. Fitness improvements are lost if too much time is allowed to pass between exercise sessions.

• *Get in shape gradually.* An exercise program can be divided into three phases: the beginning phase, during which the body adjusts to the new type and level of activity; the progress phase, during which fitness is increased; and the maintenance phase, in which the targeted level of fitness is maintained over the long term (Figure 2-4). When beginning a program, start slowly to give your body time to adapt to the stress of exercise. As you progress, increase duration and frequency before increasing intensity. If you train too much or too intensely, you are more likely to suffer injuries or become **overtrained,** a condition characterized by lack of energy, aching muscles and joints, and decreased physical performance. Injuries and overtraining slow down an exercise program and impede motivation. The goal is not to get in shape as quickly as possible but to gradually become and remain physically fit.

• *Warm up before exercising, and cool down afterward.* Warming up decreases the chances of injury by helping the body gradually progress from rest to activity. A warm-up should include low-intensity movements similar to those used in the activity that will follow. Stretching exercises are also often recommended. Cooling down after exercise is important for restoring circulation to its normal resting condition. Cool down by continuing to exercise but at a lower level of intensity.

• *Listen to your body.* Don't exercise if it doesn't feel right. Sometimes you need a few days of rest to recover enough to train with the intensity required for improving fitness. On the other hand, you can't train sporadically either. If you listen to your body and it always tells you to rest, you won't make any progress.

• *Try training with a partner.* Training partners can motivate and encourage each other through hard spots and help each other develop proper exercise techniques.

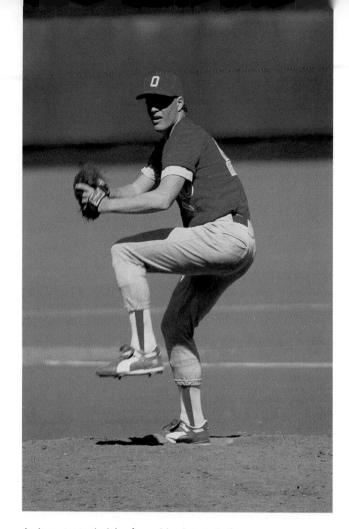

An important principle of exercising is to train the way you want your body to change. By practicing the moves used in pitching, this man is increasing the strength of specific muscles needed for playing baseball as well as improving his speed, skill, and agility.

Training with a partner can make exercising seem easier and more fun.

• *Train your mind.* This is one of the most difficult skills to acquire, but it is critical for achieving and maintaining fitness. Becoming fit requires commitment, discipline, and patience. These qualities come from understanding the importance of exercise and having clear and reachable goals. Use the lifestyle management techniques discussed in Chapter 1 to keep your program on track. Believe in yourself and your potential—and you *will* achieve your goals!

• *Keep your exercise program in perspective.* As important as physical fitness is, it is only part of a well-rounded life. You have to have time for work and school, family and friends, relaxation and hobbies. Some people become overinvolved in exercise and neglect other parts of their lives. They think of themselves as runners, dancers, swimmers, or triathletes rather than as people who participate in those activities. Balance and moderation are the key ingredients of a fit and well life.

TERMS **overtraining** A condition caused by training too much or too intensely, characterized by lack of energy, decreased physical performance, fatigue, depression, aching muscles and joints, and susceptibility to injury.

exercise stress test A test usually administered on a treadmill or cycle ergometer that involves analysis of the changes in electrical activity in the heart from an electrocardiogram (EKG or ECG) taken during exercise. Used to determine if any heart disease is present and to assess current fitness level.

graded exercise test (GXT) An exercise test that starts at an easy intensity and progresses to maximum capacity.

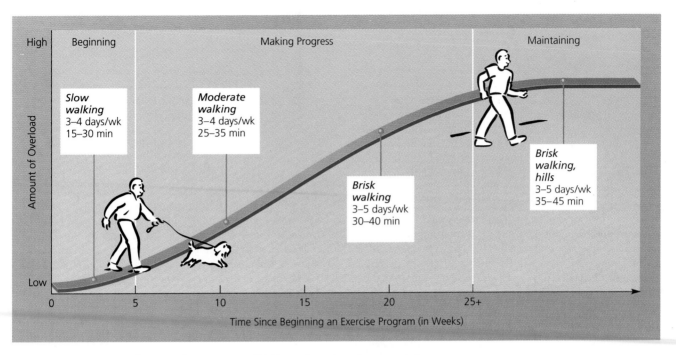

Figure 2-4 Progression of an exercise program. This figure shows how the amount of overload is increased gradually over time in a sample walking program. Regardless of the activity chosen, it is important that an exercise program begin slowly and progress gradually. Once a person achieves the desired level of fitness, she or he can maintain it by exercising 3 to 5 days a week. SOURCE: Progression data from American College of Sports Medicine. 2000. *ACSM's Guidelines for Exercise Testing and Prescription,* 6th ed. Baltimore, Md.: Lippincott Williams & Wilkins.

COMMON QUESTIONS ANSWERED

Is exercise safe for me?   People of any age who are not at high risk for serious health problems can safely exercise at a moderate intensity (60% or less of maximum heart rate) without a prior medical evaluation. (See Chapter 3 for a discussion of maximum heart rate.) Likewise, if you are male and under 40 or female and under 50 and in good health, exercise is probably safe for you. If you are over these ages or have health problems (especially high blood pressure, heart disease, muscle or joint problems, or obesity), see your physician before starting a vigorous exercise program. The Canadian Society for Exercise Physiology has developed a questionnaire called PAR-Q to help determine exercise safety. This questionnaire is included in Lab 2-2. Completing it should alert you to any potential problems you may have. If a physician isn't sure whether exercise is safe for you, he or she may recommend an **exercise stress test** or a **graded exercise test (GXT)** to see whether you show symptoms of heart disease during exercise. For most people, however, it's far safer to exercise than to remain sedentary.

You must also consider your physical safety when exercising. If you ride a bicycle or run on public streets, wear clothing that can be seen easily. Bicyclists should always wear helmets. Even though you may have the right-of-way, give cars plenty of leeway; in a collision, a car will sustain less damage than a bicycle or your unprotected body. Don't train in isolated areas unless you're with a friend. Exercising alone, you could easily be injured or become a crime victim. (See Appendix A for more information on personal safety.)

Where can I get help and advice about exercise?   Because fitness is essential to a wellness lifestyle, you need to learn as much as you can about exercise. One of the best places to get help is an exercise class. There, expert instructors can help you learn the basics of training and answer your questions. Make sure the instructor is certified by ACSM or has formal training in exercise physiology. Read articles by credible experts in fitness magazines. Because of competition among publications, these magazines include articles by leading experts in exercise science written at a layperson's level.

A qualified personal trainer can also be helpful in getting you started in an exercise program or a new form of training. Make sure this person has proper qualifications, such as a college degree in exercise physiology or physical education or ACSM or American Council on Exercise (ACE) certification. Don't seek out a person for advice simply because he or she looks fit.

(continued)

Should I follow my exercise program if I'm sick? If you have a mild head cold or feel one coming on, it is probably OK to exercise moderately. Just begin slowly and see how you feel. However, if you have symptoms of a more serious illness—fever, swollen glands, nausea, extreme tiredness, muscle aches—wait until you have fully recovered before resuming your exercise program. Continuing to exercise while suffering from an illness more serious than a cold can compromise your recovery and may even be dangerous.

How can I fit my exercise program into my day? Good time management is an important skill in creating and maintaining an exercise program. Choose a regular time to exercise, preferably the same time every day. Don't tell yourself you'll exercise "sometime during the day" when you have free time—that free time may never come. Schedule your workout, and make it a priority. Include alternative plans in your program to account for circumstances like bad weather or vacations.

You don't have to work on all fitness components in the same exercise session. The important thing is to have a regular schedule. (You'll have the chance to develop strategies for successful time management in the Behavior Change Workbook at the end of the text.)

Where can I work out? Identify accessible and pleasant places to work out. For running, find a field or park with a soft surface. For swimming, find a pool that's open at times convenient for you. For cycling, find an area with minimal traffic and air pollution. Make sure the place you exercise is safe and convenient. If you join a health club or fitness center, follow the guidelines in the box "Choosing a Health Club."

SUMMARY

- Exercising daily in moderation contributes substantially to good health. Even without a formal, vigorous exercise program, you can get many of the same health benefits by becoming more physically active.

- If you are already active, you benefit even more by increasing the intensity or duration of your activity.

- The five components of physical fitness most important for health are cardiorespiratory endurance, muscular strength, muscular endurance, flexibility, and body composition.

- Physical training is the process of bringing about long-term improvements in the body's functioning through exercise. All training is based on the fact that the body adapts to physical stress.

- According to the principle of *specificity*, bodies change specifically in response to the type of training received.

- Bodies also adapt to *progressive overload*. Therefore, when we progressively increase our amount of exercise—its frequency, intensity, and duration—we become increasingly fit.

- Bodies adjust to lower levels of activity by losing fitness, a principle known as *reversibility*. To counter the effects of reversibility we should keep training at the same intensity, even if we reduce the number or length of sessions.

- According to the principle of *individual differences*, people vary in the maximum level of fitness they can achieve.

- When designing an exercise program, assess your current level of fitness, set realistic goals, and choose activities that develop all components of fitness.

- In addition, train regularly, get in shape gradually, warm up and cool down, maintain a structured but flexible program, consider training with a partner, train your mind, and keep exercise in perspective.

FOR MORE INFORMATION

Books

American College of Sports Medicine. 2000. *ACSM's Guidelines for Exercise Testing and Prescription,* 6th ed. Baltimore, Md.: Lippincott Williams & Wilkins. *Includes the ACSM guidelines for safety of exercising, a basic discussion of exercise physiology, and information about fitness testing and prescription.*

American College of Sports Medicine. 1998. *ACSM Fitness Book,* 2d ed. Champaign, Ill.: Human Kinetics. *A brief, easy-to-use guide to creating a successful fitness program.*

Department of Health and Human Services. 1996. *Physical Activity and Health: A Report of the Surgeon General.* Atlanta, Ga.: DHHS (also available online: http://www.cdc.gov/nccdphp/sgr/sgr.htm). *Summarizes evidence for the benefits of physical activity and makes recommendations.*

Fahey, T. D. 2000. *Super Fitness for Sports, Conditioning, and Health.* Boston: Allyn & Bacon. *A brief guide to developing fitness that emphasizes training techniques for improving sports performance.*

Farquhar, J. W. 1996. *Fresh Start: The Stanford Medical School Health and Fitness Program.* San Francisco: KQED. *An excellent guide to exercising for health and prevention of disease.*

Franks, B. D., E. T. Howley, and Y. Iyriboz. 1999. *The Health Fitness Handbook.* Champaign, Ill.: Human Kinetics. *Provides basic information for beginning a fitness program, including advice for setting realistic goals and changing health-related behaviors.*

National Center for Chronic Disease Prevention and Health Promotion. 1999. *Promoting Physical Activity: A Guide for Community Action.* Champaign Ill.: Human Kinetics. *Although de-*

Health clubs or fitness centers can provide you with important benefits. Among the most important are motivation and companionship. Joining a club can help you get in some aerobic exercise with others who are similarly motivated. Other important benefits are instruction and supervision, whether you're starting out or progressing to higher levels. Finally, good equipment provides benefits. You can easily and safely isolate and develop specific muscle groups in chest, arms, hips, buttocks, and legs, or you can ride a stationary bike or train on a stair-climbing machine for overall endurance. If you're thinking of joining one of the 15,000 fitness centers currently out there, here are some guidelines to help you choose the club that's right for you.

Convenience

- Look for an established facility that's within 10–15 minutes of your home or work. If it's farther away, your chances of sticking to an exercise regimen start to diminish.

- Check out the facility's hours, then visit it at the time you would normally exercise. Will you have easy access to the equipment and exercise classes you want at that time?

Atmosphere

- Look around to see if there are others there who are your age and at about your fitness level. (If everyone seems close in age or fitness level, then the club may cater to a certain age group or lifestyle—for example, hard-core bodybuilders.)

- If you like to exercise to music, make sure the music played there is to your liking, both its type and loudness.

- Observe how the members dress. Will you fit in, or will you be uncomfortable?

Safety

- Find out if the club offers basic fitness testing that includes cardiovascular screening.

- Also determine if there is emergency equipment on the premises and if personnel are trained in CPR.

- Ask if at least one staff member on each shift is trained in first aid.

Cost

- Buy only what you need and can afford. If you want to use only workout equipment, you may not need a club that has racquetball courts and saunas.

- Check the contract. Choose the one that covers the shortest period of time possible, especially if it's your first health club experience.

- Make sure the contract permits you to extend your membership if you have a prolonged illness or go on vacation.

- Try out the club. Ask for a free trial workout, or 1-day pass, or an inexpensive 1- or 2-week trial membership.

- Find out whether there is an extra charge for the particular services you want.

Effectiveness

- Tour the facility. Does it offer what the brochure says it does?

- Don't get cheated. Check with your Better Business Bureau or Consumer Affairs office to see if others have complained.

- Make sure the facility is certified. Look for the displayed names American College of Sports Medicine (ACSM), American Council on Exercise (ACE), or Aerobics and Fitness Association of America (AFAA)

- Check the equipment. A good club will have treadmills, bikes, stair-climbers, resistance machines, and weights. Make sure these machines are up-to-date and well maintained.

Cleanliness

- Check to see that the facility is clean, including showers and lockers.

- Make sure the facility is climate controlled and well ventilated.

SOURCES: Fahey, T. D. 2000. *Basic Weight Training for Men and Women.* Mountain View, Calif.: Mayfield, pp. 36–38. Balady, G. J. 1998. Health clubs: Are they right for you? *Harvard Men's Health Watch*, November, 6. Health clubs: What to look for. 1999. *Consumer Reports*, February, 34. Keys to "safe" exercise for your patients (Choosing a fitness center). 1999. *Consultant* 39(3): 724.

signed for professionals, this guide provides a wealth of helpful advice for overcoming barriers to physical activity.

Nieman, D. C. 1999. *Exercise Testing and Prescription: A Health-Related Approach,* 4th ed. Mountain View, Calif.: Mayfield. *Comprehensive discussions of fitness testing, exercise and disease, nutrition and physical performance, and exercise prescription.*

Rippe, J. M., and M. A. Waite. 1997. *Fit over Forty: A Revolutionary Plan to Achieve Lifelong Physical and Spiritual Health and Well-Being.* New York: Morrow. *A sensible approach to incorporating exercise into a wellness lifestyle, with special emphasis on older adults.*

Schlosberg, S. 1999. *The Ultimate Workout Log: An Exercise Diary and Fitness Guide.* New York: Houghton Mifflin. *A 6-month log that also provides fitness definitions, training tips, and motivational quotes.*

Journals

ACSM Health and Fitness Journal (401 West Michigan Street, Indianapolis, IN 46202; http://www.health-fitjrnl.com)

Physician and Sportsmedicine (4530 W. 77th Street, Minneapolis, MN 55435; many of the articles are also available online at http://www.physsportsmed.com)

Organizations, Hotlines, and Web Sites

American Alliance for Health, Physical Education, Recreation, and Dance (AAHPERD). A professional organization dedicated to promoting quality health and education programs.

  800-213-7193

  http://www.aahperd.org

American College of Sports Medicine (ACSM). The principal professional organization for sports medicine and exercise science. Provides brochures, publications, and audio- and videotapes.

  317-637-9200

  http://www.acsm.org

American Council on Exercise (ACE). Promotes exercise and fitness; the Web site features fact sheets on many consumer topics, including choosing shoes, cross-training, and steroids.

  800-529-8227 (Consumer Fitness Hotline)

  http:/www.acefitness.org

American Heart Association: Just Move. Provides practical advice for people of all fitness levels plus an online fitness diary.

  http://www.justmove.org

American Medical Association/Personal Trainer. Includes a fitness assessment and guidelines for creating a safe, effective program for developing the health-related components of fitness.

  http://www.ama-assn.org/insight/gen_hlth/fitness/fitness.htm

Canada's Physical Activity Guide. Offers many suggestions for incorporating physical activity into everyday life; also includes the Physical Activity Readiness Questionnaire (PAR-Q).

  http://www.paguide.com

CDC Physical Activity Information. Provides information on the benefits of physical activity and suggestions for incorporating moderate physical activity into daily life.

  http://www.cdc.gov/nccdphp/phyactiv.htm

Disabled Sports USA. Provides sports and recreation services to people with physical or mobility disorders.

  301-217-0960

  http://www.nas.com/~dsusa

Georgia State University: Exercise and Physical Fitness Page. Provides information about the benefits of exercise and how to get started on a fitness program.

  http://www.gsu.edu/~wwwfit

Melpomene Institute. Provides information about physical activity and health for women.

  651-642-1951

  http://www.melpomene.org

The following provide links to sites with information on a wide variety of activities and fitness issues:

FitnessLink

  http://www.fitnesslink.com

Fitness Partner Connection Jumpsite

  http//www.primusweb.com/fitnesspartner

NetSweat: The Internet's Fitness Resource

  http//www.netsweat.com

Yahoo! Recreation and Sports

  http//www.dir.yahoo.com/recreation/sports

American College of Sports Medicine. 1998. ACSM position stand: The recommended quantity and quality of exercise for developing and maintaining cardiorespiratory and muscular fitness, and flexibility in healthy adults. *Medicine and Science in Sports and Exercise* 30(6): 975–991.

Beilin, L. J. 1999. Lifestyle and hypertension—An overview. *Clinical and Experimental Hypertension* 21:749-762.

Berstein, M. S., A. Morabia, and D. Sloutskis. 1999. Definition and prevalence of sedentarism in an urban population. *American Journal of Public Health* 89:862–867.

Brill, P. A., et al. 2000. Muscular strength and physical function. *Medicine and Science in Sports and Exercise* 32(2): 412–416.

Brooks, G. A., et al. 2000. *Exercise Physiology: Human Bioenergetics and Its Applications,* 3d ed. Mountain View, Calif.: Mayfield.

Department of Health and Human Services. 1996. *Physical Activity and Health: A Report of the Surgeon General.* Atlanta, Ga.: DHHS.

Emmons, K. M., et al. 1999. The Working Healthy Project: A worksite health-promotion trial targeting physical activity, diet, and smoking. *Journal of Occupational and Environmental Medicine* 41:545–555.

Francis, K. T. 1999. Status of the year 2000 health goals for physical activity and fitness. *Physical Therapy* 79:405–414.

Hu, F. B., et al. 1999. Walking compared with vigorous physical activity and risk of Type 2 diabetes in women: A prospective study. *Journal of American Medical Association* 282(15): 1433–1439.

Jaffe, L., et al. 1999. Incentives and barriers to physical activity for working women. *American Journal of Health Promotion* 13:215–218.

Mason, J. E., et al. 1999. A prospective study of walking as compared with vigorous exercise in the prevention of coronary heart disease in women. *New England Journal of Medicine* 341(9): 650–658.

Miszko, T. A., and M. E. Cross. 2000. A lifetime of fitness: Exercise in the perimenopausal and postmenopausal woman. *Clinics in Sport Medicine* 19(2): 215–232.

Nies, M. A., Vollman, and M. T. Cook. 1999. African American women's experience with physical activity in their daily lives. *Public Health and Nursing* 16:23–31.

Pereira, M. A., and M. K. Schmitz. 1999. Effects of a lifestyle exercise intervention. *Preventive Medicine* 28:101–103.

Salmon, J., et al. 2000. Leisure-time, occupational, and household physical activity among professional, skilled, and less-skilled workers and homemakers. *Preventive Medicine* 30(3): 191–199.

Shephard, R. J. 1999. How much physical activity is needed for good health? *International Journal of Sports Medicine* 20: 23–27.

Snell, P. G., and J. H. Mitchell. 1999. Physical inactivity: An easily modified risk factor? *Circulation* 100:2–4.

Sternfeld, B., B. E. Ainsworth, and C. P. Quesenberry. 1999. Physical activity patterns in a diverse population of women. *Preventive Medicine* 28:313–323.

SELECTED BIBLIOGRAPHY

American College of Sports Medicine. 2000. *ACSM's Guidelines for Exercise Testing and Prescription*, 6th ed. Baltimore, Md.: Lippincott Williams & Wilkins.

Name _____ **Section** _____ **Date** _____

 LAB 2-1 *Your Physical Activity Profile*

Complete this lab to assess your overall level of activity on an average day. The amount of time you spend on lifestyle physical activity (Part I), exercise/sports (Part II), and sleep should total 24 hours.

Part I   Lifestyle Physical Activity

Fill in the approximate amount of time you spend on activities in the following three intensity categories during a typical day. Include time spent in school- and work-related activities, home activities, and leisure activities; time spent on exercise/sports should be listed only in Part II. Light activities include most sitting and standing activities. During moderate activity, breathing rate increases, but a person is still able to carry on a conversation comfortably; during vigorous activity, a person is usually too out of breath to talk easily.

Light Activity	Moderate Activity	Vigorous Activity
___ Attending class, studying	___ Walking moderately or briskly	___ Walking briskly uphill
___ Using a computer	___ Bicycling (for transportation)	___ Heavy construction work or digging, teaching an exercise class, firefighting, or another occupational activity requiring strenuous effort and total body movement
___ Watching TV, listening to music	___ Waiting tables, washing dishes, or another occupational activity involving extended periods of moderate effort	
___ Talking on the phone		
___ Eating meals		
___ Office work, sales, or another occupational activity involving sitting or standing and movement of little more than hands	___ Active play with children; carrying a child; pushing a stroller	___ Heavy housework (moving heavy furniture, carrying heavy items up stairs)
___ Walking slowly	___ Moderate housework (scrubbing floors, heavy sweeping, washing windows, carrying heavy bags)	___ Vigorous yard work (swinging an ax, climbing and trimming trees, pushing a nonmotorized mower, shoveling snow)
___ Driving		
___ Child care (most activities)	___ Moderate yard work (planting, raking, light digging, weeding while standing, pushing a motorized mower)	
___ Light housework (ironing, cooking, light sweeping, dusting, vacuuming)		___ Vigorous home activities (carrying heavy loads, concrete or masonry work, hand-sawing)
___ Light yard work (pruning, weeding while sitting, using a riding mower	___ Moderate home repair (cleaning gutters, refinishing furniture, painting, wallpapering)	
___ Light home repair (wiring, plumbing, carpentry)	___ Hand-washing or waxing a car	*Other vigorous activities (list):*
	___ Social dancing	Also record the number of flights of stairs you climb on an average day:
Other light activities (list):	*Other moderate activities (list)*	___ flights
___ _____	___ _____	___ _____
___ _____	___ _____	___ _____
___ **Total time (hours)**	___ **Total time (hours)**	___ **Total time (hours)**

To help identify ways to incorporate more moderate physical activity into your day, break out the amount of time in each intensity category according to the type of activity:

	Light activity (hours)	Moderate activity (hours)	Vigorous activity (hours)
Transportation-related activities			
School- or job-related activities			
Home and child-care activities			
Leisure activities			

How much of your transportation and leisure time is in the light activity category? List three strategies for substituting moderate activities for light activities. Examples include walking or biking rather than driving for short errands and going for a walk with a friend rather than chatting on the phone; see p. 23 for additional suggestions.

1. _____

2. _____

3. _____

Part II   Your Exercise Index

Circle the scores that best describe your typical exercise/sports habits:

1. Frequency: How often do you exercise?

Less than 1 time a week	0
1 time a week	1
2 times a week	2
3 times a week	3
4 times a week	4
5 or more times a week	5

2. Duration: How long do you exercise?

Less than 5 minutes	0
5–14 minutes	1
15–29 minutes	2
30–44 minutes	3
45–59 minutes	4
60 minutes or more	5

3. Intensity: How hard do you exercise?

No change in pulse from resting level	0
Little change in pulse from resting level (slow walking, bowling, yoga)	1
Slight increase in pulse and breathing (table tennis, active golf with no golf cart)	2
Moderate increase in pulse and breathing (leisurely bicycling, easy continuous swimming, rapid walking)	3
Intermittent heavy breathing and sweating (tennis singles, basketball, squash)	4
Sustained heavy breathing and sweating (jogging, cross-country skiing, rope skipping)	5

To assess your exercise index, multiply your three scores and then find the appropriate classification in the table below.

Frequency _____ × Duration _____ × Intensity _____ = Exercise index _____

Exercise index	Classification
Less than 15	Sedentary
15–24	Low
25–40	Moderate
41–60	Moderately high
Over 60	High

If your exercise index is in one of the lower categories, review the components of your score (frequency, duration, intensity) to see how you can raise your score. Add to your current exercise program, or devise a new one.

To monitor your progress toward your goal, enter the results of both parts of this lab in the Preprogram Assessment column in Appendix D. After several weeks of a program to become more physically active, do this lab again, and enter the results in the Postprogram Assessment column of Appendix D. How do the results compare?

SOURCES: Part I activity classifications from CDC Division of Nutrition and Physical Activity. 1999. *Promoting Physical Activity: A Guide for Community Action.* Champaign, Ill.: Human Kinetics. Part II from Kusinitz, I., and M. Fine. 1995. *Your Guide to Getting Fit,* 3d ed. Mountain View, Calif.: Mayfield.

Name _____ Section _____ Date _____

LAB 2-2 *Safety of Exercise Participation*

PAR-Q & YOU

(A Questionnaire for People Aged 15 to 69)

Part I   Regular physical activity is fun and healthy, and increasingly more people are starting to become more active every day. Being more active is very safe for most people. However, some people should check with their doctor before they start becoming much more physically active.

If you are planning to become much more physically active than you are now, start by answering the seven questions in the box below. If you are between the ages of 15 and 69, the PAR-Q will tell you if you should check with your doctor before you start. If you are over 69 years of age, and you are not used to being very active, check with your doctor.

Common sense is your best guide when you answer these questions. Please read the questions carefully and answer each one honestly: check YES or NO.

YES	NO	
☐	☐	1. Has your doctor ever said that you have a heart condition <u>and</u> that you should only do physical activity recommended by a doctor?
☐	☐	2. Do you feel pain in your chest when you do physical activity?
☐	☐	3. In the past month, have you had chest pain when you were not doing physical activity?
☐	☐	4. Do you lose your balance because of dizziness or do you ever lose consciousness?
☐	☐	5. Do you have a bone or joint problem that could be made worse by a change in your physical activity?
☐	☐	6. Is your doctor currently prescribing drugs (for example, water pills) for your blood pressure or heart condition?
☐	☐	7. Do you know of <u>any other reason</u> why you should not do physical activity?

If

you

answered

YES to one or more questions

Talk with your doctor by phone or in person BEFORE you start becoming much more physically active or BEFORE you have a fitness appraisal. Tell your doctor about the PAR-Q and which questions you answered YES.
- You may be able to do any activity you want—as long as you start slowly and build up gradually. Or, you may need to restrict your activities to those which are safe for you. Talk with your doctor about the kinds of activities you wish to participate in and follow his/her advice.
- Find out which community programs are safe and helpful for you.

NO to all questions

If you answered NO honestly to <u>all</u> PAR-Q questions, you can be reasonably sure that you can:
- start becoming much more physically active—begin slowly and build up gradually. This is the safest and easiest way to go.
- take part in a fitness appraisal—this is an excellent way to determine your basic fitness so that you can plan the best way for you to live actively.

DELAY BECOMING MUCH MORE ACTIVE:
- if you are not feeling well because of a temporary illness such as a cold or a fever—wait until you feel better; or
- if you are or may be pregnant—talk to your doctor before you start becoming more active

Please note: If your health changes so that you then answer YES to any of the above questions, tell your fitness or health professional. Ask whether you should change your physical activity plan.

<u>Informed Use of the PAR-Q:</u> The Canadian Society for Exercise Physiology, Health Canada, and their agents assume no liability for persons who undertake physical activity, and if in doubt after completing this questionnaire, consult your doctor prior to physical activity.

You are encouraged to copy the PAR-Q but only if you use the entire form.

Note: If the PAR-Q is being given to a person before he or she participates in a physical activity program or a fitness appraisal, this section may be used for legal or administrative purposes.

I have read, understood and completed this questionnaire. Any questions I had were answered to my full satisfaction.

NAME _____

SIGNATURE _____   DATE _____

SIGNATURE OF PARENT _____   WITNESS _____
or GUARDIAN (for participants under the age of majority)

Part II General Health Profile

To help further assess the safety of exercise for you, complete as much of this health profile as possible.

General Information

Age: _____

Height: _____

Weight: _____

Are you currently trying to ____ gain or

____ lose weight? (check one if appropriate)

Blood pressure: ____ /____

Blood lipid levels

    Total cholesterol: _____

    HDL: _____

    LDL: _____

Triglycerides: _____

Blood glucose level: _____

Medical Conditions/Treatments

Do you have any of the following conditions? Check any that apply to you and add any other conditions that might affect your ability to exercise safely.

_____ heart disease

_____ lung disease

_____ diabetes

_____ allergies

_____ asthma

_____ depression, anxiety, or another psychological disorder

_____ eating disorder

_____ back pain

_____ arthritis

_____ other injury or joint problem: _____

_____ substance abuse problem

_____ other: _____

_____ other: _____

_____ other: _____

_____ Do you have a family history of cardiovascular disease (CVD) (a parent, sibling, or child who had a heart attack or stroke before age 55 for men or 65 for women)?

List any medications or supplements you are taking or any medical treatments you are undergoing. Include the name of the substance or treatment and its purpose. Include both prescription and over-the-counter drugs and any vitamin, mineral, or other dietary supplement you are taking.

_____   _____

_____   _____

_____   _____

_____   _____

Lifestyle Information

Check any of the following that is true for you, and fill in the requested information.

_____ I usually eat high-fat foods (fatty meats, cheese, fried foods, butter, full-fat dairy products) every day.

_____ I consume fewer than 5 servings of fruits and vegetables on most days.

_____ I smoke cigarettes or use other tobacco products. If true, describe your use of tobacco (type and frequency): _____

_____ I regularly drink alcohol. If true, describe your typical weekly consumption pattern: _____

_____

_____ I often feel as if I need more sleep. (I need about _____ hours per day; I get about _____ hours per day.)

_____ I feel as though stress has adversely affected my level of wellness during the past year.

Describe your current activity pattern. What types of moderate physical activity do you engage in on a daily basis? Are you involved in a formal exercise program or do you regularly participate in sports or recreational activities?

_____

_____

_____

Cardiorespiratory Endurance

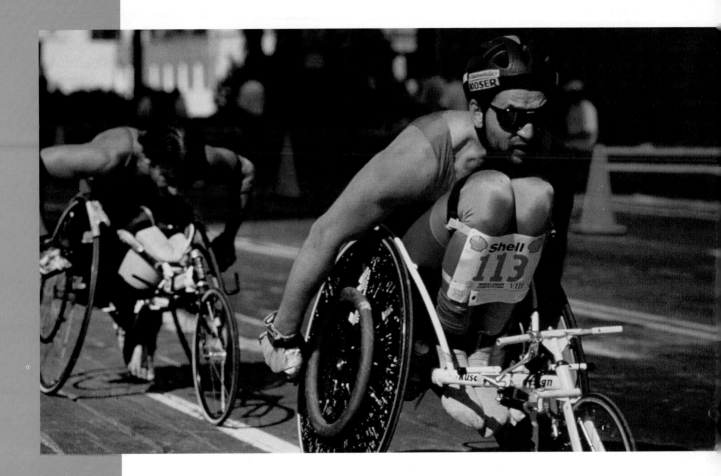

LOOKING AHEAD

After reading this chapter, you should be able to answer these questions about cardiorespiratory endurance:

- How does the body produce the energy it needs for exercise?

- What are the major effects and benefits of cardiorespiratory endurance exercise?

- How is cardiorespiratory endurance measured and assessed?

- How do type, intensity, duration, and frequency of exercise affect the development of cardiorespiratory endurance?

- What elements go into a successful cardiorespiratory fitness program?

- What are the best ways to prevent and treat exercise injuries?

Cardiorespiratory endurance—the ability of the body to perform prolonged, large-muscle, dynamic exercise at moderate-to-high levels of intensity—is a key health-related component of fitness. As explained in Chapter 2, a healthy cardiorespiratory system is essential to high levels of fitness and wellness.

This chapter reviews the short- and long-term effects and benefits of cardiorespiratory endurance exercise. It then describes several tests that are commonly used to assess cardiorespiratory fitness. Finally, it provides guidelines for creating your own cardiorespiratory endurance program, one that is geared to your current level of fitness and built around activities you enjoy.

BASIC PHYSIOLOGY OF CARDIORESPIRATORY ENDURANCE EXERCISE

A basic understanding of the body processes involved in cardiorespiratory endurance exercise can help you design a safe and effective fitness program. In this section, we'll take a brief look at how the cardiorespiratory system functions and how the body produces the energy it needs to respond to the challenge of physical activity.

The Cardiorespiratory System

The cardiorespiratory system picks up and transports oxygen, nutrients, and other key substances to the organs and tissues that need them; it also picks up waste products and carries them to where they can be used or expelled. The cardiorespiratory system consists of the heart, the blood vessels, and the respiratory system (Figure 3-1).

The Heart   The heart is a four-chambered, fist-sized muscle located just beneath the ribs under the sternum (breastbone). Its role is to pump oxygen-poor blood to the lungs and oxygenated (oxygen-rich) blood to the rest of the body. Blood actually travels through two separate circulatory systems: The right side of the heart pumps blood to the lungs in what is called **pulmonary circulation,** and the left side pumps blood through the rest of the body in **systemic circulation.**

Waste-carrying, oxygen-poor blood enters the right upper chamber, or **atrium,** of the heart through the **venae cavae,** the largest veins in the body (Figure 3-2). As the right atrium fills, it contracts and pumps blood into the right lower chamber, or **ventricle,** which, when it contracts, pumps blood through the pulmonary artery into the lungs. There, blood picks up oxygen and discards carbon dioxide. Cleaned, oxygenated blood then flows from the lungs through the pulmonary veins into the left atrium. As this chamber fills, it contracts and pumps blood into the powerful left ventricle, which pumps it

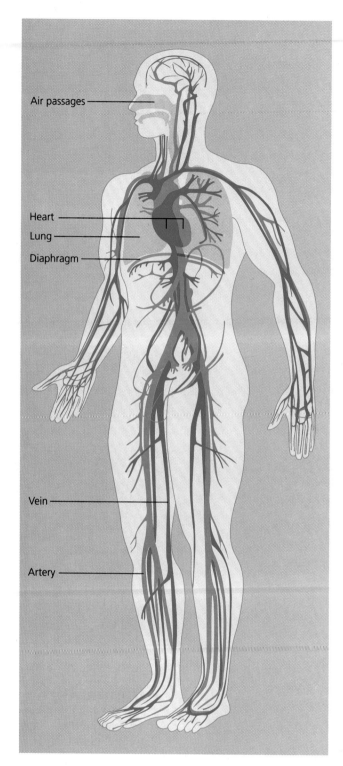

Air passages

Heart
Lung
Diaphragm

Vein

Artery

Figure 3-1   The cardiorespiratory system.

through the **aorta,** the body's largest artery, to be fed into the rest of the body's blood vessels.

The period of the heart's contraction is called **systole;** the period of relaxation is called **diastole.** During systole, the atria contract first, pumping blood into the ventricles;

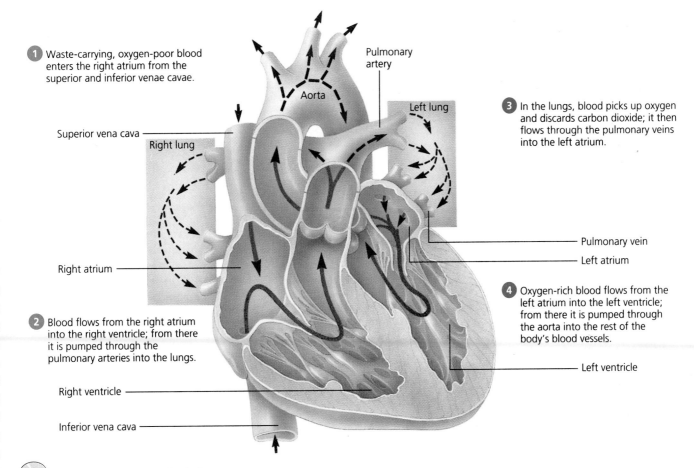

① Waste-carrying, oxygen-poor blood enters the right atrium from the superior and inferior venae cavae.

Pulmonary artery

Aorta

Left lung

③ In the lungs, blood picks up oxygen and discards carbon dioxide; it then flows through the pulmonary veins into the left atrium.

Superior vena cava

Right lung

Pulmonary vein

Left atrium

Right atrium

④ Oxygen-rich blood flows from the left atrium into the left ventricle; from there it is pumped through the aorta into the rest of the body's blood vessels.

② Blood flows from the right atrium into the right ventricle; from there it is pumped through the pulmonary arteries into the lungs.

Left ventricle

Right ventricle

Inferior vena cava

Figure 3-2 Circulation in the heart.

a fraction of a second later, the ventricles contract, pumping blood to the lungs and the body. During diastole, blood flows into the heart. A person weighing 150 pounds has about 5 quarts of blood, which are circulated about once every minute.

The heartbeat—the split-second sequence of contractions of the heart's four chambers—is controlled by nerve impulses. These signals originate in a bundle of specialized cells in the right atrium called the pacemaker (SA node). Unless it is speeded up or slowed down by the brain in response to such stimuli as danger or the tissues' need for more oxygen, the heart produces nerve impulses at a steady rate.

The Blood Vessels Blood vessels are classified by size and function. **Veins** carry blood to the heart; **arteries** carry it away from the heart. Veins have thin walls, but arteries have thick elastic walls that enable them to expand and relax with the volume of blood being pumped through them. After leaving the heart, the aorta branches into smaller and smaller vessels. The smallest arteries branch still further into **capillaries**, tiny vessels only one cell thick. The capillaries deliver oxygen and nutrient-

TERMS

pulmonary circulation The part of the circulatory system that moves blood between the heart and the lungs; controlled by the right side of the heart.

systemic circulation The part of the circulatory system that moves blood between the heart and the rest of the body; controlled by the left side of the heart.

atria The two upper chambers of the heart in which blood collects before passing to the ventricles; also called *auricles*.

venae cavae The large veins through which blood is returned to the right atrium of the heart.

ventricles The two lower chambers of the heart from which blood flows through arteries to the lungs and other parts of the body.

aorta The large artery that receives blood from the left ventricle and distributes it to the body.

systole Contraction of the heart.

diastole Relaxation of the heart.

veins Vessels that carry blood to the heart.

arteries Vessels that carry blood away from the heart.

capillaries Very small blood vessels that distribute blood to all parts of the body.

rich blood to the tissues and pass on oxygen-poor, waste-carrying blood. From the capillaries, this blood empties into small veins (venules) and then into larger veins that return it to the heart to repeat the cycle.

Blood pumped through the heart doesn't reach its cells, so the heart has its own network of arteries, veins, and capillaries. Two large vessels, the right and left coronary arteries, branch off the aorta and supply the heart muscle with oxygenated blood. Blockage of a coronary artery is a leading cause of heart attacks (see Chapter 11).

The Respiratory System The **respiratory system** supplies oxygen to the body and carries off carbon dioxide, a waste product of body processes. Air passes in and out of the lungs as a result of pressure changes brought about by the contraction and relaxation of the diaphragm and rib muscles; the lungs expand and contract about 12–20 times a minute. As air is inhaled, it passes through the nasal passages, the throat, larynx, trachea (windpipe), and bronchi into the lungs. The lungs consist of many branching tubes that end in tiny, thin-walled air sacs called **alveoli.**

Carbon dioxide and oxygen are exchanged between alveoli and capillaries in the lungs. Carbon dioxide passes from blood cells into the alveoli, where it is carried up

and out of the lungs (exhaled). Oxygen from inhaled air is passed from the alveoli into blood cells; these oxygen-rich blood cells then return to the heart and are pumped throughout the body. Oxygen is an important component of the body's energy-producing system, so the cardiorespiratory system's ability to pick up and deliver oxygen is critical for the functioning of the body—at rest and during exercise.

Energy Production

Metabolism is the sum of all the chemical processes necessary to maintain the body. Energy is required to fuel vital body functions—to build and break down tissue, contract muscles, conduct nerve impulses, regulate body temperature, and so on. The rate at which your body uses energy—its metabolic rate—depends on your level of activity. At rest, you have a low metabolic rate; if you stand up and begin to walk, your metabolic rate increases. If you jog, your metabolic rate may increase more than 800% above its resting level. Olympic-caliber distance runners can increase their metabolic rate by a whopping 2000% or more.

Energy from Food The body converts chemical energy from food into substances that cells can use as fuel. These fuels can be used immediately or stored for later use. The body's ability to store fuel is critical, because if all the energy from food were released immediately, much of it would be wasted.

The three classes of energy-containing nutrients in food are carbohydrates, fats, and proteins. During digestion, most carbohydrates are broken down into the simple sugar **glucose.** Some glucose remains circulating in the blood ("blood sugar"), where it can be used as a quick source of fuel to produce energy. Glucose may also be converted to **glycogen** and stored in the liver, muscles, and kidneys. If glycogen stores are full and the body's immediate need for energy is met, the remaining glucose is converted to fat and stored in the body's fatty tissues. Excess energy from dietary fat is also stored as body fat. Protein in the diet is used primarily to build new tissue, but it can be broken down for energy or incorporated into fat stores. Glucose, glycogen, and fat are important fuels for the production of energy in the cells; protein is a significant energy source only when other fuels are lacking. (See Chapter 8 for more on the other roles of carbohydrate, fat, and protein in the body.)

ATP: The Energy "Currency" of Cells The basic form of energy used by cells is **adenosine triphosphate,** or **ATP.** When a cell needs energy, it breaks down ATP, a process that releases energy in the only form the cell can use directly. Cells store a small amount of ATP; when they need more, they create it through chemical reactions that utilize the body's stored fuels—glucose, glycogen, and fat. When you exercise, your cells need to produce more

TERMS **respiratory system** The lungs, air passages, and breathing muscles; supplies oxygen to the body and carries off carbon dioxide.

alveoli Tiny air sacs in the lungs through whose walls gases such as oxygen and carbon dioxide diffuse in and out of blood.

glucose A simple sugar that circulates in the blood and can be used by cells to fuel adenosine triphosphate (ATP) production.

glycogen A complex carbohydrate stored principally in the liver and skeletal muscles; the major fuel source during most forms of intense exercise. Glycogen is the storage form of glucose.

adenosine triphosphate (ATP) Energy source for cellular processes.

immediate energy system Energy system that supplies energy to muscle cells through the breakdown of cellular stores of ATP and creatine phosphate (CP).

nonoxidative (anaerobic) energy system Energy system that supplies energy to muscle cells through the breakdown of muscle stores of glucose and glycogen; also called the *anaerobic system* or the *lactic acid system* because chemical reactions take place without oxygen and produce lactic acid.

anaerobic Occurring in the absence of oxygen.

lactic acid A metabolic acid resulting from the metabolism of glucose and glycogen; an important source of fuel for many tissues of the body, its accumulation may produce fatigue.

oxidative (aerobic) energy system Energy system that supplies energy to cells through the breakdown of glucose, glycogen, fats, and amino acids; also called the *aerobic system* because chemical reactions require oxygen.

aerobic Dependent on the presence of oxygen.

TABLE 3-1   *Characteristics of the Body's Energy Systems*

	Energy System*		
	Immediate	Nonoxidative	Oxidative
Duration of activity for which system predominates	0–10 seconds	10 seconds–2 minutes	>2 minutes
Intensity of activity for which system predominates	High	High	Low to moderately high
Rate of ATP production	Immediate, very rapid	Rapid	Slower but prolonged
Fuel	Adenosine triphosphate (ATP), creatine phosphate (CP)	Muscle stores of glycogen and glucose	Body stores of glycogen, glucose, fat, and protein
Oxygen used?	No	No	Yes
Sample activities	Weight lifting, picking up a bag of groceries	400-meter run, running up several flights of stairs	1500-meter run, 30-minute walk, standing in line for a long time

*For most activities, all three systems contribute to energy production; the duration and intensity of the activity determine which system predominates.

SOURCE: Adapted from Brooks, G. A., et al. 2000. *Exercise Physiology: Human Bioenergetics and Its Applications*, 3d ed. Mountain View, Calif.: Mayfield.

energy. Consequently, your body mobilizes its stores of fuel to increase ATP production.

Exercise and the Three Energy Systems

The muscles in your body use three energy systems to create ATP and fuel cellular activity. These systems use different fuels and chemical processes and perform different, specific functions during exercise (Table 3-1).

The Immediate Energy System   The **immediate energy system** provides energy rapidly but for only a short period of time. It is used to fuel activities that last for about 10 or fewer seconds—examples in sports include weight lifting and shot-putting; examples in daily life include rising from a chair or picking up a bag of groceries. The components of this energy system include existing cellular ATP stores and creatine phosphate (CP), a chemical that cells can use to make ATP. CP levels are depleted rapidly during exercise, so the maximum capacity of this energy system is reached within a few seconds. Cells must then switch to the other energy systems to restore levels of ATP and CP. (Without adequate ATP, muscles will stiffen and become unusable.)

The Nonoxidative (Anaerobic) Energy System   The **nonoxidative energy system** is used at the start of an exercise session and for high-intensity activities lasting for about 10 seconds to 2 minutes, such as the 400-meter run. During daily activities, this system may be called on to help you run to catch a bus or dash up several flights of

stairs. The nonoxidative energy system creates ATP by breaking down glucose and glycogen. This system doesn't require oxygen, which is why it is sometimes referred to as the **anaerobic** system. The capacity of this system to produce energy is limited, but it can generate a great deal of ATP in a short period of time. For this reason, it is the most important energy system for very intense exercise.

There are two key limiting factors for the nonoxidative energy system. First, the body's supply of glucose and glycogen is limited. Once these are depleted, a person may experience fatigue and dizziness, and judgment may be impaired. (The brain and nervous system rely on carbohydrates as fuel and must have a continuous supply to function properly.) Second, the nonoxidative system results in the production of **lactic acid**. Although lactic acid is an important fuel for the body, it releases substances called hydrogen ions that are thought to interfere with metabolism and muscle contraction, thereby causing fatigue. During heavy exercise, such as sprinting, the body produces large amounts of lactic acid and hydrogen ions, and muscles fatigue rapidly. Fortunately, exercise training increases the body's ability to cope with these substances.

The Oxidative (Aerobic) Energy System   The **oxidative energy system** is used during any physical activity that lasts longer than about 2 minutes, such as distance running, swimming, hiking, or even standing in line for a long time. The oxidative system requires oxygen to generate ATP, which is why it is considered an **aerobic** process.

The oxidative system cannot produce energy as quickly as the other two systems, but it can supply energy for much longer periods of time. It provides energy during most daily activities.

In the oxidative energy system, ATP production takes place in cellular structures called **mitochondria.** Because mitochondria can use carbohydrates (glucose and glycogen) or fats to produce ATP, the body's stores of fuel for this system are much greater than those for the other two energy systems. The actual fuel used depends on the intensity and duration of exercise and on the fitness status of the individual. Carbohydrates are favored during intense exercise; fats, for lower-intensity activities. During a prolonged exercise session, carbohydrates are the predominant fuel at the start of the workout, but fat utilization increases over time. Fit individuals use a greater proportion of fat as fuel, an important adaptation because glycogen depletion is one of the limiting factors for the oxidative energy system. Thus, by being able to use more fat as fuel, a fit individual can exercise for a longer duration before glycogen is depleted and muscles become fatigued.

Oxygen is another limiting factor. The oxygen requirement of this energy system is proportional to the intensity of exercise—as intensity increases, so does oxygen consumption. There is a limit to the body's ability to increase the transport and use of oxygen; this limit is referred to as **maximal oxygen consumption,** or $\dot{V}O_{2max}$. $\dot{V}O_{2max}$ is determined partly by genetics and partly by fitness status (the muscles' power-generating capacity and fatigue resistance). It depends on many factors, including the capacity of blood to carry oxygen, the rate at which oxygen is transported to the tissues, and the amount of oxygen that cells extract from the blood. $\dot{V}O_{2max}$ determines how intensely a person can perform endurance exercise and for how long, and it is considered the best overall measure of the capacity of the cardiorespiratory system. (The assessment tests described later in the chapter are designed to help you predict your $\dot{V}O_{2max}$.)

The Energy Systems in Combination   Your body typically uses all three energy systems when you exercise. The intensity and duration of the activity determine which system predominates. For example, when you play tennis, you use the immediate energy system when hitting the ball, but you replenish cellular energy stores using the nonoxidative and oxidative systems. When cycling, the oxidative system predominates. However, if you must suddenly exercise very intensely—ride up a steep hill, for example—the other systems become important because the oxidative system is unable to supply ATP fast enough to sustain high-intensity effort.

Physical Fitness and Energy Production   Physically fit people can increase their metabolic rate substantially, generating the energy needed for powerful or sustained exercise. People with lower levels of fitness cannot respond to exercise in the same way. Their bodies are less capable of delivering oxygen and fuel to exercising muscles; they are also less able to cope with lactic acid and other substances produced during intense physical activity. Because of this, they fatigue more rapidly—their legs hurt and they breathe heavily walking up a flight of stairs, for example. Regular physical training can substantially improve the body's ability to produce energy and meet the challenges of increased physical activity.

For many sports, one energy system will be most important. For weight lifters, for example, it is the immediate energy system; for sprinters, the nonoxidative system; and for endurance runners, the oxidative system. In designing an exercise program, focus on the energy system most important to your goals. Because improving the functioning of the cardiorespiratory system is critical to overall wellness, endurance exercise that utilizes the oxidative energy system—activities performed at moderate to high intensities for a prolonged duration—is a key component of any health-related fitness program.

TERMS   **mitochondria**   Intracellular structures containing enzymes used in the chemical reactions that convert the energy in food to a form the body can use.

maximal oxygen consumption ($\dot{V}O_{2max}$)   The highest rate of oxygen consumption an individual is capable of during maximum physical effort, reflecting the body's ability to transport and use oxygen; measured in milliliters used per minute per kilogram of body weight.

blood pressure   The force exerted by the blood on the walls of the blood vessels; created by the pumping action of the heart. Blood pressure increases during systole and decreases during diastole.

free radicals   Highly reactive compounds that can damage cells by taking electrons from key cellular components such as DNA or the cell membrane; produced by normal metabolic processes and through exposure to environmental factors, including sunlight.

BENEFITS OF CARDIORESPIRATORY ENDURANCE EXERCISE

Cardiorespiratory endurance exercise helps the body become more efficient and better able to cope with physical challenges. It also lowers risk for many chronic diseases. Let's take a closer look at the physiological adaptations and long-term benefits of regular endurance exercise.

Improved Cardiorespiratory Functioning

At rest, a healthy cardiorespiratory system has little difficulty keeping pace with the body's need for oxygen, fuel, and waste removal. During exercise, however, the demands on the system increase dramatically as metabolic

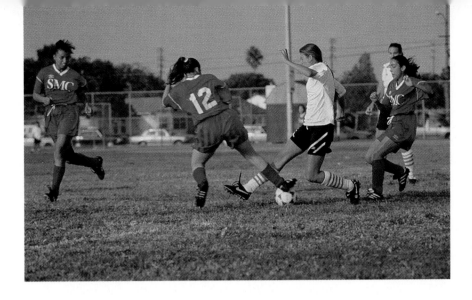

Exercise offers both long-term health benefits and immediate pleasures. Many popular sports and activities, including soccer, develop cardiorespiratory endurance.

rate goes up. The principal cardiorespiratory responses to exercise include the following:

- Increased cardiac output and **blood pressure.** More blood is pumped by the heart each minute because both heart rate and stroke volume (the amount of blood pumped with each beat) go up. Increased cardiac output speeds the delivery of oxygen and fuel and the removal of waste products.

- Increased ventilation (rate and depth of breathing).

- Increased blood flow to active skeletal muscles and to the heart; constant or slightly increased blood flow to the brain.

- Increased blood flow to the skin and increased sweating. The chemical reactions that produce energy for exercise release heat, which must be dissipated to maintain a safe body temperature.

- Decreased blood flow to the stomach, intestines, liver, and kidneys, resulting in reduced activity in the gastrointestinal tract and reduced urine output.

All of these changes help the body respond to the challenge of exercise in the short term. When performed regularly, endurance exercise also causes more permanent adaptations. It improves the functioning of the heart, the ability of the cardiorespiratory system to carry oxygen to the body's tissues, and the capacity of the cells to take up and use oxygen. These improvements reduce the effort required to carry out everyday activities and make the body better able to respond to physical challenges.

Endurance training enhances the health of the heart by maintaining or increasing its blood and oxygen supply, decreasing work and oxygen demand of the heart, and increasing the function of the heart muscle. The trained heart is more efficient and subject to less stress. It pumps more blood per beat, so heart rate is lower at rest and during exercise. The resting heart rate of a fit person is often 10–20 beats per minute lower than that of a sedentary person; this translates into as many as 10 million fewer beats in the course of one year. Improved heart efficiency results because endurance training improves heart contraction strength, increases heart cavity size (in young adults), and increases blood volume so that the heart pushes more blood into the circulation system during each of its contractions. Training also tends to reduce blood pressure, so the heart does not have to work as hard when it contracts.

Improved Cellular Metabolism

Regular endurance exercise also improves metabolism at the cellular level. It increases the number of capillaries in the muscles so that they can be supplied with more oxygen and fuel. It also trains the muscles to make the most of available oxygen and fuel so that they work more efficiently. Exercise increases the size and number of mitochondria in muscle cells, thereby increasing the energy capacity of the cells. Endurance training also helps in energy production by preventing glycogen depletion and increasing the muscles' ability to use lactic acid and fat as fuels.

Fitness programs that best develop metabolic efficiency are characterized by both long-duration, moderately intense endurance exercise and brief periods of more intense effort. For example, climbing a small hill while jogging or cycling introduces the kind of intense exercise that leads to more efficient use of lactic acid and fats.

Regular exercise may also help protect your cells from chemical damage. Many scientists believe that aging and some chronic diseases are linked to cellular damage caused by **free radicals.** Training activates antioxidant enzymes that prevent free radical damage to cell structures, thereby enhancing health. (See Chapter 8 for more on free radicals and antioxidants.) Training also improves the functional stability of cells and tissues by improving the regulation of salts and fluids in the cells. This is particularly important in the heart, where instability can lead to cardiac arrest and death.

Research has shown that most aspects of physiological functioning peak when people are about 30 years old and then decline at a rate of about 0.5–1.0% a year. This decline in physical capacity is characterized by a decrease in maximal oxygen consumption, cardiac output, muscular strength, fat-free mass, joint mobility, and other factors. However, regular exercise can substantially alter the rate of decline in functional status, and it is associated with both longevity and improved quality of life.

Regular endurance exercise can improve maximal oxygen consumption in older people by up to 15–30%—the same degree of improvement seen in younger individuals. In fact, studies have shown that Masters athletes in their 70s have $\dot{V}O_{2max}$ values equivalent to those of sedentary 20-year-olds. At any age, endurance training can improve cardiorespiratory functioning, cellular metabolism, body composition, and psychological and emotional well-being. Older people who exercise regularly have better balance and greater bone density and are less likely than their sedentary peers to suffer injuries as a result of falls. Regular endurance training also substantially reduces the risk of many chronic and disabling diseases, including heart disease, cancer, diabetes, and osteoporosis.

Other forms of exercise training are also beneficial for older adults. Resistance training is a safe and effective way to build strength and fat-free mass and can help people remain independent as they age. Lifting weights has also been shown to boost spirits in older people, perhaps because improvements in strength appear quickly and are easily applied to everyday tasks such as climbing stairs and carrying groceries. Flexibility exercises can improve the range of motion in joints and also help people maintain functional independence as they age.

Life expectancy in the United States has increased dramatically over the past century, and about 70% of Americans now live to at least age 70. A lifetime of regular exercise is one of the best age-proofing strategies available; however, it's never too late to start. Even in people over 80, beginning an exercise program can improve physical functioning and quality of life. Most older adults are able to participate in a program that includes moderate walking and strengthening and stretching exercises, and modified programs can be created for people with chronic conditions and other special health concerns (see Chapter 7). The wellness benefits of exercise are available to people of all ages and levels of ability.

SOURCES: Brooks, G. A., et al. 2000. *Exercise Physiology: Human Bioenergetics and Its Applications,* 3d ed. Mountain View, Calif.: Mayfield. American College of Sports Medicine. 1998. *ACSM's Resource Manual for Guidelines for Exercise Testing and Prescription,* 3d ed. Baltimore, Md.: Williams & Wilkins.

Reduced Risk of Chronic Disease

Regular endurance exercise lowers your risk of many chronic, disabling diseases. It can also help people with those diseases improve their health (see the box "Benefits of Exercise for Older Adults").

Cardiovascular Disease A sedentary lifestyle is one of the six major risk factors for **cardiovascular disease (CVD)** (see Chapter 11). The other primary factors are smoking, unhealthy cholesterol levels, high blood pressure, diabetes, and obesity. People who are sedentary have CVD death rates significantly higher than those of fit individuals.

Endurance exercise has a positive effect on levels of fats in the blood. High concentrations of blood fats such as cholesterol and triglycerides are linked to cardiovascular disease because they contribute to the formation of fatty deposits on the lining of arteries. If one of the coronary arteries, which supply oxygenated blood to the heart, becomes blocked by such a deposit, the result is a heart attack; blockage of a cerebral artery can cause a stroke.

Cholesterol is carried in the blood by **lipoproteins,** which are classified according to size and density. Cholesterol carried by low-density lipoproteins (LDLs) tends to stick to the walls of arteries. High-density lipoproteins (HDLs), on the other hand, pick up excess cholesterol in the bloodstream and carry it back to the liver for excretion from the body. High LDL levels and low HDL levels are associated with a high risk of CVD. High levels of HDL and low levels of LDL are associated with lower risk. More information about cholesterol and heart disease is provided in Chapter 11. For our purposes in this chapter, it is important to know only that endurance exercise influences blood fat levels in a positive way—by increasing HDL and decreasing triglycerides (and possibly LDL)—thereby reducing the risk of CVD.

Regular exercise tends to reduce high blood pressure, a contributing factor in diseases such as **coronary heart disease,** stroke, kidney failure, and blindness. It also helps prevent obesity and diabetes, both of which contribute to CVD.

Cancer Some studies have shown a relationship between increased physical activity and a reduction in a person's risk of all types of cancer, but these findings are not conclusive. There is strong evidence that exercise reduces the risk of colon cancer and promising data that it reduces the risk of cancer of the breast and reproductive organs in women. Exercise may decrease the risk of colon cancer by speeding the movement of food through the gastrointestinal tract (quickly eliminating potential carcinogens), enhancing immune function, and reducing blood fats. The protective mechanism in the case of reproductive system cancers is less clear, but physical activity during the high school and college years may be particularly important for preventing breast cancer later in life.

Diabetes   Recent studies have shown that regular exercise helps prevent the development of the most common form of diabetes (see Chapter 6 for more on diabetes). Exercise burns excess sugar and makes cells more sensitive to the hormone insulin, which is involved in the regulation of blood sugar levels. Obesity is a key risk factor for diabetes, and exercise helps keep body fat at healthy levels. For people who have diabetes, physical activity is an important part of treatment.

Osteoporosis   A special benefit of exercise, especially for women, is protection against osteoporosis, a disease that results in loss of bone density and poor bone strength. Weight-bearing exercise helps build bone during the teens and twenties. People with denser bones can better endure the bone loss that occurs with aging. With stronger bones and muscles and better balance, fit people are less likely to experience debilitating falls and bone fractures. (See Chapter 8 for more on osteoporosis.)

Better Control of Body Fat

Too much body fat is linked to a variety of health problems, including cardiovascular disease, cancer, and diabetes. Healthy body composition can be difficult to achieve and maintain because a diet that contains all essential nutrients can be relatively high in calories, especially for someone who is sedentary. Excess calories are stored in the body as fat. Regular exercise increases daily calorie expenditure so that a healthy diet is less likely to lead to weight gain. Endurance exercise burns calories directly and, if intense enough, continues to do so by raising resting metabolic rate for several hours following an exercise session. A higher metabolic rate means that a person can consume more calories without gaining weight.

Endurance exercise can also help maintain or increase metabolic rate slightly by helping people maintain a high proportion of fat-free mass. Strength training, discussed in Chapter 4, is even more effective at building muscle mass than endurance training. (Energy balance and the role of exercise in improving body composition are discussed in detail in Chapter 6.)

Improved Immune Function

Exercise can have either positive or negative effects on the immune system, the physiological processes that protect us from disease. Moderate endurance exercise boosts immune function, whereas excessive training (overtraining) depresses it. Physically fit people get fewer colds and upper respiratory tract infections than people who are not fit. In addition to regular exercise, the immune system can be strengthened by eating a well-balanced diet rich in whole grains, fruits, vegetables, and low-fat dairy and meat products; managing stress; and getting 7–8 hours of sleep every night.

Improved Psychological and Emotional Well-Being

Most people who participate in regular endurance exercise experience social, psychological, and emotional benefits. Performing physical activities provides proof of skill mastery and self-control, thus enhancing self-image. Recreational sports provide an opportunity to socialize, have fun, and strive to excel.

Endurance exercise also provides protection against the effects of stress that have been linked to poor cardiorespiratory health. Psychological stress causes increased secretion of **epinephrine** and **norepinephrine**, the so-called fight-or-flight hormones, which are thought to speed the buildup of fatty deposits in the arteries. Excessive hostility and anger are also associated with the risk of heart disease. Endurance exercise decreases the secretion of hormones triggered by emotional stress. It can diffuse hostility and alleviate depression and anxiety by providing an emotional outlet and inducing feelings of relaxation (see the box "Exercise and the Mind"). Regular exercise can also relieve sleeping problems.

Refer to Figure 3-3 for a summary of specific physiological benefits of cardiorespiratory endurance exercise. As cardiorespiratory fitness is developed, these benefits translate into both physical and emotional well-being and a much lower risk of chronic disease.

ASSESSING CARDIORESPIRATORY FITNESS

The body's ability to maintain a level of exertion (exercise) for an extended period of time is a direct reflection of cardiorespiratory fitness. It is determined by the body's ability to take up, distribute, and use oxygen during physical activity. As explained earlier, the best quantitative measure of cardiorespiratory endurance is maximal oxygen consumption, expressed as $\dot{V}O_{2max}$, the amount of oxygen the body uses when a person reaches maximum ability to supply oxygen during exercise (measured in milliliters of oxygen used per minute for each kilogram of

TERMS

cardiovascular disease (CVD)   Disease of the heart and blood vessels.

lipoproteins   Substances in blood, classified according to size, density, and chemical composition, that transport fats.

coronary heart disease   Heart disease caused by the buildup of fatty deposits on the arteries that supply oxygen to the heart; also called *coronary artery disease*.

epinephrine   A hormone secreted in response to stress that stimulates the heart, makes carbohydrates available in the liver and muscles, and releases fat from fat cells.

norepinephrine   A stress hormone with many of the same effects as epinephrine.

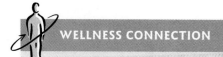
If you've ever gone for a long, brisk walk after a hard day's work, you know how refreshing exercise can be. Exercise can improve mood, stimulate creativity, clarify thinking, relieve anxiety, and provide an outlet for anger or aggression. But why does exercise make you feel good? Does it simply take your mind off your problems? Or does it cause a physical reaction that affects your mental state?

Current research indicates that exercise triggers many physical changes in the body that can alter mood. Scientists are now trying to explain how and why exercise affects the mind. One theory has to do with the physical structure of the brain. The area of the brain responsible for the movement of muscles is near the area responsible for thought and emotion. As muscles work vigorously, the resulting stimulation in the muscle center of the brain may also stimulate the thought and emotion center, producing improvements in mood and cognitive functions.

Other researchers suggest that exercise stimulates the release of opiates known as **endorphins,** chemicals in the brain that can suppress fatigue, decrease pain, and produce euphoria. Still others believe the relationship between exercise and mood to be much more complex.

A third area of research focuses on changes in brain activity during and after exercise. One change is an increase in alpha brain-wave activity. Alpha waves indicate a highly relaxed state; meditation also induces alpha wave activity. A second change is an alteration in the levels of **neurotransmitters,** brain chemicals that increase alertness and reduce stress.

Higher levels of neurotransmitters may explain how exercise improves mild-to-moderate cases of depression. Researchers have found that cardiorespiratory endurance exercise can be as effective as psychotherapy in reducing anxiety, and even more effective when used in conjunction with other therapies. In addition to boosting neurotransmitter activity, exercise has been found to block out stressful stimuli and enhance self-esteem.

Although most people don't associate exercise with mental skills, physical activity has been shown to have positive effects on cognitive functioning in both the short term and the long term; it may even regenerate brain cells. A recent study showed that mice who engaged in regular exercise grew twice as many new brain cells as mice who sat in their cages.

Exercise may also help boost creativity. In a study of college students, those who ran regularly or took aerobic dance classes scored significantly higher on standard psychological tests of creativity than did sedentary students. Over the long term, exercise can slow and possibly even reverse certain age-related declines in cognitive performance, including slowed reaction time and loss of short-term memory and nonverbal reasoning skills.

The message from all this research is that exercise is a critical factor in developing *all* the dimensions of wellness, not just physical health. Even moderate exercise like walking briskly a few times a week can significantly improve your well-being. A lifetime of physical activity can leave you with a healthier body and a sharper, happier, more creative mind.

---

body weight). Maximal oxygen consumption can be measured precisely in an exercise physiology laboratory through analysis of the air a person inhales and exhales when exercising to a level of exhaustion (maximum intensity). This procedure can be expensive and time-consuming, making it impractical for the average person.

Four Assessment Tests

Fortunately, several simple assessment tests provide reasonably good estimates of maximal oxygen consumption (within ±10–15% of the results of a laboratory test). Four methods are described here and presented in Lab 3-1: a 1-mile walk test, a 3-minute step test, a 1.5-mile run-walk test, and the Åstrand-Rhyming cycle ergometer test. To assess yourself, choose among these methods based on your access to equipment, your current physical condition, and your own preference. Don't take any of

these tests without checking with your physician if you are ill or have any of the risk factors for exercise discussed in Chapter 2 and Lab 2-2. Table 3-2 lists the fitness prerequisites and cautions recommended for each test.

You'll get more accurate results from these tests if you avoid strenuous activity the day of the test; avoid caffeine, which can affect heart rate; and don't smoke or eat a heavy meal for up to 3 hours before the test. Record your test results in Lab 3-1, and then use the appropriate formula to calculate your maximal oxygen consumption.

The 1-Mile Walk Test   The 1-mile walk test estimates your level of cardiorespiratory fitness (maximal oxygen consumption) based on the amount of time it takes you to complete 1 mile of brisk walking and your exercise heart rate at the end of your walk; age, gender, and body weight are also considered. A fast time and a low heart rate indicate a high level of cardiorespiratory endurance.

The 3-Minute Step Test   The rate at which the pulse returns to normal after exercise is also a good measure of cardiorespiratory capacity; heart rate remains lower and recovers faster in people who are more physically fit. For the step test, you step continually at a steady rate for 3 minutes and then monitor your heart rate during recovery.

TERMS   **endorphins**   Substances resembling morphine that are secreted by the brain and that decrease pain, suppress fatigue, and produce euphoria.

neurotransmitters   Brain chemicals that transmit nerve impulses.

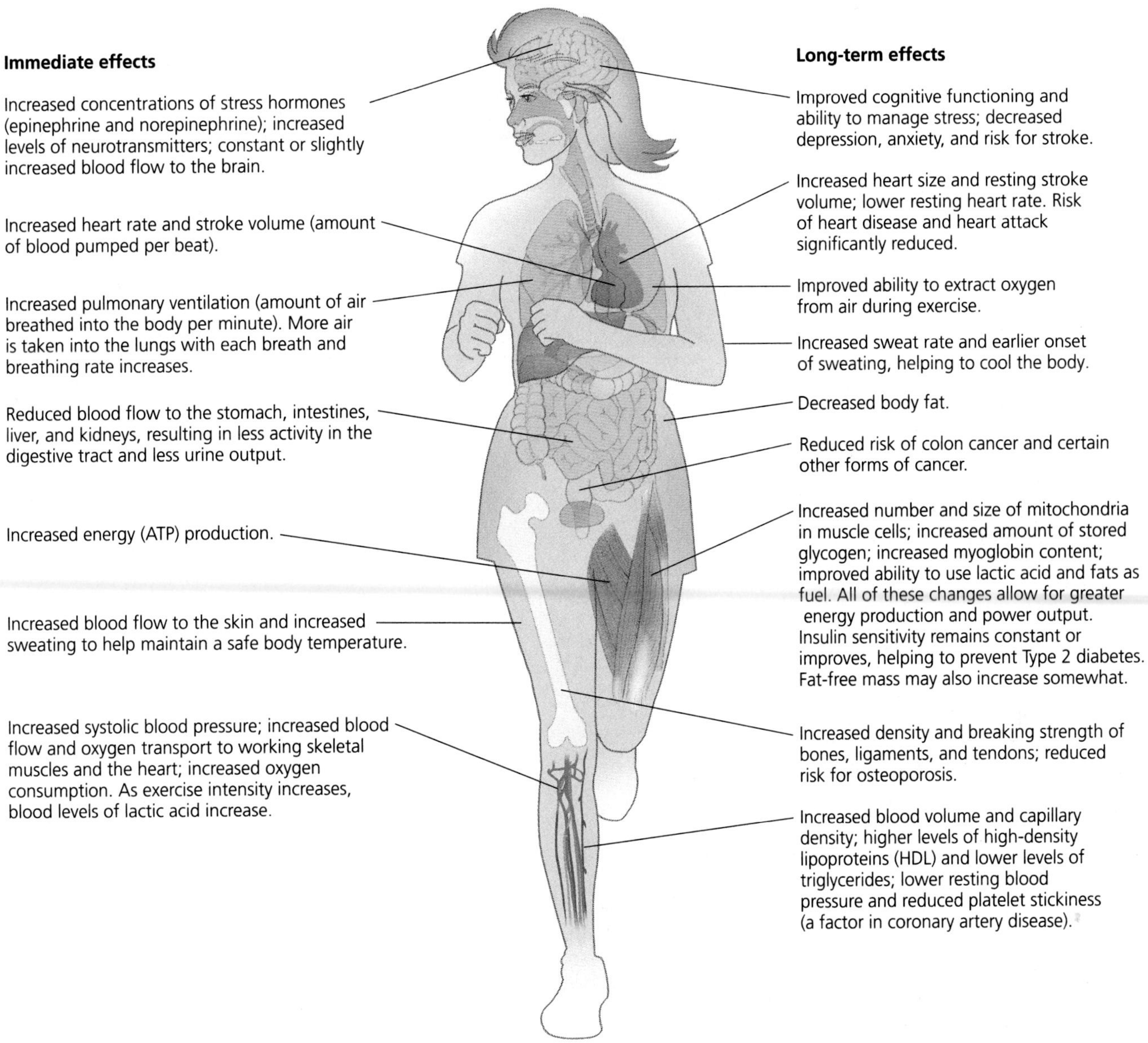

Immediate effects

Increased concentrations of stress hormones (epinephrine and norepinephrine); increased levels of neurotransmitters; constant or slightly increased blood flow to the brain.

Increased heart rate and stroke volume (amount of blood pumped per beat).

Increased pulmonary ventilation (amount of air breathed into the body per minute). More air is taken into the lungs with each breath and breathing rate increases.

Reduced blood flow to the stomach, intestines, liver, and kidneys, resulting in less activity in the digestive tract and less urine output.

Increased energy (ATP) production.

Increased blood flow to the skin and increased sweating to help maintain a safe body temperature.

Increased systolic blood pressure; increased blood flow and oxygen transport to working skeletal muscles and the heart; increased oxygen consumption. As exercise intensity increases, blood levels of lactic acid increase.

Long-term effects

Improved cognitive functioning and ability to manage stress; decreased depression, anxiety, and risk for stroke.

Increased heart size and resting stroke volume; lower resting heart rate. Risk of heart disease and heart attack significantly reduced.

Improved ability to extract oxygen from air during exercise.

Increased sweat rate and earlier onset of sweating, helping to cool the body.

Decreased body fat.

Reduced risk of colon cancer and certain other forms of cancer.

Increased number and size of mitochondria in muscle cells; increased amount of stored glycogen; increased myoglobin content; improved ability to use lactic acid and fats as fuel. All of these changes allow for greater energy production and power output. Insulin sensitivity remains constant or improves, helping to prevent Type 2 diabetes. Fat-free mass may also increase somewhat.

Increased density and breaking strength of bones, ligaments, and tendons; reduced risk for osteoporosis.

Increased blood volume and capillary density; higher levels of high-density lipoproteins (HDL) and lower levels of triglycerides; lower resting blood pressure and reduced platelet stickiness (a factor in coronary artery disease).

Figure 3-3   Immediate and long-term effects of regular cardiorespiratory endurance exercise.   When endurance exercise is performed regularly, short-term changes in the body develop into more permanent adaptations; these long-term effects include improved ability to exercise, reduced risk of many chronic diseases, and improved psychological and emotional well-being.

The 1.5-Mile Run-Walk Test   The 1.5-mile run-walk test is considered one of the best indirect measures of cardiorespiratory capacity. Oxygen consumption increases with speed in distance running; a fast time on this test indicates high maximal oxygen consumption.

The Åstrand-Rhyming Cycle Ergometer Test   A cycle ergometer measures power output, the amount of resistance the cycle exerts against a person's pedaling. A higher power output means the cyclist is applying more pressure—that is, pedaling harder or faster. The Åstrand-Rhyming test estimates maximal oxygen consumption from the exercise heart rate reached after pedaling a cycle ergometer for 6 minutes at a constant rate and resistance. A low exercise heart rate after pedaling at a high power output indicates a high maximal oxygen consumption.

Monitoring Your Heart Rate

Each time your heart beats, it pumps blood into your arteries; this surge of blood causes a pulse that you can feel by holding your fingers against an artery. Counting your pulse to determine your exercise heart rate is a key part of

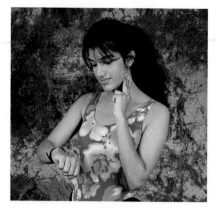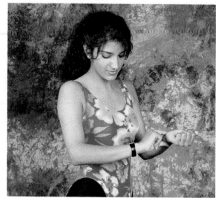

A pulse count can be used to determine exercise heart rate. The pulse can be taken at the carotid artery in the neck (left) or at the radial artery in the wrist (right).

TABLE 3-2	Fitness Prerequisites and Cautions for the Cardiorespiratory Endurance Assessment Tests

Note: The conditions for exercise safety given in Chapter 2 apply to all fitness assessment tests. If you answered yes to any question on the PAR-Q in Lab 2-2, see your physician before taking any assessment test. If you experience any unusual symptoms while taking a test, stop exercising, and discuss your condition with your instructor.

Test	Fitness Prerequisites/Cautions
1-mile walk test	Recommended for anyone who meets the criteria for safe exercise. Can be used by individuals who cannot perform other tests because of low fitness level or injury.
3-minute step test	If you suffer from joint problems in your ankles, knees, or hips or are significantly overweight, check with your physician before taking this test.
1.5-mile run-walk test	Recommended for people who are healthy and at least moderately active. If you have been sedentary, you should participate in a 4- to 8-week walk-run program before taking the test. Don't take this test in extremely hot or cold weather if you aren't used to exercising under those conditions.
Åstrand-Rhyming test	Recommended for people who are healthy and at least moderately active. It can be taken by people with some joint problems because body weight is supported by the cycle.

most assessment tests for maximal oxygen consumption. Heart rate can also be used to monitor exercise intensity during a workout. (Intensity is described in more detail in the next section.)

The two most common sites for monitoring heart rate are the carotid artery in the neck and the radial artery in the wrist. To take your pulse, press your index and middle fingers gently on the correct site. You may have to shift position several times to find the best place to feel your pulse. Don't use your thumb to check your pulse; it has a pulse of its own that can confuse your count. Be careful not to push too hard, particularly when taking your pulse in the carotid artery (strong pressure on this artery may cause a reflex that slows the heart rate).

Heart rates are usually assessed in beats per minute (bpm). But counting your pulse for an entire minute isn't practical when you're exercising. And because heart rate slows rapidly when you stop exercising, it can give inaccurate results. It's best to do a shorter count—10 seconds—and then multiply the result by 6 to get your heart rate in beats per minute. The same procedure can be used to take someone else's pulse, as in the cycle ergometer test.

Interpreting Your Score

Once you've completed one or more of the assessment tests, use the table under "Rating Your Cardiovascular Fitness" at the end of Lab 3-1 to determine your level of cardiorespiratory fitness. Find the row that corresponds to your age and gender, and then find the category that contains your score for maximal oxygen consumption. For example, a 19-year-old female with a maximal oxygen consumption score of 36 ml/kg/min would be classified as having fair cardiorespiratory fitness. You can see from the table that there are differences in ratings for $\dot{V}O_{2max}$ between men and women.

You can monitor the progress of your fitness program by repeating the cardiorespiratory assessment test(s) from time to time. Because your $\dot{V}O_{2max}$ score will vary somewhat for different types of tests, always compare scores for the *same* test.

Cardiorespiratory endurance exercises are best for developing the type of fitness associated with good health, so they should serve as the focus of your exercise program. To create a successful endurance exercise program, you must set realistic goals; choose suitable activities; set your starting frequency, intensity, and duration of exercise at appropriate levels; remember to warm up and cool down; and adjust your program as your fitness improves.

Setting Goals

You can use the results of cardiorespiratory fitness assessment tests to set a specific oxygen consumption goal for your cardiorespiratory endurance program. Your goal should be high enough to ensure a healthy cardiorespiratory system, but not so high that it will be impossible to achieve. Scores in the fair and good ranges for maximal oxygen consumption suggest good fitness; scores in the excellent and superior ranges indicate a high standard of physical performance. You can also set more general goals, such as lowering your risk for diabetes or being able to hike 5 miles.

Choosing Sports and Activities

Cardiorespiratory endurance exercises include activities that involve the rhythmic use of large-muscle groups for an extended period of time, such as jogging, walking, cycling, aerobic dancing and other forms of group exercise, cross-country skiing, and swimming. Start-and-stop sports, such as tennis and racquetball, also qualify, as long as you have enough skill to play continuously and intensely enough to raise your heart rate to target levels.

Having fun is a strong motivator; select a physical activity that you enjoy, and it will be easier to stay with your program. Exercising with a friend can also be helpful as a motivator. Consider whether you prefer competitive or individual sports, or whether starting something new would be best. Other important considerations are access to facilities, expense, and the time required to achieve an adequate skill level and workout.

Determining Frequency of Training

To build cardiorespiratory endurance, you should exercise 3–5 days per week. Beginners should start with 3 and work up to 5 days per week. Training more than 5 days per week can lead to injury and isn't necessary for the typical person on an exercise program designed to promote wellness. Training fewer than 3 days per week makes it difficult to improve your fitness (unless exercise intensity is very high) or to use exercise to lose weight. In addition, you risk injury because your body never gets a chance to fully adapt to regular exercise training.

Determining Intensity of Training

Intensity is the most important factor in achieving training effects. You must exercise intensely enough to stress your body so that fitness improves. Two methods of monitoring exercise intensity are described below; choose the method that works best for you. Be sure to make adjustments in your intensity levels for environmental or individual factors. For example, on a hot and humid day or on your first day back to your program after an illness, you should decrease your intensity level.

Target Heart Rate Zone   One of the best ways to monitor the intensity of cardiorespiratory endurance exercise is to measure your heart rate. It isn't necessary to exercise at your maximum heart rate to improve maximal oxygen consumption. Fitness adaptations occur at lower heart rates with a much lower risk of injury.

According to the American College of Sports Medicine, your **target heart rate zone**—rates at which you should exercise to experience cardiorespiratory benefits—is between 65% and 90% of your maximum heart rate. To calculate your target heart rate zone, follow these steps:

1. Estimate your maximum heart rate (MHR) by subtracting your age from 220, or have it measured precisely by undergoing an exercise stress test in a doctor's office, hospital, or sports medicine lab.

2. Multiply your MHR by 65% and 90% to calculate your target heart rate zone.

For example, a 19-year-old would calculate her target heart rate zone as follows:

$$MHR = 220 - 19 = 201$$
$$65\% \text{ training intensity} = 0.65 \times 201 = 131 \text{ bpm}$$
$$90\% \text{ training intensity} = 0.90 \times 201 = 181 \text{ bpm}$$

To gain fitness benefits, the young woman in our example would have to exercise at an intensity that raises her heart rate to between 131 and 181 bpm.

An alternative method for calculating target heart rate range uses **heart rate reserve,** the difference between maximum heart rate and resting heart rate. Using this method, target heart rate is equal to resting heart rate plus between 50% and 85% of heart rate reserve. Formulas for both methods of calculating target heart rate are given in Lab 3-2.

Use Lab 3-2 to determine your target heart rate zone. If you have been sedentary, start by exercising at the lower

target heart rate zone   The range of heart rates that should **TERMS** be reached and maintained during cardiorespiratory endurance exercise to obtain training effects.

heart rate reserve   The difference between maximum heart rate and resting heart rate; used in one method for calculating target heart rate range.

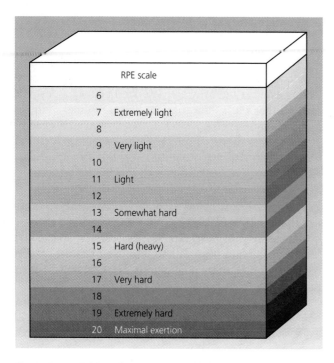

RPE scale	
6	
7	Extremely light
8	
9	Very light
10	
11	Light
12	
13	Somewhat hard
14	
15	Hard (heavy)
16	
17	Very hard
18	
19	Extremely hard
20	Maximal exertion

Figure 3-4 Ratings of perceived exertion. Experienced exercisers may use this subjective scale to estimate how near they are to their target heart rate zone. The scale was developed in the 1950s by Swedish exercise physiologist Gunnar Borg and is also known as the Borg scale. From *Psychology from Research to Practice*, edited by H. L. Pick. Reprinted with permission from Plenum Publishing Corporation.

Ratings of Perceived Exertion The second way to monitor intensity is to monitor your perceived level of exertion. Repeated pulse counting during exercise can become a nuisance if it interferes with the activity. As your exercise program progresses, you will probably become familiar with the amount of exertion required to raise your heart rate to target levels. In other words, you will know how you feel when you have exercised intensely enough. If this is the case, you can use the scale of **ratings of perceived exertion (RPE)** shown in Figure 3-4 to monitor the intensity of your exercise session without checking your pulse.

To use the RPE scale, select a rating that corresponds to your subjective perception of how hard you are exercising when you are training in your target heart rate zone. If your target zone is about 135–155 bpm, exercise intensely enough to raise your heart rate to that level, and then associate a rating—for example, "somewhat hard" or "hard" (14 or 15)—with how hard you feel you are working. To reach and maintain intensity in future workouts, exercise hard enough to reach what you feel is the same level of exertion. You should periodically check your RPE against your target heart rate zone to make sure it's correct. Research has shown RPE to be an accurate means of monitoring exercise intensity, and you may find it more convenient than pulse counting.

Determining Duration of Training

A total duration of 20–60 minutes is recommended; exercise can take place in a single session or in multiple sessions lasting 10 or more minutes. The total duration of exercise depends on its intensity. To improve cardiorespiratory endurance during a low-to-moderate-intensity activity such as walking or slow swimming, you should exercise for 45–60 minutes. For high-intensity exercise performed at the top of your target heart rate zone, a duration of 20 minutes is sufficient. Some studies have shown that 5–10 minutes of extremely intense exercise (greater than 90% of maximal oxygen consumption) improves cardiorespiratory endurance. However, training at this intensity, particularly during high-impact activities, increases the risk of injury. Also, because of the discomfort of high-intensity exercise, you are more likely to discontinue your exercise program. Longer-duration, low-to-moderate-intensity activities generally result in more gradual gains in maximal oxygen consumption. See Figure 3-5 for a summary of the relative intensities of various activities and sports. In planning your program, start off with less-vigorous activities and only gradually increase intensity.

Warming Up and Cooling Down

It's important to warm up before every session of cardiorespiratory endurance exercise and to cool down afterward. Because the body's muscles work better when their

end of your target heart rate range (65% of maximum heart rate or 50% of heart rate reserve) for at least 4–6 weeks. Fast and significant gains in maximal oxygen consumption can be made by exercising closer to the top of the range, but you may increase your risk of injury and overtraining. You *can* achieve significant health benefits by exercising at the bottom of your target range, so don't feel pressured into exercising at an unnecessarily intense level. If you exercise at a lower intensity, you can increase the duration or frequency of training to obtain as much benefit to your health, as long as you are above the 65% training threshold. (For people with a very low initial level of fitness, a lower training intensity, 55–64% of maximum heart rate or 40–49% of heart rate reserve, may be sufficient to achieve improvements in maximal oxygen consumption, especially at the start of an exercise program. Intensities of 70–85% of maximum heart rate are appropriate for average individuals.)

By monitoring your heart rate, you will always know if you are working hard enough to improve, not hard enough, or too hard. To monitor your heart rate during exercise, count your pulse while you're still moving or immediately after you stop exercising. Count beats for 10 seconds, and then multiply that number by 6 to see if your heart rate is in your target zone. If the young woman in our example were aiming for 144 bpm, she would want a 10-second count of 24 beats.

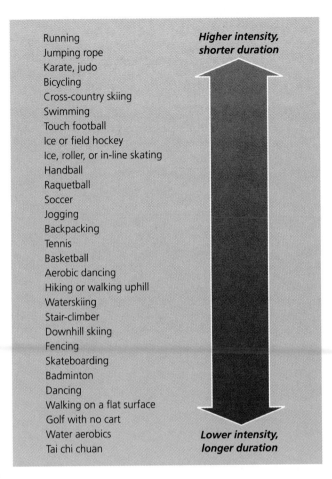

Figure 3-5 Activities and sports for developing cardiorespiratory endurance. The potential of an activity to develop cardiorespiratory endurance depends primarily on the intensity, duration, and frequency of training; the scale shown here reflects intensities. (See Table 7-1 on pp. 169–170 for more information about the fitness potential of different sports and activities.)

temperature is slightly above resting level, warming up enhances performance and decreases the chance of injury. It gives the body time to redirect blood to active muscles and the heart time to adapt to increased demands. Warming up also helps spread **synovial fluid** throughout the joints, which helps protect their surfaces from injury.

As mentioned in Chapter 2, a warm-up session should include low-intensity movements similar to those in the activity that will follow. Low-intensity movements include walking slowly before beginning a brisk walk, hitting forehands and backhands before a tennis match, and running a 12-minute mile before progressing to an 8-minute one. Some experts also recommend including stretching exercises in your warm-up; however, it's best to stretch after your body temperature has been elevated by the active part of the warm-up (see Chapter 5).

Cooling down after exercise is important for returning the body to a nonexercising state. A cool-down, consisting of 5–10 minutes of reduced activity, should follow every workout to allow heart rate, breathing, and circulation to return to normal. Stretching exercises can be part of a cool-down.

The general pattern of a safe and successful workout for cardiorespiratory fitness is illustrated in Figure 3-6.

Maintaining Cardiorespiratory Fitness

Although your fitness level will probably improve quickly at the beginning of your fitness program, this rate of progress will probably slow after 4–6 weeks. The more fit you become, the harder you will have to work to improve. But there is a limit. Increasing intensity and duration indefinitely can lead to injury. Once you reach an acceptable level of fitness, maintain it by continuing to exercise at the same intensity at least 3 nonconsecutive days every week.

EXERCISE INJURIES

Even the most careful physically active person can suffer an injury. Most injuries are annoying rather than serious or permanent. However, an injury that isn't cared for properly can escalate into a chronic problem, sometimes serious enough to permanently curtail the activity. It's important to learn how to deal with injuries so they don't derail your fitness program. Strategies for the care of common exercise injuries and discomforts appear in Table 3-3; some general guidelines are given below.

When to Call a Physician

Some injuries require medical attention. Consult a physician for head and eye injuries, possible ligament injuries, broken bones, and internal disorders such as chest pain, fainting, elevated body temperature, and intolerance to hot weather. Also seek medical attention for ostensibly minor injuries that do not get better within a reasonable amount of time. You may need to modify your exercise program for a few weeks to allow an injury to heal. A knowledgeable physician can often give you important medical advice that will speed healing and get you back to your program sooner.

Managing Minor Exercise Injuries

For minor cuts and scrapes, stop the bleeding and clean the wound. Treat injuries to soft tissue (muscles and

> **ratings of perceived exertion (RPE)** A system of monitoring exercise intensity based on assigning a number to the subjective perception of target intensity. **TERMS**
>
> **synovial fluid** Fluid found within many joints that provides lubrication and nutrition to the cells of the joint surface.

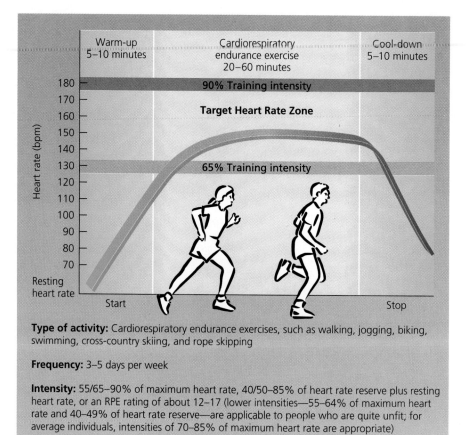

Type of activity: Cardiorespiratory endurance exercises, such as walking, jogging, biking, swimming, cross-country skiing, and rope skipping

Frequency: 3–5 days per week

Intensity: 55/65–90% of maximum heart rate, 40/50–85% of heart rate reserve plus resting heart rate, or an RPE rating of about 12–17 (lower intensities—55–64% of maximum heart rate and 40–49% of heart rate reserve—are applicable to people who are quite unfit; for average individuals, intensities of 70–85% of maximum heart rate are appropriate)

Duration: 20–60 minutes (one session or multiple sessions lasting 10 or more minutes)

Figure 3-6 A cardiorespiratory endurance workout. Longer-duration exercise at lower intensities can often be as beneficial for promoting health as shorter-duration, high-intensity exercise.

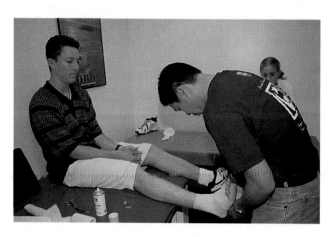

Many exercise injuries can be handled by the individual, but serious injuries, such as broken bones and torn ligaments, require medical attention.

joints) immediately with rest and ice packs. Elevate the affected part of the body, and compress it with an elastic bandage to minimize swelling. Apply ice regularly for 36–48 hours after an injury occurs or until all the swelling is gone. (Don't leave ice on one spot for more than 20 minutes.) Some experts also recommend taking an over-the-counter medication such as aspirin, ibuprofen, or naproxen to decrease inflammation.

Don't apply heat to an injury at first, because heat draws blood to the area and increases swelling. After the swelling has subsided, apply either moist heat (hot towels, heat packs, warm water immersion) or dry heat (heating pads) to speed up healing.

To rehabilitate your body, follow the steps listed in the box "Rehabilitation Following a Minor Athletic Injury."

Preventing Injuries

The best method for dealing with exercise injuries is to prevent them. If you choose activities for your program carefully and follow the training guidelines described here and in Chapter 2, you should be able to avoid most types of injuries. Important guidelines for preventing athletic injuries include the following:

- Train regularly, and stay in condition.
- Gradually increase the intensity, duration, or frequency of your workouts.
- Avoid or minimize high-impact activities.
- Get proper rest between exercise sessions.
- Warm up thoroughly before you exercise, and cool down afterward.
- Achieve and maintain a good level of flexibility.

TABLE 3-3 *Care of Common Exercise Injuries and Discomforts*

Injury	Symptoms	Treatment
Blister	Accumulation of fluid in one spot under the skin	Don't pop or drain it unless it interferes too much with your daily activities. If it does pop, clean the area with antiseptic and cover with a bandage. Do not remove the skin covering the blister.
Bruise (contusion)	Pain, swelling, and discoloration	R-I-C-E: rest, ice, compression, elevation.
Fractures and dislocations	Pain, swelling, tenderness, loss of function, and deformity	Seek medical attention, immobilize the affected area, and apply cold.
Joint sprain	Pain, tenderness, swelling, discoloration, and loss of function	R-I-C-E. Apply heat after 36–48 hours if swelling has disappeared. Stretch and strengthen affected area.
Muscle cramp	Painful, spasmodic muscle contractions	Gently stretch for 15–30 seconds at a time, and/or massage the cramped area. Drink fluids, and increase dietary salt intake if exercising in hot weather.
Muscle soreness or stiffness	Pain and tenderness in the affected muscle	Stretch the affected muscle gently; exercise at a low intensity; apply heat. Nonsteroidal anti-inflammatory drugs, such as ibuprofen, help some people.
Muscle strain	Pain, tenderness, swelling, and loss of strength in the affected muscle	R-I-C-E; apply heat after 36–48 hours if swelling has disappeared. Stretch and strengthen the affected area.
Shin splints	Pain and tenderness on the front of the lower leg; sometimes also pain in the calf muscle	Rest; apply ice to the affected area several times a day and before exercise; wrap with tape for support. Stretch and strengthen muscles in the lower legs. Purchase good-quality footwear, and run on soft surfaces.
Side stitch	Pain on the side of the abdomen	Decrease the intensity of your workout, or stop altogether; bend over in the direction of the stitch.
Tendinitis	Pain and tenderness of the affected area; loss of use	R-I-C-E; apply heat after 36–48 hours if swelling has disappeared. Stretch and strengthen the affected area.

TACTICS AND TIPS   *Rehabilitation Following a Minor Athletic Injury*

1. Reduce the initial inflammation using the R-I-C-E principle:

   Rest: Stop using the injured area as soon as you experience pain. Avoid any activity that causes pain.

   Ice: Apply ice to the injured area to reduce swelling and alleviate pain. Apply ice immediately for 10–20 minutes, and repeat every few hours until the swelling disappears. Let the injured part return to normal temperature between icings, and do not apply ice to one area for more than 20 minutes. An easy method for applying ice is to freeze water in a paper cup, peel some of the paper away, and rub the exposed ice on the injured area. If the injured area is large, you can surround it with several bags of crushed ice or ice cubes; bags of frozen vegetables can also be used. Place a thin towel between the bag and your skin. If you use a cold gel pack, limit application time to 10 minutes.

   Compression: Wrap the injured area firmly with an elastic or compression bandage between icings. If the area starts throbbing or begins to change color, the bandage may be wrapped too tightly. Do not sleep with the wrap on.

   Elevation: Raise the injured area above heart level to decrease the blood supply and reduce swelling. Pillows,

   books, or a low chair or stool can be used to raise the injured area.

2. After 36–48 hours, apply heat if the swelling has completely disappeared. Immerse the affected area in warm water or apply warm compresses, a hot water bottle, or a heating pad. As soon as it's comfortable, begin moving the affected joints slowly. If you feel pain, or if the injured area begins to swell again, reduce the amount of movement. Continue stretching and moving the affected area until you have regained normal range of motion.

3. Gradually begin exercising the injured area to build strength and endurance. Depending on the type of injury, weight training, walking, and resistance training with a partner can all be effective.

4. Gradually reintroduce the stress of an activity until you can return to full intensity. Don't progress too rapidly or you'll reinjure yourself. Before returning to full exercise participation, you should have a full range of motion in your joints, normal strength and balance among your muscles, normal coordinated patterns of movement (with no injury compensation movements, such as limping), and little or no pain.

COMMON QUESTIONS ANSWERED

What kind of clothing should I wear during exercise? Exercise clothing should be comfortable, let you move freely, and allow your body to cool itself. Avoid clothing that constricts normal blood flow or is made from nylon or rubberized fabrics that prevent evaporation of perspiration. Cotton is an excellent material for facilitating the evaporation of sweat. If you sweat heavily when you exercise and find that too much moisture accumulates in cotton clothing, try fabrics containing synthetic materials such as polypropylene that wick moisture away from the skin. Socks made with moisture-wicking compounds may be particularly helpful for people whose feet sweat heavily.

What kind of equipment should I buy? Once you have chosen activities to develop cardiorespiratory fitness, carefully consider what equipment you'll need. Good equipment enhances your enjoyment and decreases your risk of injury. The recent surge of interest in physical activity has been accompanied by a wave of new equipment, but some new products are either overpriced or of poor quality. See the box "Choosing Equipment for Fitness and Sport" for ways to make sound decisions about equipment.

Do I need a special diet for my endurance exercise program? No. For most people, a nutritionally balanced diet contains all the energy and nutrients needed to sustain an exercise program. Don't waste your money on unnecessary vitamins, minerals, and protein supplements. (Chapter 8 has information about putting together a healthy diet.)

Should I drink extra fluids before or during exercise? Yes. Your body depends on water to carry out many chemical reactions and to regulate body temperature. Sweating during exercise depletes your body's water supply and can lead to dehydration if fluids aren't replaced. Serious dehydration can cause reduced blood volume, increased heart rate, elevated body temperature, muscle cramps, heat stroke, and even death. Drinking water before and during exercise is important to prevent dehydration and enhance your performance.

Thirst alone isn't a good indication of how much you need to drink because one's sense of thirst is quickly depressed by drinking even small amounts of water. As a rule of thumb, try to drink about 8 ounces of water (more in hot weather) for every 30 minutes of heavy exercise. Bring a water bottle when you exercise so you can replace your fluids while they're being depleted. Water, preferably cold, and diluted carbohydrate drinks are the best fluid replacements. (See Chapter 8 for more on diet and fluid recommendations for active people.)

What is cross-training? Cross-training is a pattern of training in which your program centers on two or more different cardiorespiratory endurance activities. Alternating activities can make your exercise program more fun, but it may slow your development of activity-specific adaptations. For example, if you alternate jogging and tennis, you will probably not develop the coordination, speed, and upper-body strength associated with tennis as quickly as if you just played tennis. However, if you are quickly bored with a single activity, you'll be more likely to stick with your exercise program if you alternate activities to make it more interesting. Alternating activities may also reduce your risk of some types of injuries.

Is it all right to participate in cardiorespiratory endurance exercise while menstruating? Yes. There is no evidence that exercise during menstruation is unhealthy or that it has negative effects on performance. If you have headaches, backaches, and abdominal pain during menstruation, you may not feel like exercising; for some women, exercise helps relieve these symptoms. Listen to your body, and exercise at whatever intensity is comfortable for you.

What causes muscle cramps and what can I do about them? Muscle cramps are caused by local muscle fatigue that triggers the nervous system to overstimulate the muscles. Until recently, muscle cramps were thought to be caused by dehydration or salt depletion in the muscles, but scientists have found little evidence for this. Muscle cramps can occur during or after exercise performed either in heat or in cold. You can prevent cramps by improving your fitness and making sure you consume enough fluid and electrolytes during exercise

- Use proper body mechanics when lifting objects or executing sports skills.

- Don't exercise when you are ill or overtrained.

- Use proper equipment, particularly shoes, and choose an appropriate exercise surface. If you exercise on a grass field, soft track, or wooden floor, you are less likely to be injured than on concrete or a hard track.

- Don't return to your normal exercise program until your athletic injuries have healed.

SUMMARY

- The cardiorespiratory system consists of the heart, blood vessels, and respiratory system; it picks up and transports oxygen, nutrients, and waste products.
- The body takes chemical energy from food and uses it to produce ATP and fuel cellular activities. ATP is stored in the body's cells as the basic form of energy.
- During exercise, the body supplies ATP and fuels cellular activities by combining three energy sys-

and in your diet. When cramps do occur, gently stretch the cramping muscle for 15–30 seconds. Do not overstretch the cramping muscle because this can lead to serious injury.

What causes side pains during exercise, and what can I do about them? A side pain experienced during exercise is called a stitch. Exercise can wreak havoc on your stomach, intestines, and liver, causing cramping, acid indigestion, diarrhea, bleeding, and gas. Scientists have learned that exercise shocks your GI tract by restricting blood flow, traumatizing sensitive tissues (particularly the visceral ligaments), and imparing the movement of food. In most people, bending forward while tightening the abdominal muscles, tightening a belt around the waist, or breathing through pursed lips will ease side pain quickly. Stitches occur less frequently when you improve your fitness. A fit body has more capacity to distribute blood to its muscles and GI tract. Persistent side pains may be due to more serious medical problems, so seek medical advice if you continue to have them.

Is it safe to exercise in hot weather? Prolonged, vigorous exercise can be dangerous in hot and humid weather. Heat from exercise is released in the form of sweat, which cools the skin and the blood circulating near the body surface as it evaporates. The hotter the weather, the more water the body loses through sweat; the more humid the weather, the less efficient the sweating mechanism is at lowering body temperature. If you lose too much water or if your body temperature rises too high, you may suffer from a heat disorder such as heat exhaustion or heat stroke. Use caution when exercising if the temperature is above 80°F or if the humidity is above 60%. To exercise safely, watch for the signals of heat disorder, regardless of the weather, and follow the tips given in the box "Exercising in Hot Weather."

Is it safe to exercise in cold weather? If you dress warmly in layers and don't stay out in very cold temperatures for too long, exercise can be safe even in subfreezing temperatures. Take both the temperature and the wind-chill factor into account when choosing clothing. Dress in layers so you can

subtract them as you warm up and add them if you get cold. A substantial amount of heat loss comes from the head and neck, so keep these areas covered. In subfreezing temperatures, protect the areas of your body most susceptible to frostbite—fingers, toes, ears, nose, and cheeks—with warm socks, mittens or gloves, and a cap, hood, or ski mask. Wear clothing that "breathes" and will wick moisture away from your skin to avoid being overheated by trapped perspiration. Warm up thoroughly, and drink plenty of fluids.

Is it safe to exercise in a smoggy city? Do not exercise outdoors during a smog alert or if air quality is very poor (symptoms of poor air quality include eye and throat irritations and respiratory discomfort). If you have any type of cardiorespiratory difficulty, avoid exertion outdoors when air quality is poor. You can avoid smog and air pollution by exercising in parks, near water (riverbanks, lakeshores, and ocean beaches), or in residential areas with less traffic (areas with stop-and-go traffic will have lower air quality than areas where traffic moves quickly). Air quality is usually better in the early morning and late evening.

Will high altitude affect my ability to exercise? At high altitudes (above 2000 meters or about 6500 feet) there is less oxygen available in the air than at lower altitudes. High altitude doesn't affect anaerobic exercise, such as stretching and weight lifting, but it does affect aerobic activities—that is, any type of cardiovascular endurance exercise. The reason is that the heart and lungs have to work harder, even when the body is at rest, to deliver enough oxygen to body cells. The increased cardiovascular strain of exercise reduces endurance. To play it safe when at high altitudes, avoid heavy exercises—at least for the first 5 days—and drink plenty of water. And don't expect to reach your normal lower altitude exercise capacity.

tems: *immediate,* for short periods of energy; *nonoxidative (anaerobic),* for intense activity; and *oxidative (aerobic),* for prolonged activity. Which energy system predominates depends on the duration and intensity of the activity.

• Cardiorespiratory endurance exercise improves cardiorespiratory functioning and cellular metabolism; it reduces the risk of chronic disease such as heart disease, cancer, Type 2 diabetes, obesity, and osteoporosis; and it improves immune function and psychological and emotional well-being.

• Cardiorespiratory fitness is measured by seeing how well the cardiorespiratory system transports and uses oxygen. The upper limit of this measure is called maximal oxygen consumption, or $\dot{V}O_{2max}$.

• $\dot{V}O_{2max}$ can be measured precisely in a laboratory, or it can be estimated reasonably well through less expensive assessment tests. Four popular tests are the 1-mile walk test, the 3-minute step test, the 1.5-mile run-walk test, and the Åstrand-Rhyming cycle ergometer test.

Your choice of exercise equipment often affects your enjoyment, your risk of injury, and the likelihood of your continued participation. Nothing will ruin the joy of an activity more than ill-fitting or defective equipment. Following a few simple principles of equipment selection will greatly enhance your sport and exercise experiences.

Price

Try to purchase the best equipment you can afford. If you shop around, you can often find merchandise of good quality at a discount. Bargains are often available through mail-order companies and discount stores. Look in the back of sports specialty magazines for good prices on items such as tennis rackets, running shoes, and windsurf boards.

Good-quality used equipment can often be purchased at a fraction of the retail price. Used sporting goods shops have become very popular throughout the United States and Canada. Sporting goods are also often listed in newspaper classified ads.

Quality

Although price and quality generally go hand in hand, you can often buy good-quality equipment at less than premium prices. Before you invest in a new piece of equipment, investigate it. Ask coaches and instructors if the results are worth the price. Most magazines devoted to individual sports and activities review new equipment. The February 2000 issue of *Consumer Reports* rated several types of home exercise equipment. Don't buy without doing some research. It's also a good idea to buy equipment with a money-back guarantee or a free trial period; if the equipment doesn't meet your expectations, you can return it.

Fit

Equipment that fits properly will enhance your enjoyment and prevent injury. Shoes that pinch your feet will make running unbearable. The wrong size grip on a tennis racket can lead to an elbow injury. When shopping for exercise equipment, take your time and get the help you need to ensure a proper fit.

Intended Use

Many people purchase expensive home exercise equipment, only to have it sit in a corner gathering dust. Before buying an expensive home treadmill, stationary cycle, or stair-climber, try it for several weeks at a local health club or gym. Ask yourself how often you'll actually use the equipment. If you honestly will use it regularly, go ahead and buy a home treadmill or stationary cycle. If you will use a piece of equipment only occasionally, you are better off using one at a gym. Also make sure you have space to use and store it at home.

Also consider how intense your workouts will be. If you intend to push your equipment to the limit, buy a model that can handle the stress. There's nothing more frustrating than a tennis racket that breaks the first time you use it or a treadmill belt that slips when you try to run fast. Although heavy-duty equipment tends to cost more, it may be worth the extra money. But take care not to pay extra for features you don't need.

Your Skill Level

Some equipment is designed for people with superior levels of strength, fitness, and skill. Buying "advanced" equipment can actually diminish your enjoyment of an activity. For example, slalom skis designed for a racer would be extremely difficult for a beginning skier to turn. Shoes designed for competitive marathon runners may have less padding to protect the legs and feet from injury, making them inappropriate for a recreational runner (see Chapter 7 for more on choosing footwear). Buy equipment that is appropriate for your current skill level.

Safety

Don't skimp on safety equipment. For popular sports like in-line skating, failing to buy a helmet and appropriate pads can lead to a serious injury. Check your safety equipment frequently to ensure that it's in good working condition. For example, ski bindings that work perfectly one season may not release properly after sitting in your garage for a year.

- The best exercise for good health is cardiorespiratory endurance exercise. To have a successful exercise program, set realistic goals; choose suitable activities; begin slowly; always warm up and cool down; and as fitness improves, exercise more often, longer, and harder.

- Intensity of training, the most important factor in achieving cardiorespiratory benefits, can be measured through target heart rate zone and ratings of perceived exertion.

- Serious injuries require medical attention. Application of the R-I-C-E principle (rest, ice, compression, elevation) is appropriate for treating many types of muscle or joint injuries.

FOR MORE INFORMATION

Refer to Chapter 2 for resources on exercise physiology and fitness testing. Additional sources of information and programs include the YMCA/YWCA and campus or private sports medicine centers for fitness testing, health clubs for places to exercise and training advice, and physical education departments for activity classes.

Books

American Physical Therapy Association. 1999. *The American Physical Therapy Association Body Maintenance and Repair Guide.* New York: Henry Holt. *Presents solid information on anatomy, physiology, injury prevention, and rehabilitation.*

- Use caution when exercising in extreme heat or humidity (over 80°F and/or 60% humidity).
- Slow exercise or add rest breaks to maintain your prescribed target heart rate; as you become acclimatized, you can gradually increase intensity and duration.
- Exercise in the early morning or evening, when temperatures are lowest.
- Drink 2 cups of fluids 2 hours before you begin exercising, and drink 4–8 ounces of fluid every 10–15 minutes during exercise (more frequently during high-intensity activities).

- Wear clothing that "breathes," allowing air to circulate and cool the body. Wearing white or light colors will help by reflecting, rather than absorbing, heat. A hat can help keep direct sun off your face. Do not wear rubber, plastic, or other nonporous clothing.
- Rest frequently in the shade.
- Keep a record of your morning body weight to track whether weight lost through sweating is restored.
- Slow down or stop if you begin to feel uncomfortable. Watch for the signs of heat disorders listed below; if they occur, act appropriately.

Problem	Symptoms	Treatment
Heat cramps	Muscle cramps, usually in the muscles most used during exercise.	Stop exercising, drink fluids, and stretch cramped muscles.
Heat exhaustion	Paleness; headache; nausea; fainting; dizziness; profuse sweating; weakness; cold, clammy skin; and a rapid, weak pulse.	Cool the body: Stop exercising, get out of the heat, remove excess clothing, drink cold fluids, and apply cool and/or damp towels to the body.
Heat stroke	Hot, flushed skin (skin may be dry or sweaty); rapid pulse; high body temperature; dizziness; confusion or disorientation; vomiting; diarrhea; unconsciousness.	Get immediate medical attention, and try to lower body temperature: Get out of the heat, remove excess clothing, drink cold fluids, and apply cool and/or damp towels to the body or immerse it in cold water.

The Complete Idiot's Guide to Walking for Health. 1999. Indianapolis, Ind.: Macmillan General Reference. *Advice for beginning a walking program and finding time to incorporate walking into one's daily routine.*

Edwards, S. 1996. *Sally Edwards' Heart Zone Training: Exercise Smart, Stay Fit and Live Longer.* Holbrook, Mass.: Adams Media. *Describes the use of heart rate and heart rate monitors for the development of fitness; upbeat and motivational.*

Hines, E. W. 1999. *Fitness Swimming.* Champaign, Ill.: Human Kinetics. *Provides step-by-step instructions for setting up a swimming fitness program.*

Kusinitz, I., and M. Fine. 1995. *Your Guide to Getting Fit,* 3d ed. Mountain View, Calif.: Mayfield. *Includes assessment tests and a step-by-step guide to developing a cardiorespiratory endurance exercise program.*

Pryor, E., and M. Kraines. 2000. *Keep Moving! Fitness through Aerobics and Step.* 4th ed. Mountain View, Calif.: Mayfield. *The fitness principles and techniques every aerobic dancer should know.*

Sharkey, B. J. 1997. *Fitness and Health,* 4th ed. Champaign, Ill.: Human Kinetics. *An excellent guide to fitness and health for people serious about their exercise program.*

Sports Medicine Counsel Staff. 1999. *Beginning Runner's Handbook: The Proven 13-Week Walk/Run Program.* New York: Sterling. *Provides advice and training schedules for individuals who want to begin a walking or running program.*

St. John, Allen. 1999. *Bicycling for Dummies.* Indianapolis, Ind.: IDG Books Worldwide. *Includes information on equipment selection and repair as well as on fitness and safety.*

Organizations and Web Sites

American Heart Association. Provides information on cardiovascular health and disease, including the role of exercise in maintaining heart health and exercise tips for people of all ages.
    800-AHA-USA1
    http://www.americanheart.org
    http://www.justmove.org

Canada's Physical Activity Guide. Provides information on adding physical activity to your life; includes extensive material for older adults.
    http://paguide.com

Dr. Pribut's Running Injuries Page. Provides information about running and many types of running injuries.
    http://www.clark.net/pub/pribut/spsport.html

Federal Trade Commission: Consumer Protection—Diet, Health, and Fitness. Provides several brochures with consumer advice about purchasing exercise equipment.
    http://www.ftc.gov/bcp/menu-health.htm

50-Plus Fitness Association. Promotes fitness and active lifestyles for people 50 and older through a variety of activities, including walks, seminars, fitness events, and newsletters.
    http://www.50plus.org

Franklin Institute Science Museum/The Heart: An Online Exploration. An online museum exhibit with information on the structure and function of the heart, blood vessels, and respiratory system.
    http://www.fi.edu/biosci/heart.html

National Senior Games Association. Promotes healthy lifestyles for older adults through education, fitness, and sports.

http://www.nationalseniorgames.net

Physician and Sportsmedicine. Provides many articles with easy-to-understand advice about exercise injuries.

http://www.physsportsmed.com

Runner's World Online. Contains a wide variety of information about running, including tips for beginning runners, advice about training, and a shoe buyer's guide.

http://www.runnersworld.com

Shape Up America! Fitness Center. Includes fitness assessments, information on the benefits of exercise, tips for overcoming barriers, and tracking forms.

http://shapeup.org/fitness

Yahoo/Recreation. Contains links to many sites with practical advice on many sports and activities.

http://dir.yahoo.com/recreation/sports

See also the listings in Chapter 2.

SELECTED BIBLIOGRAPHY

All the right moves for stress relief. 2000. *Consumer Reports,* February.

American College of Sports Medicine. 2000. *ACSM's Guidelines for Exercise Testing and Prescription,* 6th ed. Baltimore, Md.: Lippincott Williams & Wilkins.

American College of Sports Medicine. 1998. ACSM position stand: The recommended quantity and quality of exercise for developing and maintaining cardiorespiratory and muscular fitness, flexibility in healthy adults. *Medicine and Science in Sports and Exercise* 30(6): 975–991.

American College of Sports Medicine. 1998. *ACSM's Resource Manual for Guidelines for Exercise Testing and Prescription,* 3d ed. Baltimore, Md.: Williams & Wilkins.

American College of Sports Medicine. 1997. *ACSM's Health/Fitness Facility Standards and Guidelines,* 2d ed. Champaign, Ill.: Human Kinetics.

Appel, L. J. 1999. Nonpharmacologic therapies that reduce blood pressure: A fresh perspective. *Clinical Cardiology* 22: 1111–1115.

Billings, J. H., 2000. Maintenance of behavior change in cardiorespiratory risk reduction. *Health Psychology* 19(1 Suppl.): 70–75.

Borg, G. A. V. 1982. Psychophysical bases of perceived exertion. *Medicine and Science in Sports and Exercise* 14:377–381.

Branch, J. D., et al. 2000. Moderate intensity exercise training improves cardiorespiratory fitness in women. *Journal of Women's Health and Gender-Based Medicine* 9(1): 65–73.

Brooks, G. A., et al. 2000. *Exercise Physiology: Human Bioenergetics and Its Applications,* 3d ed. Mountain View, Calif.: Mayfield.

Burke, L. 1999. Nutrition for sport: Getting the most out of training. *Australian Family Physician* 28:561–567.

Centers for Disease Control and Prevention. 1998. Heat-related mortality—United States, 1997. *Morbidity and Mortality Weekly Report* 47(23): 473–476.

Dowzer, C. N., et al. 1999. Maximal physiological responses to deep and shallow water running. *Ergonomics* 42:275–281.

Eyler, A. A., et al. 1999. Physical activity, social support, and middle- and older-aged minority women: Results from a U.S. survey. *Social Sciences and Medicine* 49:781–789.

Fleg, J. L. 1999. Silent myocardial ischemia and low aerobic capacity: An unlucky combination. *Journal of the American Geriatric Society* 47:1026–1028.

Fukuba, Y., and B. J. Whipp. 1999. A metabolic limit on the ability to make up for lost time in endurance events. *Journal of Applied Physiology* 87:853–861.

Gibbons, R. J., et al. 1997. ACC/AHA guidelines for exercise testing. A report of the American College of Cardiology/American Heart Association Task Force on Practice Guidelines (Committee on Exercise Testing). *Journal of the American College of Cardiology* 30:260–311.

Hood, S., and R. J. Northcote. 1999. Cardiac assessment of veteran endurance athletes: A 12-year follow-up study. *British Journal of Sports Medicine* 33:239–243.

Jones, A. J., and A. M. McConnell. 1999. Effect of exercise modality on oxygen uptake kinetics during heavy exercise. *European Journal of Applied Physiology* 80:213–219.

Katayama, K., et al. 2000. Cardiovascular response to hypoxia after endurance training at altitude and sea level and after detraining. *Journal of Applied Physiology* 88(4): 1221–1227.

Leaf, D. A., et al. 1999. The exercise-induced oxidative stress paradox: The effects of physical exercise training. *American Journal of Medical Science* 317:295–300.

Nakagaichi, M., and K. Tanaka. 1999. Development of a 12-min treadmill walk test at a self-selected pace for the evaluation of cardiorespiratory fitness in adult men. *Applied Human Science* 17:281–288.

Orleans, C. T. 2000. Promoting the maintenance of health behavior change. *Health Psychology* 19(1 Suppl.): 76–83.

Petrella, R. J. 1998. How effective is exercise training for the treatment of hypertension? *Clinical Journal of Sports Medicine* 8(3): 224–231.

Plunkett, B. T., and W. G. Hopkins. 1999. Investigation of the side pain "stitch" induced by running after fluid ingestion. *Medical Science and Sports Exercise* 31:1169–1175.

Sorensen, M., et al. 1999. The effect of exercise and diet on mental health and quality of life in middle-aged individuals with elevated risk factors for cardiovascular disease. *Journal of Sports Science* 17:369–377.

Talbot, L. A., E. J. Metter, and J. L. Fleg. 2000. Leisure-time physical activities and their relationship to cardiorespiratory fitness in healthy men and women 18–95 years old. *Medicine and Science in Sports and Exercise* 32(2): 417–425.

Tolfrey, K., A. M. Jones, and I. G. Campbell. 2000. The effect of aerobic exercise training on the lipid-lipoprotein profile of children and adolescents. *Sports Medicine* 29(2): 99–112.

Ward-Smith, A. J. 1999. The kinetics of anaerobic metabolism following the initiative of high-intensity exercise. *Mathematics and Bioscience* 159:33–45.

Washburn, R. A., and J. L. Ficker. 1999. Does participation in a structured high-intensity exercise program influence daily physical activity patterns in older adults? *Research Quarterly for Exercise and Sport* 70:201–205.

Weyand, P. G., et al. 1999. High-speed running performance is largely unaffected by hypoxic reductions in aerobic power. *Journal of Applied Physiology* 86:2059–2064.

Whaley, M. H., et al. 1999. Physical fitness and clustering of risk factors associated with the metabolic syndrome. *Medicine and Science in Sports and Exercise* 31:287–293.

LAB 3-1   *Assessing Your Current Level of Cardiorespiratory Endurance*

Before taking any of the cardiorespiratory endurance assessment tests, refer to the fitness prerequisites and cautions given in Table 3-2. For best results, don't exercise strenuously or consume caffeine the day of the test, and don't smoke or eat a heavy meal within about 3 hours of the test.

The 1-Mile Walk Test

Equipment

1.   A track or course that provides a measurement of 1 mile
2.   A stopwatch, clock, or watch with a second hand
3.   A weight scale

Preparation

Measure your body weight (in pounds) before taking the test.

Body weight: _____ lb

Instructions

1.   Warm up before taking the test. Do some walking, easy jogging, or calisthenics and some stretching exercises.
2.   Cover the 1-mile course as quickly as possible. Walk at a pace that is brisk but comfortable. You must raise your heart rate above 120 beats per minute (bpm).
3.   As soon as you complete the distance, note your time and take your pulse for 10 seconds.

     Walking time: _____ min _____ sec

     10-second pulse count: _____ beats

4.   Cool down after the test by walking slowly for several minutes.

Determining Maximal Oxygen Consumption

1.   Convert your 10-second pulse count into a value for exercise heart rate by multiplying it by 6.

     Exercise heart rate: _____ × 6 = _____ bpm
     10-sec pulse count

2.   Convert your walking time from minutes and seconds to a decimal figure. For example, a time of 14 minutes and 45 seconds would be 14 + (45/60), or 14.75 minutes.

     Walking time: _____ min + (_____ sec ÷ 60 sec/min) = _____ min

3.   Insert values for your age, gender, weight, walking time, and exercise heart rate in the following equation, where

     W = your weight (in pounds)

     A = your age (in years)

     G = your gender (male = 1; female = 0)

     T = your time to complete the 1-mile course (in minutes)

     H = your exercise heart rate (in beats per minute)

     $\dot{V}O_{2max} = 132.853 - (0.0769 \times W) - (0.3877 \times A) + (6.315 \times G) - (3.2649 \times T) - (0.1565 \times H)$

For example, a 20-year-old, 190-pound male with a time of 14.75 minutes and an exercise heart rate of 152 bpm would calculate maximal oxygen consumption as follows:

$$\dot{V}O_{2max} = 132.853 - (0.0769 \times 190) - (0.3877 \times 20) + (6.315 \times 1) - (3.2649 \times 14.75) - (0.1565 \times 152)$$
$$= 45 \text{ ml/kg/min}$$

$$\dot{V}O_{2max} = 132.853 - (0.0769 \times \underline{\hspace{1cm}}) - (0.3877 \times \underline{\hspace{1cm}}) + (6.315 \times \underline{\hspace{1cm}})$$
$$\text{weight (lb)} \qquad \text{age (years)} \qquad \text{gender}$$

$$- (3.2649 \times \underline{\hspace{1cm}}) - (0.1565 \times \underline{\hspace{1cm}}) = \underline{\hspace{1cm}} \text{ ml/kg/min}$$
$$\text{walking time (min)} \qquad \text{exercise heart rate (bpm)}$$

4. Copy this value for $\dot{V}O_{2max}$ into the appropriate place in the chart on the final page of this lab.

The 3-Minute Step Test

Equipment

1. A step, bench, or bleacher step that is 16.25 inches from ground level
2. A stopwatch, clock, or watch with a second hand
3. A metronome

Preparation

Practice stepping up onto and down from the step before you begin the test. Each step has four beats: up-up-down-down. Males should perform the test with the metronome set for a rate of 96 beats per minute, or 24 steps per minute. Females should set the metronome at 88 beats per minute, or 22 steps per minute.

Instructions

1. Warm up before taking the test. Do some walking, easy jogging, and stretching exercises.
2. Set the metronome at the proper rate. Your instructor or a partner can call out starting and stopping times; otherwise, have a clock or watch within easy viewing during the test.
3. Begin the test, and continue to step at the correct pace for 3 minutes.
4. Stop after 3 minutes. Remain standing, and count your pulse for the 15-second period from 5 to 20 seconds into recovery.

   15-second pulse count: _____ beats

5. Cool down after the test by walking slowly for several minutes.

Determining Maximal Oxygen Consumption

1. Convert your 15-second pulse count to a value for recovery heart rate by multiplying by 4.

   Recovery heart rate: $\underline{\hspace{2cm}}_{\text{15-sec pulse count}} \times 4 = \underline{\hspace{2cm}}$ bpm

2. Insert your recovery heart rate in the equation below, where

   H = recovery heart rate (in beats per minute)
   Males: $\dot{V}O_{2max} = 111.33 - (0.42 \times H)$
   Females: $\dot{V}O_{2max} = 65.81 - (0.1847 \times H)$

   For example, a man with a recovery heart rate of 162 bpm would calculate maximal oxygen consumption as follows:

   $$\dot{V}O_{2max} = 111.33 - (0.42 \times 162) = 43 \text{ ml/kg/min}$$

   Males: $\dot{V}O_{2max} = 111.33 - (0.42 \times \underline{\hspace{1.5cm}}) = \underline{\hspace{1.5cm}}$ ml/kg/min
   $$\text{recovery heart rate (bpm)}$$
   Females: $\dot{V}O_{2max} = 65.81 - (0.1847 \times \underline{\hspace{1.5cm}}) = \underline{\hspace{1.5cm}}$ ml/kg/min
   $$\text{recovery heart rate (bpm)}$$

3. Copy this value for $\dot{V}O_{2max}$ into the appropriate place in the chart on the final page of this lab.

The 1.5-Mile Run-Walk Test

Equipment

1. A running track or course that is flat and provides exact measurements of up to 1.5 miles
2. A stopwatch, clock, or watch with a second hand

Preparation

You may want to practice pacing yourself prior to taking the test to avoid going too fast at the start and becoming prematurely fatigued. Allow yourself a day or two to recover from your practice run before taking the test.

Instructions

1. Warm up before taking the test. Do some walking, easy jogging, and stretching exercises.
2. Try to cover the distance as fast as possible without overexerting yourself. If possible, monitor your own time, or have someone call out your time at various intervals of the test to determine whether your pace is correct.
3. Record the amount of time, in minutes and seconds, it takes you to complete the 1.5-mile distance.

   Running-walking time: _____ min _____ sec

4. Cool down after the test by walking or jogging slowly for about 5 minutes.

Determining Maximal Oxygen Consumption

1. Convert your running time from minutes and seconds to a decimal figure. For example, a time of 14 minutes and 25 seconds would be 14 + (25/60), or 14.4 minutes.

   Running-walking time: _____ min + (_____ sec ÷ 60 sec/min) = _____ min

2. Insert your running time in the equation below, where

   T = running time (in minutes)

   $\dot{V}O_{2max} = (483 \div T) + 3.5$

   For example, a person who completes 1.5 miles in 14.4 minutes would calculate maximal oxygen consumption as follows:

   $\dot{V}O_{2max} = (483 \div 14.4) + 3.5 = 37$ ml/kg/min

   $\dot{V}O_{2max} = (483 \div \underline{\hspace{1cm}}) + 3.5 = \underline{\hspace{1cm}}$ **ml/kg/min**

run-walk time (min)

3. Copy this value for $\dot{V}O_{2max}$ into the appropriate place in the chart on the final page of this lab.

The Åstrand-Rhyming Cycle Ergometer Test

Equipment

1. Cycle ergometer that allows for regulation of power output in kilopounds per meter (kpm)
2. A stopwatch, clock, or watch with a second hand
3. Weight scale
4. Metronome or meter on cycle ergometer to measure pedal revolutions
5. Partner to monitor heart rate

Preparation

Weigh yourself before taking the test. Adjust the seat height of the cycle so that your knees are almost completely extended as your foot goes through the bottom of the pedaling cycle. Practice pedaling the cycle ergometer at the speed of 50 pedal revolutions per minute. Each revolution includes a downstroke with each foot, so set your metronome at 100 beats per minute.

Body weight: _____ lb

1. Warm up before taking the test. Do some walking, easy jogging, and stretching exercises. A few minutes' practice on the cycle ergometer can also be part of your warm-up.

2. Set up the metronome to monitor your pace. If you aren't using a metronome, have a partner call out times at regular intervals.

3. Set the power output between 300 and 1200 kpm. If you are small or have been sedentary, a setting of 300–600 kpm is appropriate. If you are larger or fitter, try a setting of 600–900 kpm. Find a setting high enough to raise your heart rate to between 125 and 170 bpm, but not so high that you can't continue pedaling for 6 minutes.

   Note: If your heart rate goes above 170 or you experience any unusual symptoms, stop pedaling, rest for 15–20 minutes, and then repeat the test at a lower workload.

4. Ride the cycle ergometer for 6 minutes at a rate of 50 pedal revolutions per minute. Your partner should monitor your heart rate by counting your pulse for the last 10 seconds of each minute of your ride (see the photograph). Your heart rate should rise to a level in the target range (125–170 bpm) and then level off, staying relatively constant during the last few minutes of your ride. If your exercise heart rate stays below 125 bpm, rest for 15–20 minutes, and then repeat the test at a higher workload. If your heart rate gets too high or if it continues to rise throughout your ride (not leveling off in the last few minutes), rest for 15–20 minutes, and repeat the test at a lower workload.

5. If your heart rate levels off within the target range (125–170 bpm), your partner should make a final count during the last 10 seconds of the sixth minute of your ride.

   10-second pulse count: _____ beats

   Power output: _____ kpm

6. Cool down after the test by pedaling, walking, or jogging slowly for several minutes.

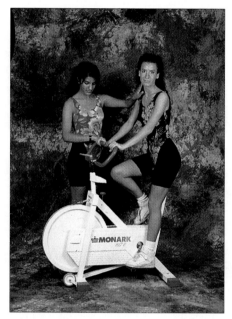

During the cycle ergometer test, a partner monitors heart rate for the last 10 seconds of every minute.

Determining Maximal Oxygen Consumption

1. Calculate your exercise heart rate by multiplying your final 10-second count by 6.

   Exercise heart rate: _____ × 6 = _____ bpm
                          10-sec pulse count

2. On the nomogram on p. 65, connect the point that represents your exercise heart rate with the point that represents the power output you used (on the scale for your sex). Read your total oxygen uptake score (in liters) at the point where the line you've drawn crosses the maximal oxygen consumption line.

   Maximal oxygen consumption (from nomogram): _____ l/min

3. Adjust your maximal oxygen consumption score for your age by multiplying it by the appropriate age-correction factor in the table below.

Age	15	20	25	30	35	40	45	50	55	60	65
Factor	1.10	1.05	1.0	0.94	0.87	0.83	0.78	0.75	0.71	0.68	0.65

   $\dot{V}O_{2max}$ corrected for age: _____ l/min × _____ = _____ l/min
                                $\dot{V}O_{2max}$ age-correction factor

4. Convert your score to one for maximal oxygen consumption (in milliliters of oxygen per minute per kilogram of body weight).

   a. Convert your weight from pounds to kilograms by dividing it by 2.2.

   b. Multiply your $\dot{V}O_{2max}$ by 1000 (to convert from liters to milliliters).

   c. Divide this number by your weight (in kilograms).

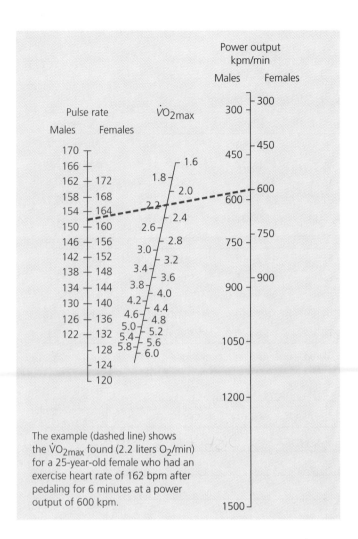

The example (dashed line) shows the $\dot{V}O_{2max}$ found (2.2 liters O_2/min) for a 25-year-old female who had an exercise heart rate of 162 bpm after pedaling for 6 minutes at a power output of 600 kpm.

Nomogram for use with the Åstrand-Rhyming cycle ergometer test.

For example, a 135-pound, 25-year-old female whose 10-second count was 27 at a workload of 600 kpm would calculate maximal oxygen consumption as follows:

1. 27 beats × 6 = 162 bpm
2. Connecting 600 kpm and 162 bpm on the nomogram gives a $\dot{V}O_{2max}$ value of 2.2 l/min
3. The age-adjustment factor for a 25-year-old is 1.00.
   2.2 l/min × 1.00 = 2.2 l/min
4. To convert 135 pounds to kilograms:
   135 lb ÷ 2.2 lb/kg = 61.4 kg

   To convert liters to milliliters:

   2.2 l/min × 1000 ml/l = 2200 ml/min

   To adjust for weight:

   2200 ml/min ÷ 61.4 kg = 35.8 ml/kg/min

Convert body weight to kg: _____ lb ÷ 2.2 lb/kg = _____ kg

Convert from liters to milliliters: _____ l/min × 1000 ml/l = _____ ml/min

age-corrected $\dot{V}O_{2max}$

Adjust for weight:

$\dot{V}O_{2max}$ = _____ ml/min ÷ _____ kg = _____ **ml/kg/min**

$\dot{V}O_{2max}$ body weight

5. Copy this value for $\dot{V}O_{2max}$ into the appropriate place in the chart on the following page.

Rating Your Cardiovascular Fitness

Record your $\dot{V}O_{2max}$ score(s) and the corresponding fitness rating from the table below.

Maximal Oxygen Consumption (ml/kg/min)

Women	Very Poor	Poor	Fair	Good	Excellent	Superior
Age: 18–29	Below 30.6	30.6–33.7	33.8–36.6	36.7–40.9	41.0–46.7	Above 46.7
30–39	Below 28.7	28.7–32.2	32.3–34.5	34.6–38.5	38.6–43.8	Above 43.8
40–49	Below 26.5	26.5–29.4	29.5–32.2	32.3–36.2	36.3–40.9	Above 40.9
50–59	Below 24.3	24.3–26.8	26.9–29.3	29.4–32.2	32.3–36.7	Above 36.7
60 and over	Below 22.8	22.8–24.4	24.5–27.1	27.2–31.1	31.2–37.4	Above 37.4
Men						
Age: 18–29	Below 37.1	37.1–40.9	41.0–44.1	44.2–48.1	48.2–53.9	Above 53.9
30–39	Below 35.4	35.4–38.8	38.9–42.3	42.4–46.7	46.8–52.4	Above 52.4
40–49	Below 33.0	33.0–36.7	36.8–39.8	39.9–44.0	44.1–50.3	Above 50.3
50–59	Below 30.2	30.2–33.7	33.8–36.6	36.7–40.9	41.0–47.0	Above 47.0
60 and over	Below 26.5	26.5–30.1	30.2–33.5	33.6–38.0	38.1–45.1	Above 45.1

SOURCE: Based on norms from the Cooper Institute for Aerobics Research, Dallas, Texas; used with permission.

	$\dot{V}O_{2max}$	Cardiovascular Fitness Rating
~~1-mile walk test~~ *12 min Run*	*47*	*Good Dist 162*
3-minute step test		
1.5-mile run-walk test		
Åstrand-Rhyming cycle ergometer test		

Is your rating as high as you want it to be? If not, what is your goal for $\dot{V}O_{2max}$? _____

_____

_____

To monitor your progress toward your goal, enter the results of this lab in the Preprogram Assessment column of Appendix D. After several weeks of a cardiorespiratory endurance exercise program, complete this lab again, and enter the results in the Postprogram Assessment column of Appendix D. How do the results compare? (For accuracy, it's best to compare $\dot{V}O_{2max}$ scores for the same test.)

SOURCES: Kline, G. M., et al. 1987. Estimation of $\dot{V}O_{2max}$ from a one-mile track walk, gender, age, and body weight. *Medicine and Science in Sports and Exercise* 19(3): 253–259. McArdle, W. D., F. I. Katch, and V. L. Katch. 1991. *Exercise Physiology: Energy, Nutrition, and Human Performance.* Philadelphia: Lea & Febiger, pp. 225–226. Brooks, G. A., and T. D. Fahey. 1987. *Fundamentals of Human Performance.* New York: Macmillan. Åstrand, P. O., and I. Rhyming. 1954. A nomogram for calculation of aerobic capacity (physical fitness) from pulse rate during submaximal work. *Journal of Applied Physiology* 7:218–221. Used with permission.

Name _____ Section _____ Date _____

LAB 3-2 *Developing an Exercise Program for Cardiorespiratory Endurance*

1. *Goals.* Determine goals for your cardiorespiratory endurance exercise program, and record them below. Goals can be specific or general, short or long term.

_____

_____

_____

_____

2. *Activities.* Refer to Figure 3.5, "Activities and Sports for Developing Cardiorespiratory Endurance (p. 55), for help in choosing one or more activities for your program. Fill in the activity names on the program plan on the following page.

3. *Duration.* Use Figure 3.5 to fill in an appropriate duration for each activity (20–60 minutes). For developing cardiorespiratory endurance, higher-intensity activities can be performed for a shorter duration; lower-intensity activities require a longer duration.

4. Intensity. Determine your exercise intensity using one of the following methods, and fill it in on the program plan.

    a. Target heart rate zone.

        Maximum heart rate: 220 − _____ = _____ bpm
                             <small>age (years)</small>

        Maximum Heart Rate Method

        65% training intensity = _____ bpm × 0.65 = _____ bpm
                                     <small>maximum heart rate</small>

        90% training intensity = _____ bpm × 0.90 = _____ bpm
                                   <small>maximum heart rate</small>

        Target heart rate zone = _____ to _____ bpm

        Heart Rate Reserve Method

        Resting heart rate: _____ bpm (taken after 10 minutes of complete rest)

        Heart rate reserve = _____ bpm − _____ bpm = _____ bpm
                      <small>maximum heart rate</small>   <small>resting heart rate</small>

        50% training intensity = (_____ bpm × 0.50) + _____ bpm = _____ bpm
                        <small>heart rate reserve</small>   <small>resting heart rate</small>

        85% training intensity = (_____ bpm × 0.85) + _____ bpm = _____ bpm
                        <small>heart rate reserve</small>   <small>resting heart rate</small>

        Target heart rate zone = _____ to _____ bpm

    b. Ratings of perceived exertion (RPE): If you prefer, determine an RPE value that corresponds to your target heart rate range (see pp. 51–52 and Figure 3–4).

5. *Frequency.* Fill in how often you plan to participate in each activity.

Activity	Duration (min)	Intensity (bpm or RPE)	Frequency (check ✓)						
			M	T	W	Th	F	Sa	Su

6. *Monitoring your program.* Complete a log like the one below to monitor your program and track your progress. Fill in the duration of exercise for each workout. To monitor your progress more closely, you can also track another variable, such as distance. For example, if your cardiorespiratory endurance program includes walking and swimming, you can keep track of miles walked and yards swum in addition to the duration of each exercise session.

Activity/Date										
1	Duration									
2	Duration									
3	Duration									
4	Duration									
5	Duration									

Activity/Date										
1	Duration									
2	Duration									
3	Duration									
4	Duration									
5	Duration									

Muscular Strength and Endurance

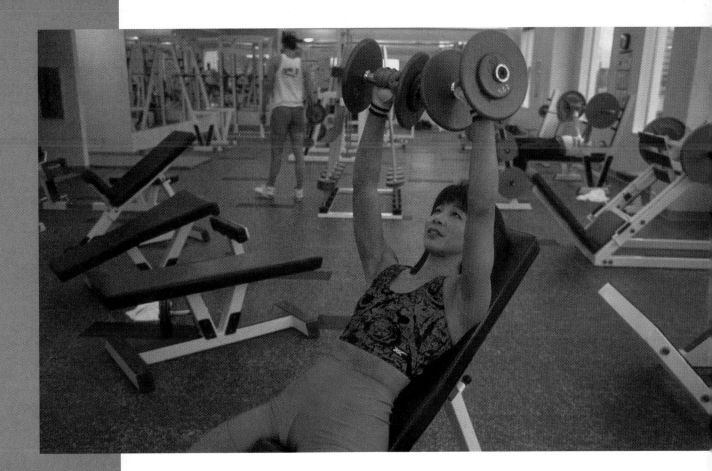

LOOKING AHEAD

After reading this chapter, you should be able to answer these questions about muscular strength and endurance:

- What are muscular strength and endurance, and how do they relate to wellness?

- How can muscular strength and endurance be assessed?

- How do weight training exercises affect muscles?

- What type, frequency, and number of weight training exercises make up a successful program?

- What supplements and drugs are being marketed to active people and athletes, and what are their effects?

- How are common weight training exercises performed using weight machines and free weights?

Exercise experts have long emphasized the importance of cardiovascular fitness. Other physical fitness factors, such as muscle strength and flexibility, were mentioned almost as an afterthought. As more was learned about how the body responds to exercise, however, it became obvious that these other factors are vital to health, wellness, and overall quality of life. Muscles make up more than 40% of your body mass. You depend on them for movement, and, because of their mass, they are the site of a large portion of the energy reactions (metabolism) that take place in your body. Strong, well-developed muscles help you perform daily activities with greater ease, protect you from injury, and enhance your well-being in other ways.

This chapter explains the benefits of strength training (also called resistance training) and describes methods of assessing muscular strength and endurance. It then explains the basics of weight training and provides guidelines for setting up your own weight training program.

BENEFITS OF MUSCULAR STRENGTH AND ENDURANCE

Enhanced muscular strength and endurance can lead to improvements in the areas of performance, injury prevention, body composition, self-image, and lifetime muscle and bone health.

Improved Performance of Physical Activities

A person with a moderate-to-high level of muscular strength and endurance can perform everyday tasks—such as climbing stairs and carrying books or groceries—with ease. Muscular strength and endurance are also important in recreational activities: People with poor muscle strength tire more easily and are less effective in activities like hiking, skiing, and playing tennis. Increased strength can enhance your enjoyment of recreational sports by making it possible to achieve high levels of performance and to handle advanced techniques.

Injury Prevention

Increased muscle strength provides protection against injury because it helps people maintain good posture and appropriate body mechanics when carrying out everyday activities like walking, lifting, and carrying. Strong muscles in the abdomen, hips, low back, and legs support the back in proper alignment and help prevent low-back pain, which afflicts more than 85% of all Americans at some time in their lives. (Prevention of low-back pain is discussed in Chapter 5.) Training for muscular strength also makes the **tendons, ligaments,** and cartilage cells stronger and less susceptible to injury.

Improved Body Composition and Metabolic Functioning

As Chapter 2 explained, healthy body composition means that the body has a high proportion of fat-free mass (primarily composed of muscle) and a relatively small proportion of fat. Strength training improves body composition by increasing muscle mass, thereby tipping the body composition ratio toward fat-free mass and away from fat. Building muscle mass through strength training also helps with losing fat because metabolic rate is related to muscle mass: The more muscle mass, the higher the metabolic rate. A high metabolic rate means that a nutritionally sound diet coupled with regular exercise will not lead to an increase in body fat. Strength training also improves glucose metabolism (an important factor in preventing diabetes) and helps to modify risk factors associated with cardiovascular disease.

Enhanced Self-Image

Weight training leads to an enhanced self-image by providing stronger, firmer-looking muscles and a toned, healthy-looking body. Men tend to build larger, stronger, more shapely muscles. Women tend to lose inches, increase strength, and develop greater muscle definition. The larger muscles in men combine with high levels of the hormone **testosterone,** the principal androgen, for a strong tissue-building effect; see the box "Gender Differences in Muscular Strength."

Because weight training involves measurable objectives (pounds lifted, repetitions accomplished), a person can easily recognize improved performance, leading to greater self-confidence. It's especially satisfying to work on improving one's personal record.

Improved Muscle and Bone Health with Aging

Research has shown that good muscle strength helps people live healthier lives. A lifelong program of regular strength training prevents muscle and nerve degeneration that can compromise the quality of life and increase the

TERMS
tendon A tough band of fibrous tissue that connects a muscle to a bone or other body part and transmits the force exerted by the muscle.

ligament A tough band of tissue that connects the ends of bones to other bones or supports organs in place.

testosterone The principal male hormone, responsible for the development of secondary sex characteristics and important in increasing muscle size.

repetition maximum (RM) The maximum amount of resistance that can be moved a specified number of times; 1 RM is the maximum weight that can be lifted once. 5 RM is the maximum weight that can be lifted five times.

repetitions The number of times an exercise is performed during one set.

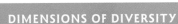
Men are generally stronger than women because they typically have larger bodies overall and larger muscles. But when strength is expressed per unit of cross-sectional area of muscle tissue, men are only 1–2% stronger than women in the upper body and about equal to women in the lower body. (Men have a larger proportion of muscle tissue in the upper body, so it's easier for them to build upper-body strength than it is for women.) Individual muscle fibers are larger in men, but the metabolism of cells within those fibers is the same in both sexes.

Two factors that help explain these disparities between the sexes are androgen levels and the speed of nervous control of muscle. Androgens are naturally occurring male hormones that are responsible for the development of secondary sex characteristics (facial hair, deep voice, and so forth). Androgens also promote the growth of muscle tissue. Androgen levels are about 6–10 times higher in men than in women, so men tend to have larger muscles. Also, because the male nervous system can activate muscles faster, men tend to have more power.

Some women are concerned that they will develop large muscles from weight training. Most studies show that women do not develop big muscles, but the evidence of top women bodybuilders suggests that they can. Some of these women may have taken drugs to increase their muscle size, but many muscular women have not. Evidence suggests, though, that it is difficult for women to gain a large amount of muscle without training intensely over many years.

The bottom line is that both men and women can increase strength through weight training. Women may not be able to lift as much weight as men, but pound for pound of muscle, they have nearly the same capacity to gain strength as men. The lifetime wellness benefits of strength training are available to everyone. Weight training is particularly beneficial for women because it helps prevent bone and muscle loss with aging and maintains fat-free weight during weight control programs.

SOURCE: Fahey, T. D. 2000. *Weight Training for Men and Women,* 4th ed. Mountain View, Calif.: Mayfield.

---

risk of hip fractures and other potentially life-threatening injuries. In the general population people begin to lose muscle mass after age 30, a condition called *sarcopenia*. At first they may notice that they can't play sports as well as they could in high school. After more years of inactivity and strength loss, people may have trouble performing even the simple movements of daily life—getting out of a bathtub or automobile, walking up a flight of stairs, or doing yard work. By age 75 about 25% of men and 75% of women can't lift more than 10 pounds. Although aging contributes to decreased strength, inactivity causes most of the loss. Poor strength makes it much more likely that a person will be injured during everyday activities.

As a person ages, motor nerves can become disconnected from the portion of muscle they control. Muscle physiologists estimate that by age 70, 15% of the motor nerves in most people are no longer connected to muscle tissue. Aging and inactivity also cause muscles to become slower and therefore less able to perform quick, powerful movements. Strength training helps maintain motor nerve connections and the quickness of muscles.

Osteoporosis is common in people over age 55, particularly postmenopausal women. Osteoporosis leads to fractures that can be life-threatening. Hormonal changes from aging account for much of the bone loss that occurs, but lack of bone stress due to inactivity and a poor diet are contributing factors. Recent research indicates that strength training can lessen bone loss even if it is taken up later in life. Increased muscle strength can also help prevent falls, which are a major cause of injury in people with osteoporosis. (Strategies for preventing osteoporosis are described in Chapter 8.)

ASSESSING MUSCULAR STRENGTH AND ENDURANCE

Muscular strength and muscular endurance are distinct but related components of fitness. Muscular strength, the maximum amount of force a muscle can produce in a single effort, is usually assessed by measuring the maximum amount of weight a person can lift one time. This single maximal movement is referred to as a **repetition maximum (RM)**. You can assess the strength of your major muscle groups by taking the one-repetition maximum (1 RM) tests for the bench press and the leg press. Refer to Lab 4-1 for guidelines on taking these tests. Instructions for assessing grip strength using a dynamometer are also included in Lab 4-1. For more accurate results, avoid any strenuous weight training for 48 hours beforehand.

Muscular endurance is the ability of a muscle to exert a submaximal force repeatedly or continuously over time. This ability depends on muscular strength because a certain amount of strength is required for any muscle movement. Muscular endurance is usually assessed by counting the maximum number of **repetitions** of a muscular contraction a person can do (such as in push-ups) or the maximum amount of time a person can hold a muscular contraction (such as in the flexed-arm hang). You can test the muscular endurance of major muscle groups in your body by taking the 60-second sit-up test or the curl-up test and the push-up test. Refer to Lab 4-2 for complete instructions on taking these assessment tests.

Record your results and your fitness rating from the assessment tests in Labs 4-1 and 4.2. If the results show that

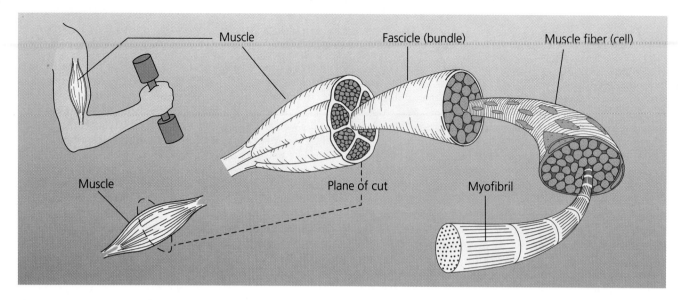

Figure 4-1   Components of skeletal muscle tissue.

improvement is needed, a weight training program will enable you to make rapid gains in muscular strength and endurance.

FUNDAMENTALS OF WEIGHT TRAINING

Weight training develops muscular strength and endurance in the same way that endurance exercise develops cardiovascular fitness: When the muscles are stressed by a greater load than they are used to, they adapt and improve their function. The type of adaptation that occurs depends on the type of stress applied.

TERMS   **muscle fiber**   A single muscle cell, usually classified according to strength, speed of contraction, and energy source.

myofibrils   Protein structures that make up muscle fibers.

hypertrophy   An increase in the size of a muscle fiber, usually stimulated by muscular overload.

hyperplasia   An increase in the number of muscle cells.

slow-twitch fibers   Red muscle fibers that are fatigue-resistant but have a slow contraction speed and a lower capacity for tension; usually recruited for endurance activities.

fast-twitch fibers   White muscle fibers that contract rapidly and forcefully but fatigue quickly; usually recruited for actions requiring strength and power.

power   The ability to exert force rapidly.

motor unit   A motor nerve (one that initiates movement) connected to one or more muscle fibers.

isometric exercise   Exercise involving a muscle contraction without a change in the length of the muscle.

Physiological Effects of Weight Training

Muscles move the body and enable it to exert force because they move the skeleton. When a muscle contracts (shortens), it moves a bone by pulling on the tendon that attaches the muscle to the bone. Muscles consist of individual muscle cells, or **muscle fibers**, connected in bundles (Figure 4-1). A single muscle is made up of many bundles of muscle fibers and is covered by layers of connective tissue that hold the fibers together. Muscle fibers, in turn, are made up of smaller units called **myofibrils.** (When your muscles are given the signal to contract, protein filaments within the myofibrils slide across one another, causing the muscle fiber to shorten.) Weight training causes the size of individual muscle fibers to increase by increasing the number of myofibrils. Larger muscle fibers mean a larger and stronger muscle. The development of large muscle fibers is called **hypertrophy.** Although not a significant method of increase in humans, muscles can also increase in size through an increase in the number of muscle cells, a process called **hyperplasia.**

Muscle fibers are classified as fast-twitch or slow-twitch fibers according to their strength, speed of contraction, and energy source. **Slow-twitch fibers** are relatively fatigue resistant, but they don't contract as rapidly or strongly as fast-twitch fibers. The principal energy system that fuels slow-twitch fibers is aerobic. **Fast-twitch fibers** contract more rapidly and forcefully than slow-twitch fibers but fatigue more quickly. Although oxygen is important in the energy system that fuels fast-twitch fibers, they rely more on anaerobic metabolism than do slow-twitch fibers (see Chapter 3 for a discussion of energy systems).

Most muscles contain a mixture of slow-twitch and fast-twitch fibers. The type of fiber that acts depends on

TABLE 4-1	Physiological Changes and Benefits from Weight Training	
Change		**Benefits**
Increased muscle mass*		Increased muscular strength
		Improved body composition
		Higher rate of metabolism
		Toned, healthy-looking muscles
Increased utilization of motor units during muscle contractions		Increased muscular strength and power
Improved coordination of motor units		Increased muscular strength and power
Increased strength of tendons, ligaments, and bones		Lower risk of injury to these tissues
Increased storage of fuel in muscles		Increased resistance to muscle fatigue
Increased size of fast-twitch muscle fibers (from a high-resistance program)		Increased muscular strength and power
Increased size of slow-twitch muscle fibers (from a high-repetition program)		Increased muscular endurance
Increased blood supply to muscles (from a high-repetition program)		Increased delivery of oxygen and nutrients
		Increased elimination of wastes
Biochemical improvements (for example, increased sensitivity to insulin)		Enhanced metabolic health

*Due to genetic and hormonal differences, men will build more muscle mass than women.

the type of work required. Endurance activities like jogging tend to use slow-twitch fibers, whereas strength and **power** activities like sprinting use fast-twitch fibers. Weight training can increase the size and strength of both fast-twitch and slow-twitch fibers, although fast-twitch fibers are preferentially increased.

To exert force, the body recruits one or more motor units to contract. A **motor unit** is made up of a nerve connected to a number of muscle fibers. The number of muscle fibers in a motor unit varies from two to hundreds. When a motor nerve calls on its fibers to contract, all fibers contract to their maximum capacity. The number of motor units recruited depends on the amount of strength required: When a person picks up a small weight, he or she uses fewer motor units than when picking up a large weight. Training with weights improves the body's ability to recruit motor units—a phenomenon called muscle learning—which increases strength even before muscle size increases.

In summary, weight training increases muscle strength because it increases the size of muscle fibers and improves the body's ability to call on motor units to exert force. The physiological changes and benefits that result from weight training are summarized in Table 4-1.

Types of Weight Training Exercises

Weight training exercises are generally classified as isometric or isotonic. Each involves a different way of using and strengthening muscles.

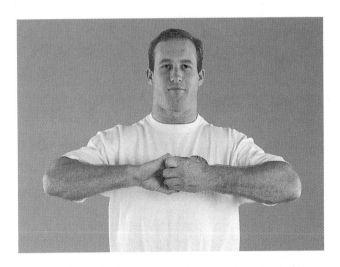

This isometric exercise for the arms and upper back involves locking the hands together and attempting to pull them apart. Isometric contractions involve force without movement.

Isometric Exercise Also called static exercise, **isometric exercise** involves a muscle contraction without a change in the length of the muscle. To perform an isometric exercise, a person can use an immovable object like a wall to provide resistance, or the individual can just tighten a muscle while remaining still (for example, tightening the abdominal muscles while sitting at a desk). In isometrics, the muscle contracts, but there is no movement.

Isometric exercises aren't as widely used as isotonic exercises because they don't develop strength throughout a

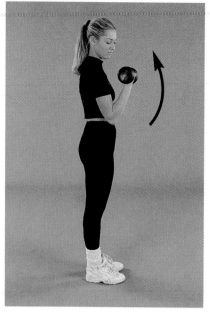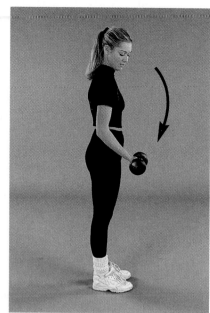

Left: A concentric contraction: The biceps muscle shortens as the arm lifts a weight toward the shoulder. **Right:** An eccentric contraction: The biceps muscle lengthens as the arm lowers a weight toward the thigh.

joint's entire range of motion. However, isometric exercises are useful in strengthening muscles after an injury or surgery, when movement of the affected joint could delay healing. Isometrics are also used to overcome weak points in an individual's range of motion. Isometrically strengthening a muscle at its weakest point will allow more weight to be lifted with that muscle during isotonic exercise. For maximum strength gains, hold the isometric contraction maximally for 6 seconds; do 5–10 repetitions.

Isotonic Exercise Also called dynamic exercise, **isotonic exercise** involves a muscle contraction with a change in the length of the muscle. Isotonic exercises are the most popular type of exercises for increasing muscle strength and seem to be most valuable for developing strength that can be transferred to other forms of physical activity. They can be performed with weight machines, free weights, or a person's own body weight (as in sit-ups or push-ups).

There are two kinds of isotonic muscle contractions: concentric and eccentric. A **concentric muscle contraction** occurs when the muscle applies force as it shortens. An **eccentric muscle contraction** occurs when the muscle applies force as it lengthens. For example, in an arm curl, the biceps muscle works concentrically as the weight is raised toward the shoulder and eccentrically as the weight is lowered.

Two of the most common isotonic exercise techniques are constant resistance exercise and variable resistance exercise. Constant resistance exercise uses a constant load (weight) throughout a joint's entire range of motion. Training with free weights is a form of constant resistance exercise. A problem with this technique is that, because of differences in leverage, there are points in a joint's range

of motion where the muscle controlling the movement is stronger and points where it is weaker. The amount of weight a person can lift is limited by the weakest point in the range. In variable resistance exercise, the load is changed to provide maximum load throughout the entire range of motion. This form of exercise uses machines that place more stress on muscles at the end of the range of motion, where a person has better leverage and is capable of exerting more force. The Nautilus pull-over machine is an example of a variable resistance exercise machine.

Four other kinds of isotonic techniques, used mainly by athletes for training and rehabilitation, are eccentric loading, plyometrics, speed loading, and isokinetics.

- **Eccentric loading** involves placing a load on a muscle as it lengthens. The muscle contracts eccentrically in order to control the weight. Eccentric loading is practiced during most types of resistance training. For example, you are performing an eccentric movement as you lower the weight to your chest during a bench press in preparation for the active movement.

- **Plyometrics** is the sudden eccentric loading and stretching of muscles followed by a forceful concentric contraction. An example would be the action of the major lower-body muscle groups when jumping from a bench to the ground and then jumping back onto the bench. This type of exercise is used to develop explosive strength.

- **Speed loading** involves moving a weight as rapidly as possible in an attempt to approach the speeds used in movements like throwing a softball or sprinting. In the bench press, for example, speed loading might involve doing 5 repetitions as fast as possible using a weight that is half the maximum load you can lift. You can gauge your progress by timing how fast you can perform the repetitions.

- **Isokinetic** exercise involves exerting force at a constant speed against an equal force exerted by a special strength training machine. The isokinetic machine provides variable resistance at different points in the joint's range of motion, matching the effort applied by the individual, while keeping the speed of the movement constant. In other words, the force exerted by the individual at any point in the range of motion is resisted by an equal force from the isokinetic machine. Isokinetic exercises are excellent for building strength and endurance, but the equipment is expensive and less commonly available than other kinds of weight machines.

Comparing the Different Types of Exercise   Isometric exercises require no equipment, so they can be done virtually anywhere. They build strength rapidly and are useful for rehabilitating injured joints. On the other hand, they have to be performed at several different angles for each joint to improve strength throughout the joint's entire range of motion. Isotonic exercises can be performed without equipment (calisthenics) or with equipment (weight lifting). They are excellent for building strength and endurance, and they tend to build strength through a joint's full range of motion.

Most people develop muscular strength and endurance using isotonic exercises. Ultimately, the type of exercise a person chooses depends on individual goals, preferences, and access to equipment.

cific muscles. You don't need a **spotter,** someone who stands by to assist when free weights are used, and you don't have to worry about dropping a weight on yourself.

Free weights require more care, balance, and coordination to use, but they strengthen your body in ways that are more adaptable to real life. Free weights are more popular with athletes for developing explosive strength for sports.

Unless you are training seriously for a sport that requires a great deal of strength, training on machines is probably safer, more convenient, and just as effective as training with free weights. However, you can increase strength either way; which to use is a matter of personal preference. The box "Exercise Machines Versus Free Weights" can help you make a decision.

Selecting Exercises

A complete weight training program works all the major muscle groups. It usually takes about 8–10 different exercises to get a complete workout. For overall fitness, you need to include exercises for your neck, upper back, shoulders, arms, chest, abdomen, lower back, thighs, buttocks, and calves. If you are also training for a particular sport, include exercises to strengthen the muscles important for optimal performance *and* the muscles most likely to be injured. A program of weight training exercises for general fitness is presented later in this chapter.

It is important to balance exercises between **agonist** and **antagonist** muscle groups. (When a muscle contracts, it is known as the agonist; the opposing muscle, which must relax and stretch to allow contraction by the

CREATING A SUCCESSFUL WEIGHT TRAINING PROGRAM

To get the most out of your weight training program, you must design it to achieve maximum fitness benefits with a low risk of injury. Before you begin, seriously consider the type and amount of training that's right for you.

Choosing Equipment: Weight Machines Versus Free Weights

Your muscles will get stronger if you make them work against a resistance. Resistance can be provided by free weights, by your own body weight, or by sophisticated exercise machines. Weight machines are preferred by many people because they are safe, convenient, and easy to use. You just set the resistance (usually by placing a pin in the weight stack), sit down at the machine, and start working. Machines make it easy to isolate and work spe-

TERMS

isotonic exercise   Exercise involving a muscle contraction with a change in the length of the muscle.

concentric muscle contraction   An isotonic contraction in which the muscle gets shorter as it contracts.

eccentric muscle contraction   An isotonic contraction in which the muscle lengthens as it contracts.

eccentric loading   Loading the muscle while it is lengthening; sometimes called *negatives*.

plyometrics   Rapid stretching of a muscle group that is undergoing eccentric stress (the muscle is exerting force while it lengthens), followed by a rapid concentric contraction.

speed loading   Moving a load as rapidly as possible.

isokinetic   The application of force at a constant speed against an equal force.

spotter   A person who assists with a weight training exercise done with free weights.

agonist   A muscle in a state of contraction, opposed by the action of another muscle, its *antagonist*.

antagonist   A muscle that opposes the action of another muscle, its *agonist*.

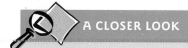
Exercise Machines

Advantages

- Safe
- Convenient
- Don't require spotters
- Don't require lifter to balance bar
- Provide variable resistance
- Require less skill
- Make it easy to move from one exercise to the next
- Allow easy isolation of individual muscle groups
- Support back (on many machines)

Disadvantages

- Limited availability
- Inappropriate for performing dynamic movements
- Allow a limited number of exercises

Free Weights

Advantages

- Allow dynamic movements
- Allow the user to develop control of the weights
- Allow a greater variety of exercises
- Widely available
- Truer to real-life situations; strength transfers to daily activities

Disadvantages

- Not as safe
- Require spotters
- Require more skill
- Cause more blisters and calluses

---

agonist, is known as the antagonist.) Whenever you do an exercise that moves a joint in one direction, also select an exercise that works the joint in the opposite direction. For example, if you do knee extensions to develop the muscles on the front of your thighs, also do leg curls to develop the antagonistic muscles on the back of your thighs.

The order of exercises can also be important. Do exercises for large-muscle groups or for more than one joint before you do exercises that use small-muscle groups or single joints. This allows for more effective overload of the larger, more powerful muscle groups. Small-muscle groups fatigue more easily than larger ones, and small-muscle fatigue limits your capacity to overload larger-muscle groups. For example, lateral raises, which work the shoulder muscles, should be performed after bench presses, which work the chest and arms in addition to the shoulders. If you fatigue your shoulder muscles by doing lateral raises first, you won't be able to lift as much weight and effectively fatigue all the key muscle groups used during the bench press.

Resistance

The amount of weight (resistance) you lift in weight training exercises is equivalent to intensity in cardiorespiratory endurance training. It determines the way your body will adapt to weight training and how quickly these adaptations will occur. Choose weights based on your current level of muscular fitness and your fitness goals. To build strength rapidly, you should lift weights as heavy as 80%

of your maximum capacity (1 RM). If you're more interested in building endurance, choose a lighter weight (perhaps 40–60% of 1 RM) and do more repetitions. For example, if your maximum capacity for the leg press is 160 pounds, you might lift 130 pounds to build strength and 80 pounds to build endurance. For a general fitness program to develop both strength and endurance, choose a weight in the middle of this range, perhaps 70% of 1 RM.

Because it can be tedious and time-consuming to continually reassess your maximum capacity for each exercise, you might find it easier to choose a weight based on the number of repetitions of an exercise you can perform with a given resistance.

Repetitions and Sets

To improve fitness, you must do enough repetitions of each exercise to fatigue your muscles. The number of repetitions needed to cause fatigue depends on the amount of resistance: the heavier the weight, the fewer repetitions to reach fatigue. In general, a heavy weight and a low number of repetitions (1–5) build strength, whereas a light weight and a high number of repetitions (15–20) build endurance (Figure 4-2). For a general fitness program to build both strength and endurance, try to do about 8–12 repetitions of each exercise; a few exercises, such as abdominal crunches and calf raises, may require more. Choose a weight heavy enough to fatigue your muscles but light enough for you to complete the repetitions with good form. To avoid risk of injury, older (approximately 50–60 years of age and above) and more frail people should perform more repetitions (10–15) using a lighter weight.

TERMS   set   A group of repetitions followed by a rest period.

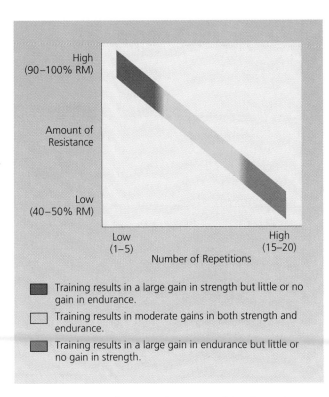

Figure 4-2 Training for strength versus training for endurance.

Legend for figure:
- Training results in a large gain in strength but little or no gain in endurance.
- Training results in moderate gains in both strength and endurance.
- Training results in a large gain in endurance but little or no gain in strength.

Graph axes: Vertical axis — Amount of Resistance, from Low (40–50% RM) to High (90–100% RM). Horizontal axis — Number of Repetitions, from Low (1–5) to High (15–20).

In weight training, a **set** refers to a group of repetitions of an exercise followed by a rest period. Surprisingly, exercise scientists have not identified the optimal number of sets for increasing strength. For developing strength and endurance for general fitness, a single set of each exercise is sufficient, provided you use enough resistance to fatigue your muscles. (You should just barely be able to complete the 8–12 repetitions for each exercise.) Doing more than 1 set of each exercise may increase strength development, and most serious weight trainers do at least 3 sets of each exercise (see below for additional guidelines for more advanced programs).

If you perform more than 1 set of an exercise, you need to rest long enough between sets to allow your muscles to work at a high enough intensity to increase fitness. The length of the rest interval depends on the amount of resistance. In a program to develop a combination of strength and endurance for wellness, a rest period of 1–3 minutes between sets is appropriate; if you are lifting heavier loads to build maximum strength, rest 3–5 minutes between sets. You can save time in your workouts if you alternate sets of different exercises. Each muscle group can rest between sets while you work on other muscles.

The Warm-Up and Cool-Down

As with cardiorespiratory endurance exercise, you should warm up before every weight training session and cool down afterward. You should do both a general warm-up—several minutes of walking or easy jogging—and a warm-up for the weight training exercises you plan to perform. For example, if you plan to do 1 or more sets of 10 repetitions of bench presses with 125 pounds, you might do 1 set of 10 repetitions with 50 pounds as a warm-up. Do similar warm-up exercises for each exercise in your program.

To cool down after weight training, relax for 5–10 minutes after your workout. Although controversial, a few studies have suggested that including a period of post-exercise stretching may help prevent muscle soreness; warmed-up muscles and joints make this a particularly good time to work on flexibility.

Frequency of Exercise

For general fitness, the American College of Sports Medicine recommends a frequency of 2–3 days per week for weight training. Allow your muscles at least 1 day of rest between workouts; if you train too often, your muscles won't be able to work at a high enough intensity to improve their fitness, and soreness and injury are more likely to result. If you enjoy weight training and would like to train more often, try working different muscle groups on alternate days. For example, work your arms and upper body one day, work your lower body the next day, and then return to upper-body exercises on the third day. Refer to the box "A Sample Weight Training Program for General Fitness" for suggestions on beginning a program.

Making Progress

The first few sessions of weight training should be devoted to learning the exercises. You need to learn the movements, and your nervous system needs to practice communicating with your muscles so you can develop strength effectively. To start, choose a weight that you can move easily through 8–12 repetitions, and do only 1 set of each exercise. Gradually add weight and (if you want) sets to your program over the first few weeks until you are doing 1–3 sets of 8–12 repetitions of each exercise.

As you progress, add weight when you can do more than 12 repetitions of an exercise. If adding weight means you can do only 7 or 8 repetitions, stay with that weight until you can again complete 12 repetitions per set. If you can do only 4–6 repetitions after adding weight, you've added too much and should take some off.

You can expect to improve rapidly during the first 6–10 weeks of training: a 10–30% increase in the amount of weight lifted. Gains will then come more slowly. Your rate of improvement will depend on how hard you work and how your body responds to resistance training. There will be individual differences in the rate of improvement. Factors such as age, motivation, and heredity will affect your progress.

Your ultimate goal depends on you. After you have achieved the level of strength and muscularity that you

Guidelines

Type of activity: 8–10 weight training exercises that focus on major muscle groups

Frequency: 2–3 days per week

Resistance: Weights heavy enough to cause muscle fatigue when exercises are performed for the selected number of repetitions

Repetitions: 8–12 of each exercise (10–15 with a lower weight for people over age 50–60)

Sets: 1 (Doing more than 1 set per exercise may result in faster and greater strength gains.)

Sample Program

1. Warm-up (5–10 minutes)
2. Weight training exercises (see table at right)
3. Cool-down (5–10 minutes)

Exercises

Exercise	Muscle Groups Developed	Resistance (lb)	Repetitions	Sets
Bench press	Chest, shoulders, triceps	60	10	1
Shoulder press	Shoulders, trapezius, triceps	40	10	1
Pull-ups	Lats, biceps	—	5	1
Lateral raises	Shoulders	5	10	1
Biceps curls	Biceps	25	10	1
Squats	Gluteals, quadriceps	30	10	1
Toe raises	Calves	25	15	1
Abdominal curls	Abdominals	—	30	1
Spine extensions	Low- and mid-back spine extensors	—	10	1
Neck flexion	Neck flexors	—	10	1

want, you can maintain your gains by training 2–3 days per week. You can monitor the progress of your program by recording the amount of resistance and the number of repetitions and sets you perform on a workout card like the one shown in Figure 4-3.

More Advanced Strength Training Programs

The weight training program described in this section—1 set of 8–12 repetitions of 8–10 exercises, performed 2–3 days per week—is sufficient to develop and maintain muscular strength and endurance for general fitness. If you have a different goal, you may need to adjust your program accordingly. As described above, performing more sets of a smaller number of repetitions with a heavier load will cause greater increases in strength. A program designed to build strength might include 3–5 sets of 4–6 repetitions each; the load used should be heavy enough to cause fatigue with the smaller number of repetitions. Be sure to rest long enough after a set to allow your muscles to recover and to work intensely during the next set.

Experienced weight trainers often engage in some form of cycle training, in which the exercises, number of sets and repetitions, and intensity are varied within a workout and/or between workouts. For example, you might do a particular exercise more intensely during some sets or on some days than others; you might also vary the exercises you perform for particular muscle groups. For information on these more advanced training techniques, consult a strength coach certified by the National Strength and Conditioning Association. Several of the books listed in the For More Information section at the end of the chapter also provide information on program design. If you decide to adopt a more advanced training regimen, start off slowly to give your body a chance to adjust and to minimize the risk of injury.

Weight Training Safety

Injuries do happen in weight training. Maximum physical effort, elaborate machinery, rapid movements, and heavy weights can combine to make the weight room a dangerous place if proper precautions aren't taken. To help ensure that your workouts are safe and productive, follow the guidelines in the box "Safe Weight Training" and the suggestions given below.

Use Proper Lifting Technique Every exercise has a proper technique that is important for obtaining maximum benefits and preventing injury. Your instructor or weight room attendant can help explain the specific techniques for performing different exercises and using different weight machines. Perform exercises smoothly and with good form. Lift or push the weight forcefully during the active phase of the lift and then lower it slowly with control. Perform all lifts through the full range of motion.

Use Spotters and Collars with Free Weights Spotters are necessary when an exercise has potential for danger: A weight that is out of control or falls can cause a serious injury. A spotter can assist you if you cannot complete a lift or if the weight tilts. A spotter can also help you move a weight into position before a lift and provide help or ad-

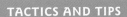

- Lift weights from a stabilized body position.

- Be aware of what's going on around you. Stay away from other people when they're doing exercises. If you bump into someone, you could cause an injury.

- Don't use defective equipment. Report any equipment malfunctions immediately.

- Protect your back by maintaining control of your spine (protect your spine from dangerous positions). Observe

proper lifting techniques, and use a weight-lifting belt when doing heavy lifts.

- Don't hold your breath while doing weight training exercises.

- Always warm up before training, and cool down afterward.

- Don't exercise if you're ill, injured, or overtrained.

WORKOUT CARD FOR   Scott Peterson

Exercise/Date		9/14	9/16	9/18	9/21	9/23	9/25	9/28	9/30	10/2	10/5	10/7	10/9	10/12	10/14	10/16								
Bench press	Wt.	70	70	70	75	75	75	80	80	80	90	90	95	105	105	105								
	Sets	1	1	1	1	1	1	1	1	1	1	1	1	1	1	1								
	Reps.	10	10	12	10	12	12	10	9	12	12	12	12	8	7	8								
Shoulder press	Wt.	40	40	40	55	55	60	60	60	70	70	75	75	75	80	85								
	Sets	1	1	1	1	1	1	1	1	1	1	1	1	1	1	1								
	Reps.	10	10	12	10	12	10	10	12	10	12	8	11	12	12	8								
Pull-ups	Wt.	–	–	–	–	–	–	–	–	–	–	–	–	–	–	–								
	Sets	1	1	1	1	1	1	1	1	1	1	1	1	1	1	1								
	Reps.	2	2	2	2	3	3	4	4	4	4	4	5	5	6	6								
Lateral raises	Wt.	5	5	5	7.5	7.5	7.5	7.5	7.5	7.5	7.5	7.5	7.5	10	10	10								
	Sets	1	1	1	1	1	1	1	1	1	1	1	1	1	1	1								
	Reps.	10	10	10	7	8	7	10	8	8	11	12	12	7	7	8								
Biceps curls	Wt.	35	35	35	40	40	40	45	45	45	50	50	50	50	50	50								
	Sets	1	1	1	1	1	1	1	1	1	1	1	1	1	1	1								
	Reps.	10	10	10	10	12	12	10	12	12	10	8	8	10	10	10								
Squats	Wt.	–	–	–	45	45	85	85	105	115	125	135	135	145	145	145								
	Sets	1	1	1	1	1	1	1	1	1	1	1	1	1	1	1								
	Reps.	10	10	10	12	15	10	12	12	15	12	10	12	9	8	9								
Toe raises	Wt.	–	–	–	45	45	85	85	105	115	125	135	135	145	145	145								
	Sets	1	1	1	1	1	1	1	1	1	1	1	1	1	1	1								
	Reps.	15	15	15	15	15	15	15	15	15	15	15	15	15	15	15								
Abdominal curls	Wt.	–	–	–	–	–	–	–	–	–	–	–	–	–	–	–								
	Sets	1	1	1	1	1	1	1	1	1	1	1	1	1	1	1								
	Reps.	20	20	20	20	20	20	25	25	25	30	30	30	30	30	30								
Spine extensions	Wt.	–	–	–	–	–	–	–	–	–	–	–	–	–	–	–								
	Sets	1	1	1	1	1	1	1	1	1	1	1	1	1	1	1								
	Reps.	5	5	5	8	8	8	10	10	10	10	10	10	10	10	10								
Neck flexion	Wt.	–	–	–	–	–	–	–	–	–	–	–	–	–	–	–								
	Sets	1	1	1	1	1	1	1	1	1	1	1	1	1	1	1								
	Reps.	5	5	5	10	10	10	10	10	10	10	10	10	10	10	10								

Figure 4-3 A sample workout card.

ditional resistance during a lift. Spotting requires practice and coordination between the lifter and the spotter(s).

Collars are devices that secure weights to a barbell or dumbbell. Although people lift weights without collars, doing so is dangerous. It is easy to lose your balance or to raise one side of the weight faster than the other. Without collars, the weights on one side of the bar will slip off, and the weights on the opposite side will crash to the floor.

Proper lifting technique for free weights also includes the following:

- Keep weights as close to your body as possible.

- Do most of your lifting with your legs. Keep your hips and buttocks tucked in.

- When you pick a weight up from the ground, keep your back straight and your head level or up. Don't bend at the waist with straight legs.

- Don't twist your body while lifting.

- Lift weights smoothly and slowly; don't jerk them. Control the weight through the entire range of motion.

- Don't bounce weights against your body during an exercise.

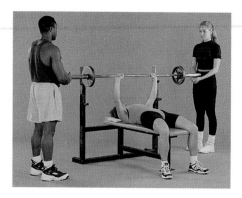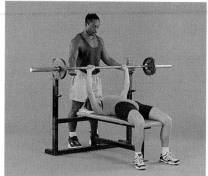

Spotters should be present when a person trains with free weights. **(a)** If two spotters are used, one spotter should stand at each end of the barbell. **(b)** If one spotter is present, he or she should stand behind the lifter.

- Never hold your breath when you lift. Exhale when exerting the greatest force, and inhale when moving the weight into position for the active phase of the lift. (Holding your breath causes a decrease in blood returning to the heart and can make you become dizzy and faint.)

- Rest between sets if you perform more than 1 set of each exercise. Fatigue hampers your ability to obtain maximum benefits from your program and is a prime cause of injury.

- When lifting barbells and dumbbells, wrap your thumbs around the bar when gripping it. You can easily drop the weight when using a "thumbless" grip.

- Gloves are not mandatory but may prevent calluses on your hands.

- When doing standing lifts, maintain a good posture so that you protect your back.

- Don't lift beyond the limits of your strength.

Use Common Sense When Exercising on Weight Machines Although notable for their safety, weight machines are not completely danger-free. The following strategies can help prevent injuries.

- Keep away from moving weight stacks. Pay attention when you're changing weights. Someone may jump on the machine ahead of you and begin an exercise while your fingers are close to the weight stack.

- Stay away from moving parts of the machine that could pinch your skin.

- Adjust each machine for your body so that you don't have to work in an awkward position. Lock everything in place before you begin.

- Beware of broken bolts, frayed cables, broken chains, or loose cushions that can give way and cause serious injury. If you notice a broken or frayed part, tell an instructor immediately.

- Make sure the machines are clean. Dirty vinyl is a breeding ground for germs that can cause skin diseases. Carry a towel around with you, and place it on the machine where you will sit or lie down.

- Be aware of what's happening around you. Talking between exercises is a great way to relax and have fun, but inattention can lead to injury.

Be Alert for Injuries Report any obvious muscle or joint injuries to your instructor or physician, and stop exercising the affected area. Training with an injured joint or muscle can lead to a more serious injury. Make sure you get the necessary first aid. Even minor injuries heal faster if you use the R-I-C-E principle of treating injuries described in Chapter 3.

Consult a physician if you're having any unusual symptoms during exercise or if you're uncertain whether weight training is a proper activity for you. Conditions such as heart disease and high blood pressure can be aggravated during weight training. Symptoms such as headaches; dizziness; labored breathing; numbness; vision disturbances; and chest, neck, or arm pains should be reported immediately.

A Caution About Supplements and Drugs

Many active people use a wide variety of nutritional supplements and drugs in the quest for improved performance and appearance. They take these substances to enhance muscle size; speed recovery from injury and prevent the effects of overtraining; increase training intensity and aggressiveness; and control fat, body water, and appetite. Most of these substances are ineffective and expensive and many are dangerous. A selective summary of "performance aids" is given in Table 4-2, along with their potential side effects.

Supplements Taken to Increase Muscle Growth The most popular category of supplements are those taken to increase muscle growth. They constitute the most significant area of abuse.

- **Anabolic steroids** are a group of synthetic derivatives of testosterone. People take them in hope of gaining

TERMS **anabolic steroids** Synthetic male hormones taken to enhance athletic performance and body composition.

TABLE 4-2 Performance Aids Marketed to Weight Trainers

Substance	Supposed Effects	Actual Effects	Selected Potential Side Effects
Adrenal androgenes: DHEA, androstenedione	Increased testosterone, muscle mass, and strength; decreased body fat	Increased testosterone, strength, and fat-free mass and decreased fat in older subjects (more studies needed in younger people)	Gonadal suppression, prostate hypertrophy, breast development in males, masculinization in women and children. Long-term effects unknown
Amino acids	Increased muscle mass	No effects if dietary protein intake is adequate	Minimal side effects; unbalanced amino acid intake can cause problems with protein metabolism
Anabolic steroids	Increased muscle mass, strength, power, psychological aggressiveness, and endurance	Increased strength, power, fat-free mass, and aggression; no effects on endurance	Minor to severe: gonadal suppression, liver disease, acne, breast development in males, masculinization in women and children, heart disease, cancer. Steroids are controlled substances[a]
Chromium picolinate	Increased muscle mass; decreased body fat	Well-controlled studies show no significant effect on fat-free mass or on body fat	Moderate doses (50–200 μg) appear safe; higher doses may cause DNA damage and other serious effects. Long-term effects unknown
Creatine monohydrate	Increased muscle creatine phosphate, muscle mass, and capacity for high-intensity exercise	Increased muscle mass and performance in some types of high-intensity exercise	Minimal side effects; some reports of muscle cramping. Long-term effects unknown
Ephedrine	Decreased body fat; increased training intensity due to stimulant effect	Decreased appetite, particularly when taken with caffeine; no evidence for increased training intensity	Abnormal heart rhythms, nervousness, headache, and gastrointestinal distress. Not recommended
Ginseng	Decreased effects of physical and emotional stress; increased oxygen consumption	Most well-controlled studies show no effect on performance	No serious side effects; high doses can cause high blood pressure, nervousness, and insomnia
Growth hormone	Increased muscle mass, strength, and power; decreased body fat	Increased muscle mass and strength	Diabetes, acromegaly (disease characterized by increased growth of bones in hands and face), enlarged heart and other organs. An extremely expensive controlled substance[a]
HMB (beta-hydroxy-beta-methylbutyrate)	Increased strength and muscle mass; decreased body fat	Some studies show increased fat-free mass and decreased fat; more research needed	No reported side effects. Long-term effects unknown
"Metabolic-optimizing" meals for athletes	Increased muscle mass; energy supply; decreased body fat	No proven effects beyond those of balanced meals	No reported side effects; extremely expensive
Protein	Increased muscle mass	No effects if dietary protein intake is adequate	Can be dangerous for people with liver or kidney disease

[a]Possession of a controlled substance is illegal without a prescription, and physicians are not allowed to prescribe controlled substances for the improvement of athletic performance. In addition, the use of anabolic steroids, growth hormone, or any of several other substances listed in this table is banned for athletic competition.

SOURCES: Brooks, G. A., et al. 2000. *Exercise Physiology: Human Bioenergetics and Its Applications*, 3d ed. Mountain View, Calif.: Mayfield. Volek, J. S. 1999. What we now know about creatine. *ACSM's Health and Fitness Journal* 3(3). Williams, M. H. 1998. *The Ergogenics Edge: Pushing the Limits of Sports Performance*. Champaign, Ill.: Human Kinetics.

weight and muscle size and improving strength, power, speed, endurance, aggressiveness, and appearance. The word *anabolic* means growing, or building. In 1988, a federal law made it illegal to distribute anabolic steroids in the United States for nontherapeutic uses. This has led to a thriving black market for illegal anabolic steroids in the United States. Despite drug testing, anabolic steroids are taken by some strength-trained athletes in sports such as bodybuilding, track and field, and football. Several studies, including one under the direction of the Centers for Disease Control and Prevention, have shown that use of anabolic steroids has filtered down to high school students; about 6% of all high school students have used them.

Anabolic steroids increase protein synthesis, which enhances fat-free weight, muscle mass, and strength. Anabolic steroids work by triggering the cells to make new proteins, blocking protein breakdown, and increasing aggressiveness, all of which help people train harder. Side effects include liver damage and tumors, decreased levels of high-density lipoprotein (good cholesterol), heart disease, depressed sperm and testosterone production, high blood pressure, increased risk of AIDS (through shared needles), depressed immune function, problems with sugar metabolism, psychological disturbances, masculinization in women and children, premature closure of bone growth centers, and an increased risk of cancer. Side effects are greatest in people who take high doses of drugs for prolonged periods.

• Human chorionic gonadotrophin (HCG) is sometimes taken by anabolic steroid users to boost natural testosterone production, which is suppressed by steroids, and to prevent the muscle atrophy common during withdrawal from steroids. HCG is a hormone that is secreted by the placenta during pregnancy. Although HCG tends to increase testosterone levels, it sometimes interferes with normal testosterone regulation, which causes additional deterioration in health and well-being. Use of HCG is not recommended and is banned in most sports.

• Growth hormone is popular with many athletes, who use it to increase muscle mass and strength. Reports in the news media suggest that, as with anabolic steroids, its general use has filtered down to high school students. Although advances in genetics have made human growth hormone more widely available, it is extremely expensive and has serious side effects.

Growth hormone speeds protein synthesis and stimulates other muscle growth factors. It affects carbohydrate and fat metabolism and stimulates sugar uptake in muscle and fat. It also stimulates fat release from adipose tissue. Although growth hormone builds muscles, the few studies on the hormone in humans have shown no beneficial effects on muscle or exercise performance. Prolonged growth hormone administration may result in elevated blood sugar, high insulin levels, heart enlargement, and increased blood fat levels. Prolonged use could also lead to acromegaly, characterized by enlarged bones in the head, face, and hands, as well as diseases of the heart, nerves, bones, and joints.

Some bodybuilders also take drugs that increase the body's growth hormone secretion. These drugs include propranolol, vasopressin, clonidine, and levodopa. There is no evidence that these substances enhance muscle growth.

• Insulin-like growth factor (IGF-1) has recently become a popular drug among some athletes. IGF-1 is produced by the pituitary gland and is stimulated by growth hormone. It speeds delivery of amino acids and sugar into cells, stimulates protein and glycogen synthesis, and helps build bone and cartilage. Although IGF-1 is a powerful anabolic agent, its effects in healthy, active people are unknown. Side effects are thought to be similar to those of growth hormone. Long-term use is known to promote cancer. IGF-1 is a potentially dangerous substance that should never be used without a physician's supervision.

• Dehydroepiandrosterone (DHEA) and androstenedione are two relatively weak male hormones produced in the adrenal glands of both men and women. Both are broken down into testosterone. People take these drugs to stimulate muscle growth and aid in weight control. Because they are promoted as food supplements, they are sold widely in health food stores and supermarkets. The few studies in humans show that they are of little value in improving athletic performance. These substances have side effects similar to those of anabolic steroids, particularly when taken in high doses. Like anabolic steroids, they increase the risk of heart disease and cancer and interfere with normal testosterone metabolism.

• Insulin is used by the body to help control carbohydrate, fat, and protein metabolism. Some athletes take insulin injections to promote muscle hypertrophy, but its effectiveness in stimulating muscle growth is not known. Insulin supplementation is an extremely dangerous practice because it can cause insulin shock (characterized by extremely low blood sugar), which can lead to unconsciousness and death.

• Protein, amino acid, and polypeptide supplements are taken to accelerate muscle development, decrease body fat, and stimulate the release of growth hormone. By a wide margin, these products are the most popular supplements taken by active people. Still, there is little scientific proof to support their use, even in athletes on extremely heavy training routines. The protein requirements of these athletes is not much higher than that of sedentary individuals. Also, most athletes take in more than enough protein in their diets. Although there appear to be few side effects from using these products, substituting amino acid or polypeptide supplements for protein-rich food can cause deficiencies in important nutrients, such as iron and the B vitamins.

• Clenbuterol (a beta agonist) is used to prevent and treat symptoms of exercise-induced asthma. Some athletes take beta agonists to enhance performance. They hope to prevent muscle atrophy, increase fat-free weight, and decrease body fat. Side effects include insomnia, heart arrhythmias, anxiety, anorexia, and nausea. More serious side effects include heart enlargement and myocardial infarction (particularly if used with anabolic steroids).

• So-called metabolic-optimizing meals contain a wide variety of individual supplemental components and are widely used by athletes and active people. Some studies suggest that these meals may increase the hormone concentrations necessary for the development of fitness, but their effects on muscle growth and performance have not been demonstrated.

• Other substances used to promote muscle growth include cyproheptadine (Periactin), conjugated linoleic acid (CLA), vanadyl sulfate, dibencozide, and organ extracts. These agents are much less popular, and their effectiveness and safety are both questionable.

Supplements Taken to Speed Recovery from Training
The primary purpose of taking these agents is to replenish depleted body fuel supplies that are important during exercise and recovery.

• Creatine monohydrate is one of the most popular athletic supplements. It is used in an effort to enhance recovery, power, strength, and muscle size. Creatine monohydrate supplements increase creatine phosphate levels in muscle. As discussed in Chapter 3, creatine phosphate is a critical fuel source in the body. Several, but not all, studies have shown that creatine monohydrate supplementation improves performance in short-term, high-intensity, repetitive exercise, which would make it a valuable supplement for people who play strength-speed sports, such as football, basketball, soccer, sprinting, and volleyball. It may help to enlarge muscles in people who lift weights by allowing them to train harder. On the other hand, in 2000, a panel of ACSM experts concluded that there is no evidence that creatine supplements increase the aerobic power of muscle. Creatine may increase water retention in muscles, giving the feeling of increased muscularity without an actual increase in muscle size. The long-term effects of creatine monohydrate supplementation are unknown, so people should take this substance with caution.

• Chromium picolinate is used to enhance the action of insulin and to improve carbohydrate metabolism. Although a few studies have shown benefits, the efficacy of this supplement is extremely controversial.

• Other substances in this category include carbohydrate beverages that athletes use during and immediately following exercise to help them recover from intense training; these beverages speed the replenishment of liver and muscle glycogen. The use of other substances to speed recovery—such as vitamin C, N-acetyl-L-cysteine (NAC), inosine, and beta-hydroxy-beta-methylbutyrate (HMB)—is not currently supported by enough positive research findings to warrant a recommendation.

Substances Taken to Increase Training Intensity and Overcome Fatigue
Active people often spend many hours a day training in the gymnasium or on the playing field, and monotony and fatigue sometimes impede significant improvement. Many bodybuilders use stimulants to help them increase training intensity and overcome fatigue.

• Amphetamines are sometimes used by athletes to prevent fatigue and to increase confidence and training intensity. Examples of amphetamines include benzedrine, dexedrine, dexamyl, and methedrine. These drugs stimulate the nervous system, causing increased arousal, wakefulness, confidence, and the feeling of an enhanced capability to make decisions. They also increase blood pressure, heart rate, oxygen consumption in the brain, and blood flow to the muscles. These drugs mask fatigue, so users feel energized, but once the drug wears off, depression or fatigue sets in. Because amphetamines can cause extreme confusion, they are of little use in sports requiring rapid decisions. Amphetamines can cause severe neural and psychological effects that include aggressiveness, paranoia, hallucinations, compulsive behavior, restlessness, irritability, heart arrhythmias, high blood pressure, and chest pains.

• Caffeine, found naturally in many plant species, is a favorite stimulant among many active people. Caffeine stimulates the nervous system and helps increase fat levels in the blood. Although there is some evidence that caffeine may improve endurance, the drug does not appear to enhance short-term maximal exercise capacity. Caffeine increases the incidence of abnormal heart rhythms and insomnia and is addictive.

• Other agents in this category include cocaine, ephedrine, and ginseng. Cocaine use is not thought to be widespread in sports, but some athletes reportedly use it to increase training intensity. Ephedrine, a weak stimulant, is widely used by weight trainers during workouts but has no effect on exercise capacity. Ginseng is also very popular with active people, but there is little evidence that it boosts exercise capacity.

Substances Taken to Aid Weight Control
Substances used in weight control include drugs that suppress appetite, thermogenic drugs, and diuretics to control weight and increase muscle definition.

• Anorectic drugs suppress appetite, and thermogenic drugs affect metabolic rate. Appetite suppressants include amphetamine, diethylpropion, fenfluramine, and phenylpropanolamine. Some of these drugs have serious side

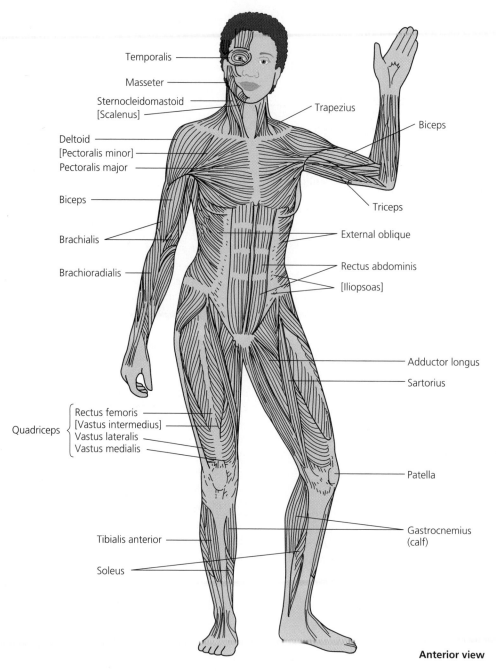

Temporalis
Masseter
Sternocleidomastoid
[Scalenus]
Deltoid
[Pectoralis minor]
Pectoralis major
Biceps
Brachialis
Brachioradialis
Trapezius
Biceps
Triceps
External oblique
Rectus abdominis
[Iliopsoas]
Adductor longus
Sartorius

Quadriceps {
Rectus femoris
[Vastus intermedius]
Vastus lateralis
Vastus medialis
}

Patella

Tibialis anterior
Soleus
Gastrocnemius
(calf)

Anterior view

Figure 4-4   The muscular system.   The muscle names enclosed in brackets refer to deep muscles.

effects, including addiction, heart rhythm disturbances, heart valve damage, and psychiatric disturbances.

Thermogenic drugs reduce lean body mass and cause an increased incidence of cardiac arrhythmias. They include thyroid hormone, ephedrine, and dinitrophenol. These drugs are extremely dangerous and are not recommended.

• Diuretics and potassium supplements are sometimes taken by people in an attempt to accentuate muscle definition. Others take potassium supplements to promote fluid retention in their muscle cells, thus in-

creasing muscle size. Athletes combine these practices with very-low-calorie diets and dehydration in the quest for leanness. There is no evidence that these unhealthy practices improve appearance or muscle size. Serious complications have developed from these practices, including muscle cell destruction, low blood pressure, blood chemistry abnormalities, and heart problems.

Supplement and Drug Use by Active People   The variety and combinations of supplements and drugs used by physically active people make it extremely difficult to de-

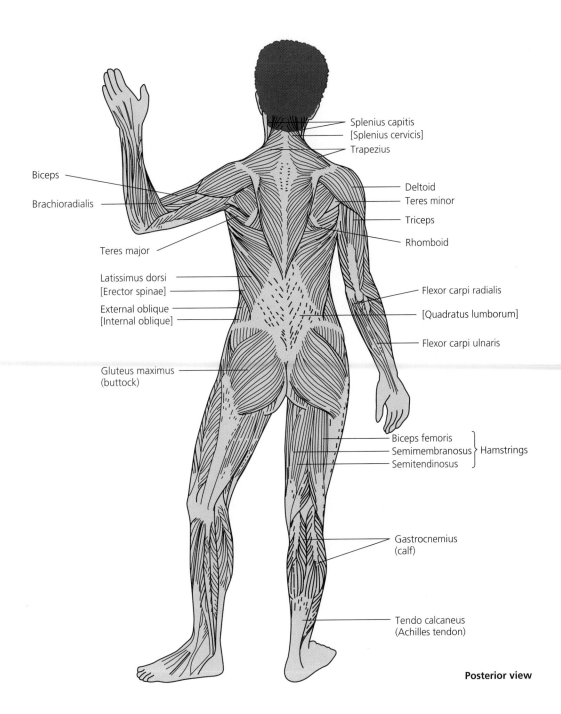

Biceps

Brachioradialis

Teres major

Latissimus dorsi
[Erector spinae]

External oblique
[Internal oblique]

Gluteus maximus
(buttock)

Splenius capitis
[Splenius cervicis]

Trapezius

Deltoid

Teres minor

Triceps

Rhomboid

Flexor carpi radialis

[Quadratus lumborum]

Flexor carpi ulnaris

Biceps femoris
Semimembranosus } Hamstrings
Semitendinosus

Gastrocnemius
(calf)

Tendo calcaneus
(Achilles tendon)

Posterior view

termine the efficacy of these practices or to predict their side effects. Many medical studies describe catastrophic side effects from use of unsafe drugs and nutritional supplements. Most supplements simply don't work.

Keep in mind that no nutritional supplement or drug will change a weak, untrained person into a strong, fit person. Those changes require regular training that stresses the muscles, heart, lungs, and metabolism and causes the body to adapt. They also require a healthy, balanced diet, as described in Chapter 8. In the next section, weight training exercises that can help you reach your goals are described.

Weight Training Exercises

A general book on fitness and wellness cannot include a detailed description of all weight training exercises. Here we present a basic program for developing muscular strength and endurance for general fitness using free weights and weight machines. Instructions for each exercise are accompanied by photographs and a listing of the muscles being trained. (Figure 4-4 is a diagram of the muscular system.) Table 4-3 lists alternative and additional exercises that can be performed on Cybex, Nautilus, or Universal machines or with free weights. If you

TABLE 4-3   *Weight Training Exercises for Machines and Free Weights*

Body Part	Cybex	Nautilus	Universal Gym	Free Weights
Neck	4-way neck	4-way neck	Neck conditioning station	Neck harness Manual exercises
Trapezius ("traps")	Chest/incline press Incline press Overhead press	Overhead press Lateral raise Reverse pull-over Compound row Shoulder shrug Rowing back	Shoulder press Shoulder shrug Upright row Bent-over row Rip-up Front raise Pull-up	Overhead press Lateral raise Shoulder shrug Power clean Upright row
Chest (Pectoralis major)	Incline press Chest/incline press Fly Chest press	Vertical chest Incline press Bench press Pec fly 10° chest	Bench press	Bench press Incline press Dumbbell fly
Deltoids	Chest/incline press Incline press Row/rear delt Overhead press Lateral raise Chest press	Lateral raise Overhead press Reverse pull-over Double chest 10° chest 50° chest Seated dip Bench press Compound row Rotary shoulder	Bench press Shoulder shrug Shoulder press Upright row Rip-up Front raise Pull-up	Raise Bench press Shoulder press Upright row Pull-up
Biceps	Row/rear delt Pull-down Arm curl	Biceps curl Lat pull	Biceps curl Lat pull	Biceps curl Lat pull Pull-up
Triceps	Chest/incline press Chest press Incline press Overhead press Arm extension	Triceps extension Seated dip Triceps extension (lat machine) Bench press Overhead press	French curl Dip Triceps extension (lat machine) Bench press Seated press	French curl Dip Triceps extension (lat machine) Bench press Military press
Latissimus dorsi ("lats")	Row/rear delt Pull-down Lat pull-down	Pull-over Behind neck Torso arm Lat pull Seated dip Compound row	Pull-up Lat pull Bent-over row Pull-over Dip	Pull-up Pull-over Dip Bent-over row Lat pull
Abdominals	Torso rotation Ab crunch	Abdominal Rotary torso	Hip flexor Leg raise Crunch Sit-up Side-bend	Hip flexor Leg raise Crunch Sit-up Side-bend Isometric tightener
Lower back	Torso rotation Back extension	Lower back	Back extension Back leg raise	Back extension Good-morning
Thigh and buttocks	Seated leg press Leg extension Prone leg curl Seated leg curl Hip adduction Hip abduction	Leg press Leg extension Prone leg curl Seated leg curl Hip extension Hip adduction Hip abduction	Leg press Leg curl Leg extension Adductor kick Abductor kick Back hip extension	Squat Leg press Leg extension Leg curl Power clean Snatch Dead lift
Calf	Rotary calf	Seated calf Heel raise: multiexercise	Calf press	Heel raise

TABLE 4-4 *Weight Training for Sports and Activities*

Emphasize these muscle groups when training for the following sports and activities. Although it is important to condition all major muscle groups, specific activities require extra conditioning in specific muscles.

Activity or Sport	Neck	Shoulders	Chest	Arms	Forearms	Upper Back	Lower Back	Abdominals	Thighs	Hamstrings	Calves
Badminton		✔	✔	✔	✔	✔			✔	✔	✔
Basketball		✔	✔	✔		✔	✔	✔	✔	✔	✔
Billiards		✔		✔	✔	✔	✔				
Canoeing		✔	✔	✔	✔	✔	✔	✔			
Cycling		✔		✔	✔	✔	✔	✔	✔	✔	✔
Dancing						✔	✔	✔	✔	✔	✔
Field hockey	✔	✔	✔	✔	✔	✔	✔	✔	✔	✔	✔
Fishing			✔	✔					✔	✔	✔
Football	✔	✔	✔	✔	✔	✔	✔	✔	✔	✔	✔
Golf	✔		✔	✔	✔	✔	✔	✔	✔	✔	
Gymnastics	✔	✔	✔	✔	✔	✔	✔	✔	✔	✔	✔
Jogging		✔		✔		✔	✔	✔	✔	✔	✔
Rock climbing		✔	✔	✔	✔	✔	✔	✔	✔	✔	✔
Scuba diving			✔			✔	✔	✔	✔	✔	
Skating, in-line		✔				✔	✔	✔	✔	✔	✔
Skiing, cross-country		✔		✔	✔	✔	✔	✔	✔	✔	✔
Skiing, downhill		✔		✔		✔	✔	✔	✔	✔	✔
Squash		✔	✔	✔	✔	✔	✔	✔	✔	✔	✔
Swimming		✔	✔	✔	✔	✔	✔	✔	✔	✔	
Table tennis		✔		✔	✔	✔			✔	✔	✔
Tennis		✔	✔	✔	✔	✔	✔	✔	✔	✔	✔
Triathlon		✔	✔	✔	✔	✔	✔	✔	✔	✔	✔
Volleyball		✔	✔	✔	✔	✔	✔	✔	✔	✔	✔
Waterskiing	✔	✔		✔	✔	✔	✔	✔	✔	✔	✔
Wrestling	✔	✔	✔	✔	✔	✔	✔	✔	✔	✔	✔

are interested in learning how to do these exercises, ask your instructor or coach for assistance.

If you want to develop strength for a particular activity, your program should contain exercises for general fitness, exercises for the muscle groups most important for the activity, and exercises for muscle groups most often injured. To create a weight training program for your favorite sport or activity, choose from among the exercises listed in Table 4-4, as well as from those listed in Table 4-3. In addition, Labs 4-2, 4-3, and 4-4 will help you assess your current level of muscular endurance, design your own weight training program, and apply it in the fitness facility you plan to use. Regardless of the goals of your program or the type of equipment you use, your program should be structured so that you obtain maximum results without risking injury. You should train at least 2 days per week, and each exercise session should contain a warm-up, 1 or more sets of 8–12 repetitions of 8–10 exercises, and a period of rest.

WEIGHT TRAINING EXERCISES
Free Weights

EXERCISE 1

BENCH PRESS

Muscles developed: Pectoralis major, triceps, deltoids

Instructions: (a) Lying on a bench on your back with your feet on the floor, grasp the bar with palms upward and hands shoulder-width apart. **(b)** Lower the bar to your chest. Then return it to the starting position. The bar should follow an elliptical path, during which the weight moves from a low point at the chest to a high point over the chin. If your back arches too much, try doing this exercise with your feet on the bench.

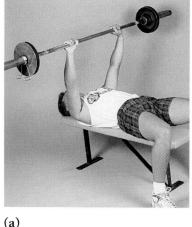 **(a)**

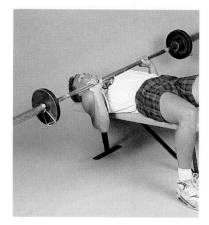 **(b)**

EXERCISE 2

**SHOULDER PRESS
(Overhead or Military Press)**

Muscles developed: Deltoids, triceps, trapezius

Instructions: This exercise can be done standing or seated, with dumbbells or barbells. The shoulder press begins with the weight at your chest, preferably on a rack. **(a)** Grasp the weight with your palms facing away from you. **(b)** Push the weight overhead until your arms are extended. Then return to the starting position (weight at chest). Be careful not to arch your back excessively.

If you are a more advanced weight trainer, you can "clean" the weight to your chest (lift it from the floor to your chest). The clean should be attempted only after instruction from a knowledgeable coach; otherwise, it can lead to injury.

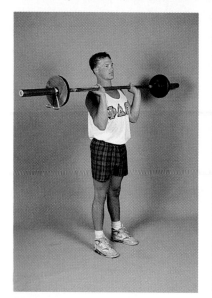 **(a)**

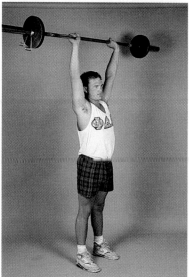 **(b)**

Although a spotter does not appear in these demonstration photographs, spotters should be used for most exercises with free weights.

PULL-UP

Muscles developed: Latissimus dorsi, biceps

Instructions: (a) Begin by grasping the pull-up bar with both hands, palms facing forward and elbows extended fully. **(b)** Pull yourself upward until your chin goes above the bar. Then return to the starting position.

Assisted pull-up: (c) This is done as described above for a pull-up, except that a spotter assists the person by pushing upward at the waist, hips, or legs during exercise.

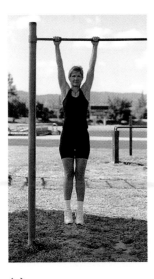

(a)

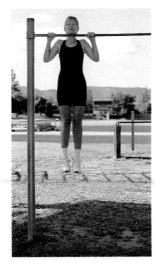

(b)

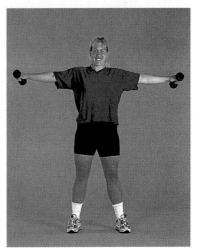

(c)

LATERAL RAISE

Muscles developed: Deltoids

Instructions: (a) Stand with feet shoulder-width apart and a dumbbell in each hand. Hold the dumbbells parallel to each other. **(b)** With elbows slightly bent, slowly lift both weights until they reach shoulder level. Keep your wrists in a neutral position, in line with your forearms. Return to the starting position.

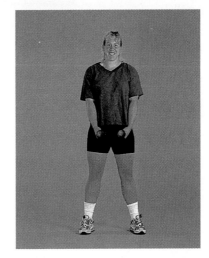

(a)

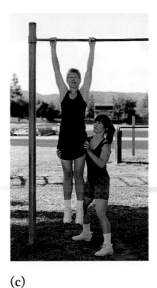

(b)

BICEPS CURL

Muscles developed: Biceps, brachialis

Instructions: (a) From a standing position, grasp the bar with your palms upward and your hands shoulder-width apart. **(b)** Keeping your upper body rigid, flex (bend) your elbows until the bar reaches a level slightly below the collarbone. Return the bar to the starting position.

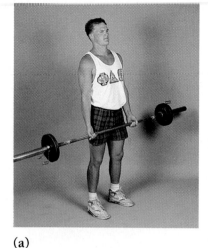 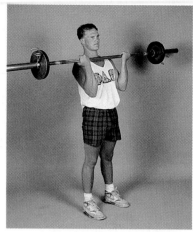

(a)   (b)

SQUAT

Muscles developed: Quadriceps, gluteus maximus, hamstrings, gastrocnemius

Instructions: Stand with feet shoulder-width apart and toes pointed slightly outward. **(a)** Rest the bar on the back of your shoulders, holding it there with hands facing forward. **(b)** Keeping your head up and lower back straight, squat down until your thighs are almost parallel with the floor. Drive upward toward the starting position, keeping your back in a fixed position throughout the exercise.

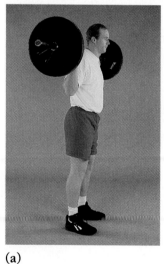 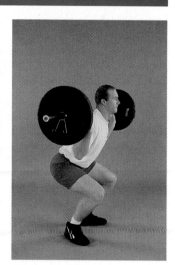

(a)   (b)

Although a spotter does not appear in these demonstration photographs, spotters should be used for most exercises with free weights.

TOE RAISE

Muscles developed: Gastrocnemius, soleus

Instructions: Stand with feet shoulder-width apart and toes pointed straight ahead. **(a)** Rest the bar on the back of your shoulders, holding it there with hands facing forward. **(b)** Press down with your toes while lifting your heels. Return to the starting position.

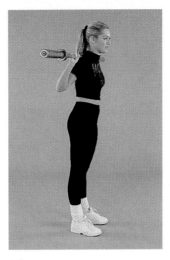 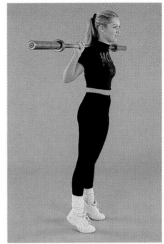

(a) (b)

CURL-UP OR CRUNCH

Muscles developed: Rectus abdominis, obliques

Instructions: **(a)** Lie on your back on the floor with your arms folded across your chest and your feet on the floor or on a bench. **(b)** Curl your trunk up and forward by raising your head and shoulders from the ground. Lower to the starting position.

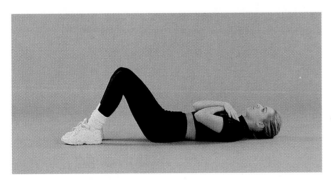 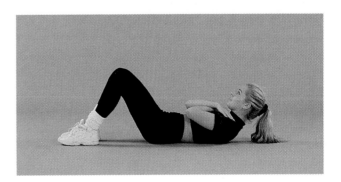

(a) (b)

SPINE EXTENSION (Isometric Exercises)

Muscles developed: Erector spinae, gluteus maximus, hamstrings, deltoids

Instructions: Begin on all fours with your knees below your hips and your hands below your shoulders.

Unilateral spine extension: (a) Extend your right leg to the rear, and reach forward with your right arm. Keep your neck neutral and your raised arm and leg in line with your torso. Don't arch your back or let your hip or shoulder sag. Hold this position for 10–30 seconds. Repeat with your left leg and left arm.

Bilateral spine extension: (b) Extend your left leg to the rear, and reach forward with your right arm. Keep your neck neutral and your raised leg in line with your torso. Don't arch your back or let your hip or shoulder sag. Hold this position for 10–30 seconds. Repeat with your right leg and left arm.

You can make this exercise more difficult by attaching weights to your ankles and wrists.

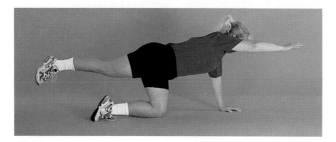

(a)

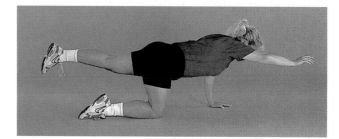

(b)

NECK FLEXION AND LATERAL FLEXION (Isometric Exercises)

Muscles developed: Sternocleidomastoids, scaleni

Instructions

Neck Flexion: (a) Place your hand on your forehead with fingertips pointed up. Using the muscles at the back of your neck, press your head forward and resist the pressure with the palm of your hand.

Lateral flexion: (b) Place your hand on the right side of your face, fingertips pointed up. Using the muscles on the left side of your neck, press your head to the right and resist the pressure with the palm of your hand. Repeat on the left side.

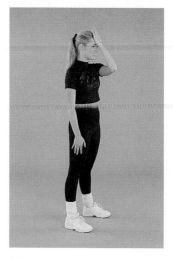

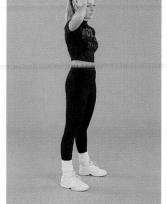

(a)

(b)

Weight Machines

BENCH PRESS

Muscles developed: Pectoralis major, anterior deltoids, triceps

Instructions: Lie on the bench so the tops of the handles are aligned with the tops of your armpits. Place your feet flat on the floor; if they don't reach, place them on the bench. **(a)** Grasp the handles with your palms facing away from you. **(b)** Push the bars until your arms are fully extended. Return to the starting position.

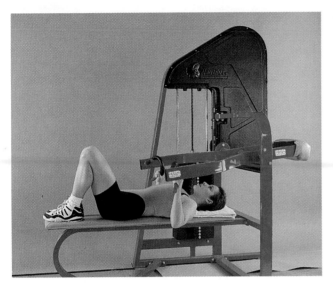
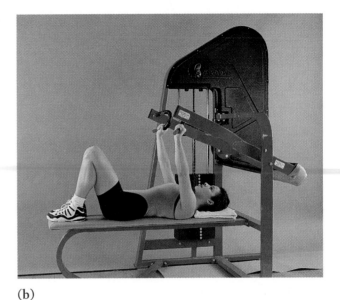

(a)   (b)

OVERHEAD PRESS (Shoulder Press)

Muscles developed: Deltoids, trapezius, triceps

Instructions: Adjust the seat so the two bars are slightly above your shoulders. **(a)** Sit down, facing away from the machine, and grasp the bars with your palms facing inward. **(b)** Press the weight upward until your arms are extended. Return to the starting position.

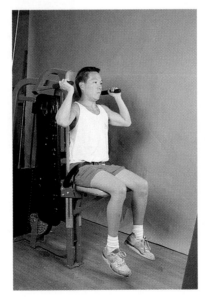
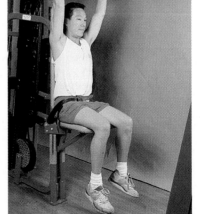

(a)   (b)

LAT PULL

Muscles developed: Latissimus dorsi, biceps

Instructions: Begin in a seated or kneeling position, depending on the type of lat machine and the manufacturer's instructions. **(a)** Grasp the bar of the machine with arms fully extended. **(b)** Slowly pull the weight down until it reaches the top of your chest. Slowly return to the starting position.

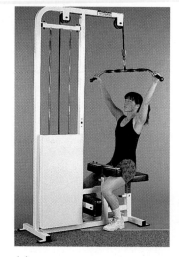 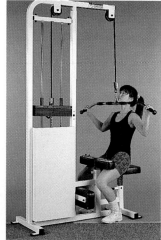

(a)   (b)

PULLOVER

Muscles developed: Latissimus dorsi, pectoralis major and minor, triceps, abdominals

Instructions: Adjust the seat so your shoulders are aligned with the cams. Push down on the foot pads with your feet to bring the bar forward until you can place your elbows on the pads. Rest your hands lightly on the bar. If possible, place your feet flat on the floor. **(a)** To get into the starting position, let your arms go backward as far as possible. **(b)** Pull your elbows forward until the bar almost touches your abdomen. Return to the starting position.

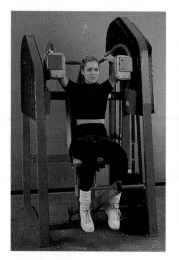 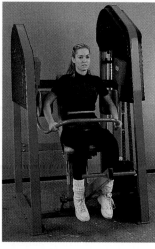

(a)   (b)

LATERAL RAISE

Muscles developed: Deltoids, trapezius

Instructions: (a) Adjust the seat so the pads rest just above your elbows when your upper arms are at your sides, your elbows are bent, and your forearms are parallel to the floor. (b) Lightly grasp the handles and push outward and up with your arms until the pads are shoulder height. Lead with your elbows rather than trying to lift the bars with your hands. Return to the starting position.

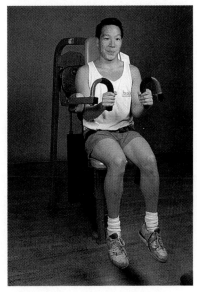

(a)

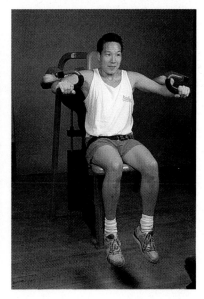

(b)

MULTITRICEPS

Muscles developed: Triceps

Instructions: Adjust the seat so your elbows are slightly lower than your shoulders when you sit down. (a) Place your elbows on the support cushions and your forearms on the bar pads. (b) Extend your elbows as much as possible. Return to the starting position.

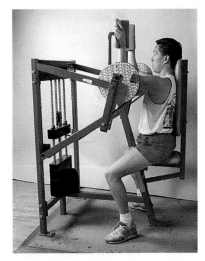

(a)

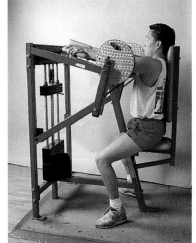

(b)

LEG PRESS

Muscles developed: Gluteus maximus, quadriceps, hamstrings

Instructions: (a) Adjust the seat so your knees are bent at a 90-degree angle. **(b)** Sit with your hands on the side handles, your feet on the pedals, and your legs fully extended. **(c)** From this position, bend your right leg 90 degrees, and then forcefully extend it. Repeat with your left leg. Alternate between right and left legs.

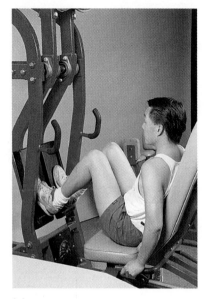

(a)

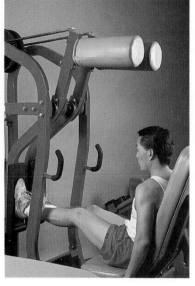

(b)

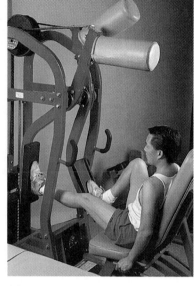

(c)

LEG EXTENSION (Knee Extension)

Muscles developed: Quadriceps

Instructions: (a) Sit on the seat with your shins under the knee-extension pads. **(b)** Extend your knees until they are straight. Return to the starting position.

Knee extensions cause kneecap pain in some people. If you have kneecap pain during this exercise, check with an orthopedic specialist before repeating it.

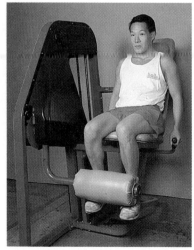

(a)

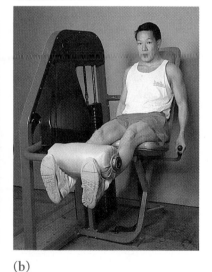

(b)

PRONE LEG CURL (Knee Flexion)

Muscles developed: Hamstrings

Instructions: (a) Lie on the front of your body, resting the pads of the machine just below your calf muscles and with your knees just off the edge of the bench. (b) Flex your knees until they approach your buttocks. Return to the starting position.

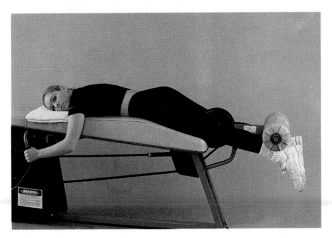

(a)

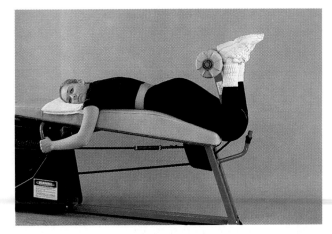

(b)

TOE RAISE

Muscles developed: Gastrocnemius, soleus

Instructions: (a) Stand with your head between the pads and one pad on each shoulder. (b) Press down with your toes while lifting your heels. Return to the starting position. Changing the direction your feet are pointing (straight ahead, inward, and outward) will work different portions of your calf muscles.

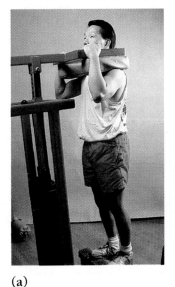

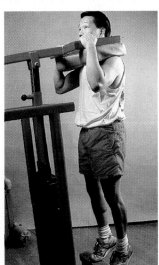

(a)   (b)

ABDOMINAL CURL

Muscles developed: Rectus abdominis, internal and external obliques, hip flexors (rectus femoris and iliopsoas muscle group) as stabilizers

Instructions: (a) Adjust the seat so the machine rotates at the level of your navel, the pad rests on your upper chest, and your feet can rest comfortably on the floor. **(b)** Move your trunk forward as far as possible. Return to the starting position.

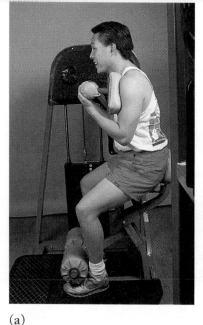 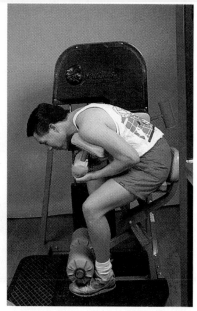

(a) (b)

LOW-BACK MACHINE (Back Extensions)

Muscles developed: Erector spinae, quadratus lumborum

Instructions: (a) Sit on the seat with your upper legs under the thigh-support pads, your back on the back roller pad, and your feet on the platform. **(b)** Extend backward until your back is straight. Return to the starting position. Try to keep your spine rigid during the exercise.

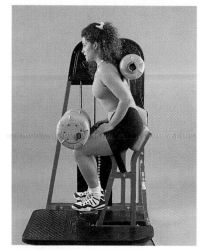 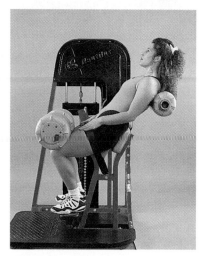

(a) (b)

FOUR-WAY NECK MACHINE

Muscles developed: Sternocleidomastoids, scaleni (flexion and lateral flexion); splenius capitis, splenius cervicis, trapezius (extension)

Instructions

Flexion: (a) Adjust the seat so the front of your forehead rests in the center of the two pads. Bend your head forward as far as possible, using your neck muscles, and then return to the starting position.

Lateral flexion: (b) Adjust the seat so the side of your head rests in the center of the two pads. Bend your head sideways toward your shoulder as far as possible, and then return to the starting position. Perform the exercise for both the right and left sides of your head.

Extension: (c) Adjust the seat so the back of your head rests in the center of the two pads. Bend your head backward as far as possible, and then return to the starting position.

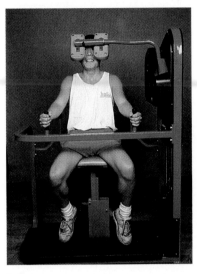

(a)

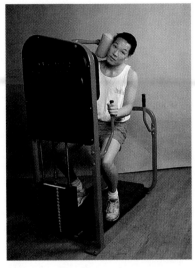

(b)

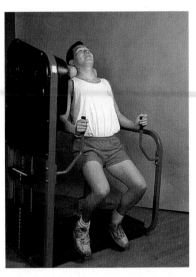

(c)

COMMON QUESTIONS ANSWERED

How do I know that my strength coach or fitness leader is knowledgeable and is properly certified?   The best coach, fitness leader, or personal trainer has formal training and practical experience. Ideally, look for someone who has a degree in exercise physiology or physical education and who is certified by either the American College of Sports Medicine or the National Strength Coaches' Association. Practical experience as an athlete and a coach is also important but should not be the determining factor assessing competence.

How long must I weight train before I begin to see changes in my body?   You will increase strength very rapidly during the early stages of a weight training program, primarily the result of muscle learning (the increased ability of the nervous system to recruit muscle fibers to exert force). Actual changes in muscle size usually begin after about 6–8 weeks of training.

I am concerned about my body composition. Will I gain weight if I do resistance exercises?   Your weight probably will not change significantly as a result of a recreational-type weight training program: 1 set of 8–12 repetitions of 8–10 exercises. You will tend to increase muscle mass and lose body fat, so your weight will stay about the same. (Men will tend to build larger muscles than women because of the tissue-building effects of male hormones.) Increased muscle mass will help you control body fat. Muscle increases your metabolism, which means you burn more calories every day. If you combine resistance exercises with endurance exercises, you will be on your way to developing a healthier body composition. Concentrate on fat loss rather than weight loss.

(continued)

Do I need more protein in my diet when I train with weights?
No. Although there is some evidence that power athletes involved in heavy training have a higher-than-normal protein requirement, there is no reason for most people to consume extra protein. Most Americans take in more protein than they need, so even if there is an increased protein need during heavy training, it is probably supplied by the average diet. (See Chapter 8 for more on dietary needs of athletes.)

What causes muscle soreness the day or two following a weight training workout? The muscle pain you feel a day or two after a heavy weight training workout is caused by injury to the muscle fibers and surrounding connective tissue. Contrary to popular belief, delayed-onset muscle soreness is not caused by lactic acid buildup. Scientists believe that injury to muscle fibers causes inflammation, which in turn causes the release of substances called **proteases.** Proteases break down part of the muscle tissue and cause pain. After a bout of intense exercise that causes muscle injury and delayed-onset muscle soreness, the muscles produce protective proteins that prevent soreness during future workouts. If you don't work out regularly, you lose these protective proteins and become susceptible to muscle soreness again.

Will strength training improve my sports performance?
Strength developed in the weight room does not automatically increase your power in sports such as skiing, tennis, or cycling. Hitting a forehand in tennis or making a turn on skis is highly specific and requires precise coordination between your nervous system and muscles. In skilled people, movements become reflex—you don't think about them when you do them. Increasing strength can disturb this coordination. Only by simultaneously practicing a sport and improving fitness can you expect to become more powerful in the skill. Practice helps you integrate your new strength with your skills, which makes you more powerful. Consequently, you can hit the ball harder in tennis or make more graceful turns on the ski slopes. (Refer to Chapter 2 for more on the concept of specificity of physical training.)

Will I improve faster if I train every day? No. Your muscles need time to recover between training sessions. Doing resistance exercises every day will cause you to become overtrained, which will increase your chance of injury and impede your progress. If you find that your strength training program has reached a plateau, try one of these strategies:

- Train less frequently. If you are currently training the same muscle groups three or more times per week, you may not be allowing your muscles to fully recover from intense workouts.

- Change exercises. Using different exercises for a particular muscle group may stimulate further strength development.

- Vary the load and number of repetitions. Try increasing or decreasing the loads you are using and changing the number of repetitions accordingly.

- Vary the number of sets. If you have been performing 1 set of each exercise, add sets.

- If you are training alone, find a motivated training partner. A partner can encourage you and assist you with difficult lifts, forcing you to work harder.

If I stop weight training, will my muscles turn to fat? No. Fat and muscle are two different kinds of tissue, and one cannot turn into the other. Muscles that aren't used become smaller (atrophy), and body fat may increase if caloric intake exceeds calories burned. Although the result of inactivity may be smaller muscles and more fat, the change is caused by two separate processes.

SUMMARY

- Improvements in muscular strength and endurance lead to enhanced physical performance, protection against injury, improved body composition, better self-image, and improved muscle and bone health with aging.

- Muscular strength can be assessed by determining the amount of weight that can be lifted in one repetition of an exercise; muscular endurance can be assessed by determining the number of repetitions of a particular exercise that can be performed.

- Hypertrophy, or increased muscle fiber size, occurs when weight training causes the number of myofibrils to increase; total muscle size thereby increases. Strength also increases through muscle learning.

- Isometric exercises (contraction without movement) are most useful when a person is recovering from an injury or surgery or needs to overcome weak points in a range of motion.

- Isotonic exercises involve contraction that results in movement. The two most common types are constant resistance (free weights) and variable resistance (weight machines).

- Supplements or drugs that are promoted as instant or quick "cures" usually don't work and are either dangerous or expensive or both.

TERMS **proteases** Enzymes that break down proteins.

- Free weights and weight machines are basically equally effective in producing fitness, although machines tend to be safer.
- Lifting heavy weights for only a few repetitions helps develop strength. Lifting lighter weights for more repetitions helps develop muscular endurance.
- A weight training program for general fitness includes at least 1 set of 8–12 repetitions (enough to cause fatigue) of 8–10 exercises, along with warm-up and cool-down periods; the program should be carried out 2–3 times a week.
- Safety guidelines for weight training include using proper technique, using spotters and collars when necessary, using common sense and remaining alert, and taking care of injuries.

FOR MORE INFORMATION

Information on and programs in weight training are available through physical education and athletics departments, private health clubs, and weight-lifting clubs.

Books

Fahey, T. D. 2000. *Basic Weight Training for Men and Women,* 4th ed. Mountain View, Calif.: Mayfield. *A practical guide to developing training programs, using free weights, tailored to individual needs.*

Fleck, S. J., and W. J. Kraemer. 1997. *Designing Resistance Training Programs.* Champaign, Ill.: Human Kinetics. *A book aimed at personal trainers or serious weight trainers who want a thorough discussion of program design methods for weight training.*

Nelson, M. 1999. *Strong Women Stay Slim.* New York: Bantam Books. *A program of strengthening exercises and diet geared toward first-time exercisers, written by a Tufts University professor.*

Ward, P. E., and R. D. Ward. 1997. *The Encyclopedia of Weight Training.* Los Angeles: Q P T Publishing. *An authoritative guide to weight training for athletes and bodybuilders written by two of America's top strength coaches.*

Williams, M. H. 1998. *The Ergogenics Edge: Pushing the Limits of Sports Performance.* Champaign, Ill.: Human Kinetics. *An excellent book on the scientific basis of substances and techniques used to improve athletic performance; written by one of the world's top sports nutrition researchers.*

Organizations and Web Sites

Biomechanics World Wide. A resource site with links to many other sites relating to biomechanics; topics include muscle mechanics and sports techniques.

http://www.per.ualberta.ca/biomechanics

Exercise: A Guide from the National Institute on Aging and the National Aeronautics and Space Administration. Provides practical advice on fitness for seniors; include animated instructions for specific weight training exercises.

http://weboflife.arc.nasa.gov/exerciseandaging

Georgia State University: Strength Training. Provides information about the benefits of strength training and how to develop a safe and effective program; also includes illustrations of a variety of exercises.

http://www.gsu.edu/~wwwfit/strength.html

Human Anatomy On-line. Provides text, illustrations, and animation about the muscular system, nerve-muscle connections, muscular contraction, and other topics.

http://www.innerbody.com/htm/body.html

University of California, San Diego/Muscle Physiology Home Page. Provides an introduction to muscle physiology, including information about types of muscle fibers and energy cycles.

http://muscle.ucsd.edu

University of Michigan/Muscles in Action. Interactive descriptions of muscle movements.

http://www.med.umich.edu/lrc/Hypermuscle/Hyper.html

Workout.Com: Exercise Zone. Includes illustrated sample programs for developing strength training programs as well as programs for specific sports- and skill-related fitness components.

http://www.workout.com/exercises/exercises.asp?nav-1

See also the listings in Chapter 2.

SELECTED BIBLIOGRAPHY

American College of Sports Medicine. 2000. *ACSM's Guidelines for Exercise Testing and Prescription,* 6th ed. Baltimore, Md.: Lippincott Williams & Wilkins.

American College of Sports Medicine. 1998. Position stand: The recommended quantity and quality of exercise for developing and maintaining cardiorespiratory and muscular fitness, and flexibility in healthy adults. *Medicine and Science in Sports and Exercise* 30(6): 975–991.

Bassey, E. J. 1998. Longitudinal changes in selected physical capabilities: Muscle strength, flexibility, and body size. *Age and Ageing* 3(Suppl.): 12–16.

Bishop, D., et al. 1999. The effect of strength training on endurance performance and muscle characteristics. *Medical Science and Sports Exercise* 31(6): 886–891.

Brooks, G. A., et al. 2000. *Exercise Physiology: Human Bioenergetics and Its Applications,* 3d ed. Mountain View, Calif.: Mayfield.

Charteris, J. 1999. Effects of velocity on upper to lower extremity muscular work and power output ratios of intercollegiate athletes. *British Journal of Sports Medicine* 33:250–254.

Demant, T. W., and E. C. Rhodes. 1999. Effects of creatine supplementation on exercise performance. *Sports Medicine* 28: 49–60.

Fahey, T. 1997. Pharmacology of bodybuilding. In Reilly, T., and M. Orme, eds., *The Clinical Pharmacology of Sport and Exercise.* Amsterdam: Elsevier.

Faigenbaum, A. D., et al. 1999. The effects of different resistance training protocols on muscular strength and endurance development in children. *Pediatrics* 104(1): 5.

Foster-Burns, S. B. 2000. Sarcopenia and decreased muscle strength in the elderly woman: Resistance training as a safe and effective intervention. *Journal of Women Aging* 11(4): 75–85.

Francaux, M., and J. R. Poortmans. 1999. Effects of training and creatine supplement on muscle strength and body mass. *European Journal of Applied Physiology* 80:165–168.

Frisch, H. 1999. Growth hormone and body composition in athletes. *Journal of Endocrinological Investigations* 22(Suppl.): 106–109.

Gajdosik, R. L., D. W. Linden, and A. K. Williams. 1999. Concentric isokinetic torque characteristics of the calf muscles of active women aged 20 to 84 years. *Journal of Orthopaedic and Sports Physical Therapy* 29:181–189.

Hahn, T., A. Foldspang, and T. Ingemann-Hansen. 1999. Dynamic strength of the quadriceps muscle and sports activity. *British Journal of Sports Medicine* 33:117–120.

Hass, C. J., et al. 2000. Single versus multiple sets in long-term recreational weightlifters. *Medicine and Science in Sports and Exercise* 32(1): 235–242.

Helewa, A., et al. 1999. Does strengthening the abdominal muscles prevent low back pain—A randomized controlled trial. *Journal of Rheumatology* 26:1808–1815.

Kadi, F., and L. E. Thornell. 1999. Training affects myosin heavy chain phenotype in the trapezius muscle of women. *Histochemistry and Cell Biology* 112:73–78.

Kadi, F., et al. 1999. Cellular adaptation of the trapezius muscle in strength-trained athletes. *Histochemistry and Cell Biology* 111:189–195.

Kawazu, T., et al. 1999. Isokinetic strength of elbow extensor muscles correlates with race time in wheelchair half-marathon racers. *Sangyo Ika Daigaku Zasshi* 21:13–21.

Kent-Braun, J. A., and A. V. Ng. 1999. Specific strength and voluntary muscle activation in young and elderly women and men. *Journal of Applied Physiology* 87:22–29.

King, D. S., et al. 1999. Effect of oral androstenedione on serum testosterone and adaptations to resistance training in young men: A randomized controlled trial. *Journal of the American Medical Association* 281(21): 2020–2028.

Kukolj, M., et al. 1999. Anthropometric, strength, and power predictors of sprinting performance. *Journal of Sports Medicine and Physical Fitness* 39:120–122.

Mannion, A. F., et al. 1999. Prediction of maximal back muscle strength from indices of body mass and fat-free body mass. *Rheumatology* (Oxford) 38:652–655.

Mero, A. 1999. Leucine supplementation and intensive training. *Sports Medicine* 27:347–358.

Metzl, J. D. 1999. Strength training and nutritional supplement use in adolescents. *Current Opinion in Pediatrics* 11: 292–296.

Musaro, A., et al. 1999. IGF-1 induces skeletal myocyte hypertrophy through calcineurin in association with GATA-2 and NF-ATc1. *Nature* 400:581–585.

Noonan, T. J. 1999. Muscle strain injury: Diagnosis and treatment. *Journal of the American Academy of Orthopaedic Surgeons* 7:262–269.

Pollock, M. L., et al. 2000. Resistance exercise in individuals with and without cardiovascular disease. *Circulation* 101: 828–833.

Pollock, M. L., et al. 1997. Twenty-year follow-up of aerobic power and body composition of older track athletes. *Journal of Applied Physiology* 82:1508–1516.

Roos, M. R., et al. 1999. Quadriceps muscle strength, contractile properties, and motor unit firing rates in young and old men. *Muscle and Nerve* 22:1094–1103.

Ryan, A. S., et al. 2000. Changes in plasma leptin and insulin action with resistive training in postmenopausal women. *International Journal of Obesity and Related Metabolic Disorders* 24(1): 27–32.

Seger, J. Y., B. Arvidsson, and A. Thorstensson. 1999. Specific effects of eccentric and concentric training on muscle strength and morphology in humans. *European Journal of Applied Physiology* 79:49–57.

Shephard, R. J. 2000. Exercise and training in women, part 1: Influence of gender on exercise and training responses. *Canadian Journal of Applied Physiology* 25(1):19–34.

Short, K. R., and K. S. Nair. 1999. Mechanisms of sarcopenia of aging. *Journal of Endocrinological Investigations* 22(Suppl.): 95–105.

Supplement watch: Breakfast of champions? 1999. *Consumer Reports on Health*, August, 8.

Taaffe, D. R., et al. 1999. Once-weekly resistance exercise improves muscle strength and neuromuscular performance in older adults. *Journal of the American Geriatrics Society* 47(10): 1208–1214.

Terjung, R. L., et al. 2000. American College of Sports Medicine roundtable. The physiological and health effects of oral creatine supplementation. *Medicine and Science in Sports and Exercise* 32(3): 706–717.

Volek, J. S. 1999. Update: What we now know about creatine. *ACSM's Health and Fitness Journal* 3(3): 27–33.

Wang, C. H., et al. 1999. Stretching and strengthening exercises: Their effect on three-dimensional scapular kinematics. *Archives of Physical Medicine and Rehabilitation* 80:923–929.

Williams, M. H. 1999. Facts and fallacies of purported ergogenic amino acid supplements. *Clinics in Sports Medicine* 18:633–649.

LAB 4-1 *Assessing Your Current Level of Muscular Strength*

For best results, don't do any strenuous weight training within 48 hours of any test.

The Maximum Bench Press Test

Equipment

1. Universal Gym Dynamic Variable Resistance machine
2. Weight scale

The ratings for this test were developed using the Universal Gym Dynamic Variable Resistance machine; results will be somewhat less accurate if the test is performed on another type of machine or with free weights.

If free weights are used, the following equipment is needed:

1. Flat bench (with or without racks)
2. Barbell
3. Assorted weight plates
4. Collars to hold weight plates in place
5. One or two spotters
6. Weight scale

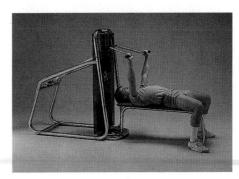

Maximum bench press test.

Preparation

Try a few bench presses with a small amount of weight so you can practice your technique, warm up your muscles, and, if you use free weights, coordinate your movements with those of your spotters. Weigh yourself, and record the results.

Body weight: _____ lb

Instructions

1. Set the machine (or place weights on the barbell) for a weight that is lower than the amount you believe you can lift.
2. Lie on the bench with your feet firmly on the floor. If you are using a weight machine, grasp the handles with palms away from you; the tops of the handles should be aligned with the tops of your armpits.
    If you are using free weights, grasp the bar at shoulder width with your palms away from you. If you have one spotter, she or he should stand directly behind the bench; if you have two spotters, they should stand to the side, one at each end of the barbell. Lower the bar to your chest in preparation for the lift.
3. Push the bars or barbell until your arms are fully extended. Exhale as you lift. If you are using free weights, the bar should follow an elliptical path, during which the weight moves from a low point at the chest to a high point over the chin. Keep your feet firmly on the floor, don't arch your back, and push the weight evenly with your right and left arms. Don't bounce the weight on your chest.
4. Rest for several minutes, then repeat the lift with a heavier weight. It will probably take several attempts to determine the maximum amount of weight you can lift (1 RM).

    1 RM: _____ lb

Rating Your Bench Press Result

1. Divide your 1 RM value by your body weight.

    1 RM _____ lb ÷ body weight _____ lb = _____

2. Find this ratio in the table below to determine your bench press strength rating. Record the result here and in the chart at the end of this lab.

Bench press strength rating: _____

Strength Ratings for the Maximum Bench Press Test

Pounds Lifted/Body Weight (lb)

Men	*Very Poor*	*Poor*	*Fair*	*Good*	*Excellent*	*Superior*
Age: Under 20	Below 0.89	0.89–1.05	1.06–1.18	1.19–1.33	1.34–1.75	Above 1.75
20–29	Below 0.88	0.88–0.98	0.99–1.13	1.14–1.31	1.32–1.62	Above 1.62
30–39	Below 0.78	0.78–0.87	0.88–0.97	0.98–1.11	1.12–1.34	Above 1.34
40–49	Below 0.72	0.72–0.79	0.80–0.87	0.88–0.99	1.00–1.19	Above 1.19
50–59	Below 0.63	0.63–0.70	0.71–0.78	0.79–0.89	0.90–1.04	Above 1.04
60 and over	Below 0.57	0.57–0.65	0.66–0.71	0.72–0.81	0.82–0.93	Above 0.93
Women						
Age: Under 20	Below 0.53	0.53–0.57	0.58–0.64	0.65–0.76	0.77–0.87	Above 0.87
20–29	Below 0.51	0.51–0.58	0.59–0.69	0.70–0.79	0.80–1.00	Above 1.00
30–39	Below 0.47	0.47–0.52	0.53–0.59	0.60–0.69	0.70–0.81	Above 0.81
40–49	Below 0.43	0.43–0.49	0.50–0.53	0.54–0.61	0.62–0.76	Above 0.76
50–59	Below 0.39	0.39–0.43	0.44–0.47	0.48–0.54	0.55–0.67	Above 0.67
60 and over	Below 0.38	0.38–0.42	0.43–0.46	0.47–0.53	0.54–0.71	Above 0.71

SOURCE: Based on norms from the Cooper Institute for Aerobics Research, Dallas, Texas; used with permission.

The Maximum Leg Press Test

Equipment

1. Universal Gym Dynamic Variable Resistance leg press machine (If you're using a Universal Gym leg press with two sets of pedals, use the lower pedals.)
2. Weight scale

The ratings for this test were developed using the Universal Gym Dynamic Variable Resistance machine; results will be somewhat less accurate if the test is performed on another type of machine.

Preparation

Try a few leg presses with the machine set for a small amount of weight so you can practice your technique and warm up your muscles. Weigh yourself, and record the results.

Body weight: _____ lb

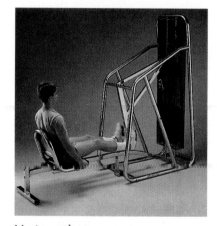

Maximum leg press test.

Instructions

1. Set the machine for a weight that is lower than the amount you believe you can press.
2. Adjust the seat so that your knees are bent at a 70-degree angle to start.
3. Grasp the side handlebars, and push with your legs until your knees are fully extended.
4. Rest for several minutes, then repeat the press with a higher weight setting. It will probably take several attempts to determine the maximum amount of weight you can press.

1 RM: _____ lb

Rating Your Leg Press Result

1. Divide your 1 RM value by your body weight.

   1 RM _____ lb ÷ body weight _____ lb 5 _____

2. Find this ratio in the table below to determine your leg press strength rating. Record the result below and in the chart at the end of this lab.

   Leg press strength rating: _____

Strength Ratings for the Maximum Leg Press Test

	Pounds Lifted/Body Weight (lb)					
Men	Very Poor	Poor	Fair	Good	Excellent	Superior
Age: Under 20	Below 1.70	1.70–1.89	1.90–2.03	2.04–2.27	2.28–2.81	Above 2.81
20–29	Below 1.63	1.63–1.82	1.83–1.96	1.97–2.12	2.13–2.39	Above 2.39
30–39	Below 1.52	1.52–1.64	1.65–1.76	1.77–1.92	1.93–2.19	Above 2.19
40–49	Below 1.44	1.44–1.56	1.57–1.67	1.68–1.81	1.82–2.01	Above 2.01
50–59	Below 1.32	1.32–1.45	1.46–1.57	1.58–1.70	1.71–1.89	Above 1.89
60 and over	Below 1.25	1.25–1.37	1.38–1.48	1.49–1.61	1.62–1.79	Above 1.79
Women						
Age: Under 20	Below 1.22	1.22–1.37	1.38–1.58	1.59–1.70	1.71–1.87	Above 1.87
20–29	Below 1.22	1.22–1.36	1.37–1.49	1.50–1.67	1.68–1.97	Above 1.97
30–39	Below 1.09	1.09–1.20	1.21–1.32	1.33–1.46	1.47–1.67	Above 1.67
40–49	Below 1.02	1.02–1.12	1.13–1.22	1.23–1.36	1.37–1.56	Above 1.56
50–59	Below 0.88	0.88–0.98	0.99–1.09	1.10–1.24	1.25–1.42	Above 1.42
60 and over	Below 0.85	0.85–0.92	0.93–1.03	1.04–1.17	1.18–1.42	Above 1.42

SOURCE: Based on norms from the Cooper Institute for Aerobics Research, Dallas, Texas; used with permission.

Hand Grip Strength Test

Equipment

Grip strength dynamometer

Preparation

If necessary, adjust the hand grip size on the dynamometer into a position that is comfortable for you; then lock the grip in place. The second joint of your fingers should fit snugly under the handle of the dynamometer.

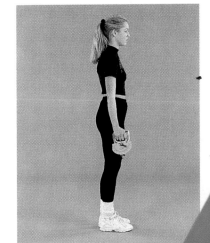

Hand grip strength test.

Instructions

1. Stand with the hand to be tested first at your side, away from your body. The dynamometer should be in line with your forearm and held at the level of your thigh. Squeeze the dynamometer as hard as possible without moving your arm; exhale as you squeeze. During the test, don't let the dynamometer touch your body or any other object.

2. Perform two trials with each hand. Rest for about a minute between trials. Record the scores for each hand to the nearest kilogram.

   Right hand: Trial 1: _____ kg   Trial 2: _____ kg

   Left hand: Trial 1: _____ kg   Trial 2: _____ kg

(Scores on the dynamometer should be given in kilograms. If the dynamometer you are using gives score~~~ convert pounds to kilograms by dividing your score by 2.2.)

Rating Your Hand Grip Strength

Your total score is the sum of the best trial for each hand.

Right hand best trial _____ kg

Left hand best trial _____ kg

Total score _____ kg

Refer to the table below for a rating of your grip strength. Record the result below and in the chart at the end of this lab.

Rating for hand grip strength: _____

Grip Strength* (kg)

Men	Needs Improvement	Fair	Good	Very Good	Excellent
Age: 15–19	Below 84	84–94	95–102	103–112	Above 112
20–29	Below 97	97–105	106–112	113–123	Above 123
30–39	Below 97	97–104	105–112	113–122	Above 122
40–49	Below 94	94–101	102–109	110–118	Above 118
50–59	Below 87	87–95	96–101	102–109	Above 109
60–69	Below 79	79–85	86–92	93–101	Above 101
Women					
Age: 15–19	Below 54	54–58	59–63	64–70	Above 70
20–29	Below 55	55–60	61–64	65–70	Above 70
30–39	Below 56	56–60	61–65	66–72	Above 72
40–49	Below 55	55–58	59–64	65–72	Above 72
50–59	Below 51	51–54	55–58	59–64	Above 64
60–69	Below 48	48–50	51–53	54–59	Above 59

*Combined right and left hand grip strength.

SOURCE: *The Canadian Physical Activity, Fitness and Lifestyle Appraisal: CSEP's Plan for Healthy Active Living, Second Edition 1998.* Reprinted by permission from the Canadian Society for Exercise Physiology.

Summary of Results

Maximum bench press test

Weight pressed: _____ lb   Rating: _____

Maximum leg press test

Weight pressed: _____ lb   Rating: _____

Hand grip strength test

Total score: _____ kg   Rating: _____

Remember that muscular strength is specific: Your ratings may vary considerably for different parts of your body. You can use these results to guide you in planning a weight training program.

To monitor your progress toward your goal, enter the results of this lab in the Preprogram Assessment column of Appendix D. After several weeks of a weight training program, do this lab again, and enter the results in the Postprogram Assessment column of Appendix D. How do the results compare?

Name _____ Section _____ Date _____

LAB 4-2 *Assessing Your Current Level of Muscular Endurance*

For best results, don't do any strenuous weight training within 48 hours of any test. To assess endurance of the abdominal muscles, perform the sit-up test or the curl-up test. The push-up test assesses endurance of muscles in the upper body.

The 60-Second Sit-Up Test

Do not take this test if you suffer from low-back pain.

Equipment

1. Stopwatch, clock, or watch with a second hand
2. Partner to hold your ankles
3. Mat or towel to lie on (optional)

Preparation

Try a few sit-ups to get used to the proper technique and warm up your abdominal muscles.

Instructions

1. Lie flat on your back on the floor with knees bent, feet flat on the floor, and your fingers interlocked behind your neck. Your partner should hold your ankles firmly so that your feet stay on the floor as you do the sit-ups.

2. When someone signals you to begin, raise your head and chest off the floor until your elbows touch your knees or thighs, and then return to the starting position. Keep your neck neutral. Keep your breathing as normal as possible; don't hold your breath.

3. Perform as many sit-ups as you can in 60 seconds.

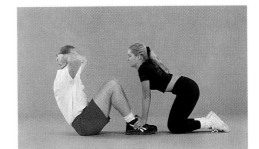

The 60-second sit-up test.

   Note: The norms for this test were established with subjects interlocking their fingers behind their neck; your results will be most accurate if you use this technique. However, some experts feel that sit-ups done in this position can cause injury to the neck. If this is a concern, perform the test with your hands cupped over your ears rather than behind your neck. Alternatively, complete the curl-up test described later in this lab. If you perform sit-ups with your hands behind your neck, take care not to force your neck forward, and stop if you feel any pain in your neck.

   Number of sit-ups: _____

Rating Your Muscular Endurance

Refer to the table below for a rating of your abdominal muscle endurance. Record your rating below and in the chart at the end of this lab.

Rating: _____

Ratings for the 60-Second Sit-Up Test

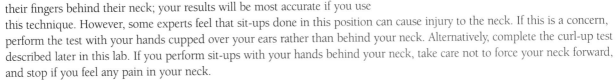

	Number of Sit-Ups					
Men	*Very Poor*	*Poor*	*Fair*	*Good*	*Excellent*	*Superior*
Age: Under 20	Below 36	36–40	41–46	47–50	51–61	Above 61
20–29	Below 33	33–37	38–41	42–46	47–54	Above 54
30–39	Below 30	30–34	35–38	39–42	43–50	Above 50
40–49	Below 24	24–28	29–33	34–38	39–46	Above 46
50–59	Below 19	19–23	24–27	28–34	35–42	Above 42
60 and over	Below 15	15–18	19–21	22–29	30–38	Above 38

(continued)

Women	Very Poor	Poor	Fair	Good	Excellent	Superior
Age: Under 20	Below 28	28–31	32–35	36–45	46–54	Above 54
20–29	Below 24	24–31	32–37	38–43	44–50	Above 50
30–39	Below 20	20–24	25–28	29–34	35–41	Above 41
40–49	Below 14	14–19	20–23	24–28	29–37	Above 37
50–59	Below 10	10–13	14–19	20–23	24–29	Above 29
60 and over	Below 3	3–5	6–10	11–16	17–27	Above 27

SOURCE: Based on norms from the Cooper Institute for Aerobics Research, Dallas, Texas; used with permission.

The Curl-Up Test

The curl-up test is preferred by some exercise scientists as a test of abdominal endurance. In a full sit-up, part of the lift is provided by the hip flexor muscles. Curl-ups optimize the use of the abdominal muscles without involving the hip flexors.

Equipment

1. Metronome
2. Stopwatch, clock, or watch with a second hand
3. Heavy tape
4. Ruler
5. Partner
6. Mat (optional)

Preparation

1. Set the metronome at a rate of 50 beats per minute.
2. Place a tape strip approximately 1 meter long on the floor or mat. Place another strip of tape 10 centimeters away from the first one.

Instructions

1. Start by lying on your back on the floor, arms by your sides, palms down and on the floor, elbows locked, and fingers straight. The longest fingertip of each hand should touch the edge of the near strip of tape. Your knees should be bent at about 90 degrees, with your feet 12–18 inches away from your buttocks.
2. To perform a curl-up, curl your head and upper back upward, keeping your arms straight. Slide your fingertips forward along the floor until you touch the other strip of tape, 10 centimeters from the starting position. Then curl back down so that your upper back and head touch the floor. Palms, feet, and buttocks should stay on the floor throughout the curl-up. (For this test, your partner does not hold your feet.) Maintain the 90-degree angle in your knees. Exhale during the lift phase of the curl-up.

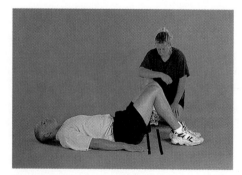

Curl-up test: (a) starting position.

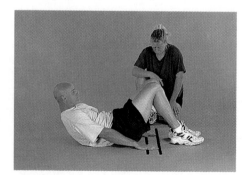

(b) Curl-up.

3. Start the metronome at the correct cadence. You will perform curl-ups at the steady, continuous rate of 25 per minute. Curl up on one beat and curl down on the next. Your partner counts the number of curl-ups you complete and makes sure that you maintain correct form.

4. Perform as many curl-ups as you can in 1 minute. If at any point during the test you can no longer maintain proper form and keep up with the rhythm set by the metronome, stop the test and record the number of curl-ups you performed up to that point.

Number of curl-ups: _____

Rating Your Muscular Endurance

Your score is the number of completed curl-ups. Refer to the appropriate portion of the table below for a rating of your abdominal muscular endurance. Record your rating below and in the chart at the end of this lab.

Rating: _____

Ratings for the Curl-Up Test

	Number of Curl-Ups				
Men	*Needs Improvement*	*Fair*	*Good*	*Very Good*	*Excellent*
Age: 15–19	Below 16	16–20	21–22	23–24	25
20–29	Below 13	13–20	21–22	23–24	25
30–39	Below 13	13–20	21–22	23–24	25
40–49	Below 11	11–15	16–21	22–24	25
50–59	Below 9	9–13	14–19	20–24	25
60–69	Below 4	4–9	10–15	16–24	25
Women					
Age: 15–19	Below 16	16–20	21–22	23–24	25
20–29	Below 13	13–18	19–22	23–24	25
30–39	Below 11	11–15	16–21	22–24	25
40–49	Below 6	6–12	13–20	21–24	25
50–59	Below 4	4–8	9–15	16–24	25
60–69	Below 2	2–5	6–10	11–17	18–25

SOURCE: *The Canadian Physical Activity, Fitness and Lifestyle Appraisal: CSEP's Plan for Healthy Active Living, Second Edition 1998*. Reprinted by permission of the Canadian Society for Exercise Physiology.

The Push-Up Test

Equipment

Mat or towel (optional)

Preparation

In this test, you will perform either standard push-ups or modified push-ups, in which you support yourself with your knees. The Cooper Institute developed the ratings for this test with men performing push-ups and women performing modified push-ups. (Biologically, males tend to be stronger than females; the modified technique reduces the need for upper-body strength in a test of muscular endurance.) Therefore, for an accurate assessment of upper-body endurance, men should perform standard push-ups and women should perform modified push-ups.

Instructions

1. *For push-ups:* Start in the push-up position with your body supported by your hands and feet. *For modified push-ups:* Start in the modified push-up position with your body supported by your hands and knees. *For both positions,* your arms and your back should be straight and your fingers pointed forward.

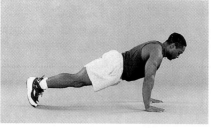

(a) Push-up.

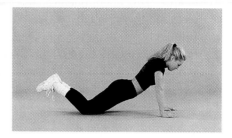

(b) Modified push-up.

2. Lower your chest to the floor with your back straight, and then return to the starting position.

3. Perform as many push-ups or modified push-ups as you can without stopping.

   Number of push-ups: _____ or number of modified push-ups: _____

Rating Your Push-Up Test Result

Your score is the number of completed push-ups or modified push-ups. Refer to the appropriate portion of the table below for a rating of your upper-body endurance. Record your rating below and in the chart at the end of this lab.

Rating: _____

Ratings for the Push-Up and Modified Push-Up Tests

Number of Push-Ups

Men	Very Poor	Poor	Fair	Good	Excellent	Superior
Age: 18–29	Below 22	22–28	29–36	37–46	47–61	Above 61
30–39	Below 17	17–23	24–29	30–38	39–51	Above 51
40–49	Below 11	11–17	18–23	24–29	30–39	Above 39
50–59	Below 9	9–12	13–18	19–24	25–38	Above 38
60 and over	Below 6	6–9	10–17	18–22	23–27	Above 27

Number of Modified Push-Ups

Women	Very Poor	Poor	Fair	Good	Excellent	Superior
Age: 18–29	Below 17	17–22	23–29	30–35	36–44	Above 44
30–39	Below 11	11–18	19–23	24–30	31–38	Above 38
40–49	Below 6	6–12	13–17	18–23	24–32	Above 32
50–59	Below 6	6–11	12–16	17–20	21–27	Above 27
60 and over	Below 2	2–4	5–11	12–14	15–19	Above 19

SOURCE: Based on norms from the Cooper Institute for Aerobics Research, Dallas, Texas; used with permission.

Summary of Results

60-second sit-up test

   Number of sit-ups: _____ Rating: _____

Curl-up test

   Number of curl-ups: _____ Rating: _____

Push-up test

   Number of push-ups: _____ Rating: _____

Remember that muscular endurance is specific: Your ratings may vary considerably for different parts of your body. You can use these results to guide you in planning a weight training program.

   To monitor your progress toward your goal, enter the results of this lab in the Preprogram Assessment column of Appendix D. After several weeks of a weight training program, do this lab again, and enter the results in the Postprogram Assessment column of Appendix D. How do the results compare?

LAB 4-3 *Designing and Monitoring a Weight Training Program*

1. *Set goals.* List the goals of your weight training program. Goals can be general, such as developing greater muscle definition, or specific, such as increasing the power in a golf swing. If your goals involve the development of a specific muscle group, note that also.

a. _____

b. _____

c. _____

d. _____

2. *Choose exercises.* Based on your goals, choose 8–10 exercises to perform during each weight training session. If your goal is general training for wellness, use the sample program in the box "A Sample Weight Training Program for General Fitness" on p. 78. If your goals relate to a specific sport, use Table 4-4 to put together a program to develop the important muscle groups. List your exercises and the muscles they develop in the space provided in the program plan below.

3. *Choose starting weights.* Experiment with different amounts of weight until you settle on a good starting weight, one that you can lift easily for 10–12 repetitions. As you progress in your program, you can add more weight. Fill in the starting weight for each exercise on the program plan.

4. *Choose a starting number of sets and repetitions.* Include at least 1 set of 8–12 repetitions of each exercise. (As you add weight, you may have to decrease the number of repetitions slightly until your muscles adapt to the heavier load.) If your program is focusing on strength alone, your sets can contain fewer repetitions using a heavier load. If you are over approximately 50–60 years of age, your sets should contain more repetitions (10–15) using a lighter load. Fill in the starting number of sets and repetitions of each exercise on the program plan.

5. *Choose the number of training sessions per week.* Work out at least 2 days per week. Indicate the days you will train on your program plan; be sure to include days of rest to allow your body to recover.

6. *Monitor your progress.* Use the workout card on the next page to monitor program progress and keep track of exercises, weights, sets, and repetitions. (A more extensive series of weight training logs is included in the Daily Fitness Log booklet.)

Program Plan for Weight Training

Exercise	Muscle(s) Developed	Weight (lb)	Repetitions	Sets	Frequency (check ✓)						
					M	T	W	Th	F	Sa	Su

WORKOUT CARD FOR _____

Exercise/Date	Wt	Sets	Reps	Wt	Sets	Reps	Wt	Sets	Reps	Wt	Sets	Reps	Wt	Sets	Reps	Wt	Sets	Reps	Wt	Sets	Reps	Wt	Sets	Reps	Wt	Sets	Reps	Wt	Sets	Reps	Wt	Sets	Reps	Wt	Sets	Reps	Wt	Sets	Reps

Name _____ **Section** _____ **Date** _____

LAB 4-4 *Getting to Know Your Fitness Facility*

To help create a successful training program, take time out to learn more about the fitness facility you plan to use.

Basic Information

Name and location of facility: _____

Hours of operation: _____

Times available for general use: _____

Times most convenient for your schedule: _____

Can you obtain an initial session or consultation with a trainer to help you create a program? ____ yes ____ no

If so, what does the initial planning session involve? _____

_____

Are any of the staff certified? Do any have special training? If yes, list/describe: _____

_____

What types of weight training equipment are available for use?_____

_____

Are other types of equipment available, such as treadmills or stair-climbers for the development of cardiorespiratory endurance? If so, briefly list/describe: _____

_____

_____

Are any group activities or classes available? If so, briefly describe: _____

_____

_____

Yes	No	
____	____	Is there a fee for using the facility? If so, how much? $_____
____	____	Is a student ID required for access to the facility?
____	____	Do you need to sign up in advance to use the facility or any of the equipment?
____	____	Is there typically a line or wait to use the equipment during the times you use the facility?
____	____	Is there a separate area with mats for stretching and/or cool-down?
____	____	Do you need to bring your own towel?
____	____	Are lockers available? If so, do you need to bring your own lock? ____ yes ____ no
____	____	Are showers available? If so, do you need to bring your own soap and shampoo?____ yes ____ no
____	____	Is drinking water available? (If not, be sure to bring your own bottle of water.)

Describe any other amenities, such as vending machines or saunas, that are available at the facility.

_____

_____

Information About Equipment

Fill in the specific equipment and exercise(s) that you can use to develop each of the following major muscles and muscle groups; in many instances, one exercise can be used to develop several muscles. If you would like to incorporate additional exercises for other muscles, list those in the bottom portion of the chart. Finally, number the exercises to indicate the order in which you'll complete them during a workout session (see p. 76 and the box "A Sample Weight Training Program for General Fitness" on page 78 for suggestions on order of exercises).

Order	Muscles and Muscle Groups	Equipment	Exercise(s)
	Pectoralis major and minor (chest)		
	Deltoids and trapezius (shoulders)		
	Latissimus dorsi, teres major and minor, rhomboid (upper back)		
	Biceps, brachialis (front of arms)		
	Triceps (back of arms)		
	Gluteus maximus (buttocks)		
	Quadriceps (front of thighs)		
	Hamstrings (back of thighs)		
	Gastrocnemius, soleus (calves)		
	Rectus abdominis, obliques (abdomen)		
	Erector spinae, quadratus lumborum (lower back)		
	Sternocleidomastoids, scaleni, splenii (neck)		

Flexibility

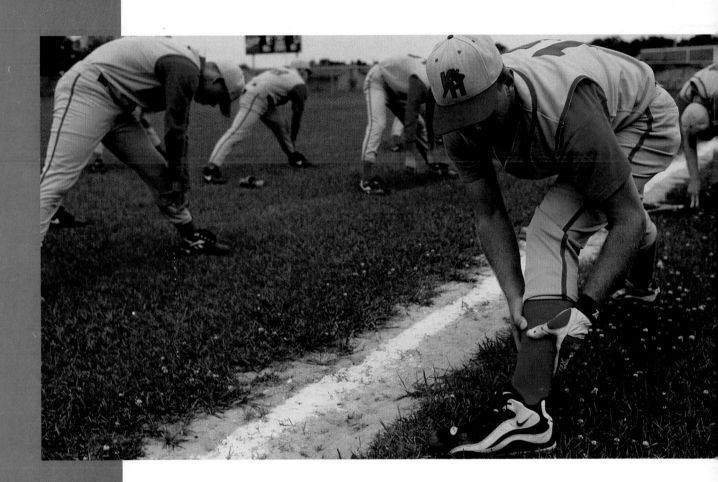

LOOKING AHEAD

After reading this chapter, you should be able to answer these questions about flexibility and stretching exercises:

- What are the potential benefits of flexibility and stretching exercises?

- What determines the amount of flexibility in each joint?

- What are the different types of stretching exercises, and how do they affect muscles?

- What type, intensity, duration, and frequency of stretching exercises will develop the greatest amount of flexibility with the lowest risk of injury?

- What are some common stretching exercises for major joints?

- How can low-back pain be prevented and managed?

Flexibility—the ability of a joint to move through its full **range of motion**—is extremely important for general fitness and wellness. The smooth and easy performance of everyday and recreational activities is impossible if flexibility is poor. Flexibility is a highly adaptable physical fitness component. It increases in response to a regular program of stretching exercises and decreases with inactivity. Flexibility is also specific: Good flexibility in one joint doesn't necessarily mean good flexibility in another. Flexibility can be increased through stretching exercises for all major joints.

There are two basic types of flexibility: static and dynamic. Static flexibility refers to the ability to assume and maintain an extended position at one end or point in a joint's range of motion; it is what most people mean by the term *flexibility*. Dynamic flexibility, unlike static flexibility, involves movement; it is the ability to move a joint through its range of motion with little resistance. For example, static shoulder flexibility would determine how far you could extend your arm across the front of your body or out to the side. Dynamic shoulder flexibility would affect your ability to pitch a softball, swing a golf club, or swim the crawl stroke. When gymnasts perform a split on the balance beam, they must have good static flexibility in their legs and hips; to perform a split leap, they must have good dynamic flexibility.

Static flexibility depends on many factors, including the structure of a joint and the tightness of muscles, tendons, and ligaments that are attached to it. Dynamic flexibility is dependent on static flexibility, but it also involves such factors as strength, coordination, and resistance to movement. Dynamic flexibility can be important for both daily activities and sports. However, because static flexibility is easier to measure and better researched, most assessment tests and stretching programs—including those presented in this chapter—target static flexibility.

This chapter describes the factors that affect flexibility and the benefits of maintaining good flexibility. It provides guidelines for assessing your current level of flexibility and putting together a successful stretching program. It also examines the common problem of low-back pain.

Good flexibility provides benefits for the entire musculoskeletal system; it may also prevent injuries and soreness and improve performance in all physical activities.

Joint Health

Good flexibility is essential to good joint health. When the muscles and other tissues that support a joint are tight, the joint is subject to abnormal stresses that can cause joint deterioration. For example, tight thigh muscles cause excessive pressure on the kneecap, leading to pain in the knee joint. Tight shoulder muscles can compress sensitive soft tissues in the shoulder, leading to pain and disability in the joint. Poor joint flexibility can also cause abnormalities in joint lubrication, leading to deterioration of the sensitive cartilage cells lining the joint; pain and further joint injury can result.

Improved flexibility can greatly improve your quality of life, particularly as you get older. Aging decreases the natural elasticity of muscles, tendons, and joints, resulting in stiffness. The problem is compounded if you have arthritis. Flexibility exercises improve the elasticity in your tissues, making it easier to move your body. When you're flexible, everything from tying your shoes to reaching for a jar on an upper shelf becomes easier.

Low-Back Pain and Injuries

Low-back pain can be related to poor spinal alignment, which puts pressure on the nerves leading out from the spinal column. Strength and flexibility in the back, pelvis, and thighs may help prevent this type of back pain. Unfortunately, research studies have not yet clearly defined the relationship between back pain and lack of flexibility. However, many back exercises help improve low-back flexibility and empirically seem to work.

Poor flexibility does increase one's risk for injury. A general stretching program has been shown to be effective in reducing the frequency of injuries as well as their severity. When injuries do occur, flexibility exercises can be used in treatment: They reduce symptoms and help restore normal range of motion in affected joints.

Overstretching—stretching muscles to extreme ranges of motion—may actually decrease the stability of a joint. Although some activities, such as gymnastics and ballet, require extreme joint movements, such flexibility is not recommended for the average person. In fact, extreme flexibility may increase the risk of injury in activities such as skiing, basketball, and volleyball. Again, as with other types of exercise, moderation is the key to safe training.

Additional Potential Benefits

- *Reduction of postexercise muscle soreness.* **Delayed-onset muscle soreness,** occurring 1–2 days after exercise, is thought to be caused by damage to the muscle fibers and supporting connective tissue. Some studies, though not all, have shown that stretching after exercise decreases the degree of muscle soreness.

- *Relief of aches and pains.* Flexibility exercises help relieve pain that develops from stress or prolonged sitting. Studying or working in one place for a long time can cause your muscles to become tense. Stretching helps relieve tension, so you can go back to work refreshed and effective.

- *Improved body position and strength for sports (and life).*

Good flexibility lets a person assume more efficient body positions and exert force through a greater range of motion. For example, swimmers with more flexible shoulders have stronger strokes because they can pull their arms through the water in the optimal position. Flexible joints and muscles let you move more fluidly. Some studies also suggest that flexibility training enhances strength development.

- *Maintenance of good posture.* Good flexibility also contributes to body symmetry and good posture. Bad posture can gradually change your body structures. Sitting in a slumped position, for example, can lead to tightness in the muscles in the front of your chest and overstretching and looseness in the upper spine, causing a rounding of the upper back. This condition, called kyphosis, is common in older people. It may be prevented by stretching regularly.

- *Relaxation.* Flexibility exercises are a great way to relax. Studies have shown that doing flexibility exercises reduces mental tension, slows your breathing rate, and reduces blood pressure.

Flexibility and Lifetime Wellness

Part of wellness is being able to move without pain or hindrance. Flexibility exercises are an important part of this process. Sedentary people often effectively lose their mobility at an early age. Even relatively young people are often handicapped by back, shoulder, knee, and ankle pain. As they age, the pain can become debilitating, leading to injuries and a lower quality of life. Good flexibility helps keep your joints and muscles moving without pain so that you can do all the things you enjoy.

WHAT DETERMINES FLEXIBILITY?

The flexibility of a joint is affected by its structure, by muscle elasticity and length, and by nervous system activity. Some factors—joint structure, for example—can't be changed. Other factors, such as the length of resting muscle fibers, can be changed through exercise; these factors should be the focus of a program to develop flexibility.

Joint Structure

The amount of flexibility in a joint is determined in part by the nature and structure of the joint. Hinge joints such as those in your fingers and knees allow only limited forward and backward movement; they lock when fully extended. Ball-and-socket joints like the hip enable movement in many different directions and have a greater range of motion. Major joints are surrounded by **joint capsules,** semielastic structures that give joints strength and stability but limit movement. Heredity also plays a part in joint structure and flexibility; for example, al-

though everyone has a broad range of motion in the ball-and-socket hip joint, not everyone can do a split.

Muscle Elasticity and Length

Soft tissues, including skin, muscles, tendons, and ligaments, also limit the flexibility of a joint. Muscle tissue is the key to developing flexibility because it can be lengthened if it is regularly stretched. As described in Chapter 4, muscles contain proteins that create movement by causing muscles to contract. These contractile proteins can also stretch, and they are involved in the development of flexibility. However, the most important component of muscle tissue related to flexibility is the connective tissue that surrounds and envelops every part of muscle tissue, from individual muscle fibers to entire muscles. Connective tissue provides structure, elasticity, and bulk and makes up about 30% of muscle mass. Two principal types of connective tissue are **collagen,** white fibers that provide structure and support, and **elastin,** yellow fibers that are elastic and flexible. Muscles contain both collagen and elastin, closely intertwined, so muscle tissue exhibits the properties of both types of fibers. A recently discovered structural protein in muscles called **titin** also has elastic properties and contributes to flexibility.

When a muscle is stretched, the wavelike elastin fibers straighten; when the stretch is relieved, they rapidly snap back to their resting position. If gently and regularly stretched, connective tissues will lengthen and flexibility will improve (Figure 5-1). Without regular stretching, the process reverses: these tissues shorten, resulting in decreased flexibility. Regular stretching also contributes to flexibility by lengthening muscle fibers through the addition of contractile units called sarcomeres.

The stretch characteristics of connective tissue in muscle are important considerations for a stretching program. The amount of stretch a muscle will tolerate is limited, and as the limits of its flexibility are reached, connective tissue becomes more brittle and may rupture if overstretched (Figure 5-2). A safe and effective program

range of motion The full motion possible in a joint.   **TERMS**

delayed-onset muscle soreness Soreness that occurs 1–2 days after exercising, probably caused by tissue damage and inflammation that leads to further tissue damage.

joint capsules Semielastic structures, composed primarily of connective tissue, that surround major joints.

soft tissues Tissues of the human body that include skin, fat, linings of internal organs and blood vessels, connective tissues, tendons, ligaments, muscles, and nerves.

collagen White fibers that provide structure and support in connective tissue.

elastin Yellow fibers that make connective tissue flexible.

titin A filament in muscle that helps align proteins that cause muscle contraction; titin has elastic properties and also plays a role in flexibility.

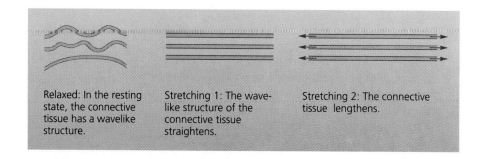

Relaxed: In the resting state, the connective tissue has a wavelike structure.

Stretching 1: The wave-like structure of the connective tissue straightens.

Stretching 2: The connective tissue lengthens.

Figure 5-1   Relaxed versus stretched connective tissue in muscle.

stretches muscles enough to slightly elongate the tissues but not so much that they are damaged. Research has shown that flexibility is improved best by stretching when muscles are warm (following exercise or the application of heat) and the stretch is applied gradually and conservatively. Sudden, high-stress stretching is less effective and can lead to muscle damage.

Nervous System Activity

Muscles contain **stretch receptors** that control their length. If a muscle is stretched suddenly, stretch receptors send signals to the spinal cord, which then sends a signal back to the same muscle, causing it to contract. These reflexes occur frequently in active muscles. They help the body know what the muscles are doing and allow for fine control of muscle length.

Small movements that only slightly stimulate these receptors cause small reflex actions. Rapid, powerful, and sudden movements that strongly stimulate the receptors cause large, powerful reflex muscle contractions. Stretches that involve rapid, bouncy movements are considered dangerous because they may stimulate a reflex muscle contraction during a stretch. A muscle that contracts at the same time it's being stretched can be easily injured, so slow, gradual stretches are always safest.

Strong muscle contractions produce a reflex of the opposite type—one that causes muscles to relax and keeps them from contracting too hard. This inverse stretch re

flex has recently been introduced as an aid to improving flexibility: Contracting a muscle prior to stretching it causes it to relax, allowing it to stretch farther. The contraction-stretch technique for developing flexibility is called **proprioceptive neuromuscular facilitation (PNF)**. More research needs to be done, however, to determine precisely the degree to which PNF techniques cause muscle relaxation and help develop flexibility.

Doing each stretching exercise several times in a row can "reset" the sensitivity of muscle stretch receptors. Stretching a muscle, relaxing, and then stretching it again cause the stretch receptors to become slightly less sensitive, thereby enabling the muscle to stretch farther. It is not known if stretch receptor sensitivity continues to change following prolonged flexibility training, but it's likely that neural changes do occur to help increase flexibility.

ASSESSING FLEXIBILITY

Because flexibility is specific to each joint, there are no tests of general flexibility. The most commonly used flexibility test is the sit-and-reach test. This test rates the flexibility of the muscles in the lower back and hamstrings; flexibility in these muscles may be important in preventing low-back pain. To assess your flexibility and identify inflexible joints, complete Lab 5-1.

CREATING A SUCCESSFUL PROGRAM TO DEVELOP FLEXIBILITY

A successful program for developing flexibility contains safe exercises executed with the most effective techniques.

Types of Stretching Techniques

Stretching techniques vary from simply stretching the muscles during the course of normal activities to sophisticated methods based on patterns of muscle reflexes. Improper stretching techniques can do more harm than good, so it's important to understand the different types of stretching exercises and how they affect the muscles.

TERMS   **stretch receptors**   Sense organs in skeletal muscles that initiate a nerve signal to the spinal cord in response to a stretch; a contraction follows.

proprioceptive neuromuscular facilitation (PNF)   A technique for stretching and strengthening muscles; PNF relies on neuromuscular reflexes to stimulate training effects.

static stretching   A technique in which a muscle is slowly and gently stretched and then held in the stretched position.

ballistic stretching   A technique in which muscles are stretched by the force generated as a body part is repeatedly bounced, swung, or jerked.

passive stretching   A technique in which muscles are stretched by force applied by an outside source.

active stretching   A technique in which muscles are stretched by the contraction of the opposing muscles.

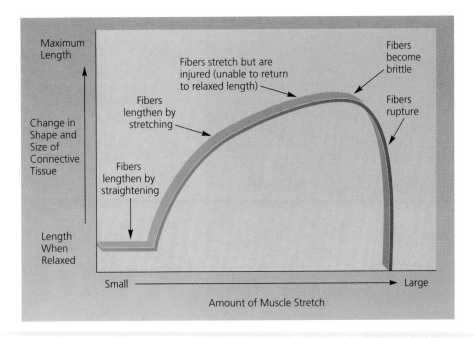

Figure 5-2 **The effect of stretch on connective tissue.**

Three common techniques are static stretches, ballistic stretches, and PNF.

Static Stretching In **static stretching**, each muscle is gradually stretched, and the stretch is held for 10–30 seconds. (Holding the stretch longer than 30 seconds will not further improve flexibility, whereas stretching for less than 10 seconds will provide little benefit.) A slow stretch prompts less reaction from stretch receptors, and the muscles can safely stretch farther than usual. Static stretching is the type most often recommended by fitness experts because it's safe and effective. The key to this technique is to stretch the muscles and joints to the point where a pull is felt, but not to the point of pain.

Ballistic Stretching In **ballistic stretching**, the muscles are stretched suddenly in a bouncing movement. For example, touching the toes repeatedly in rapid succession is a ballistic stretch for the hamstrings. The problem with this technique is that the heightened activity of stretch receptors caused by the rapid stretches can continue for some time, possibly causing injuries during any physical activities that follow. For this reason, ballistic stretching is not recommended.

Proprioceptive Neuromuscular Facilitation (PNF) PNF techniques use reflexes initiated by both muscle and joint receptors to cause greater training effects. The most popular PNF stretching technique is the contract-relax stretching method, in which a muscle is contracted before it is stretched. For example, in a seated stretch of calf muscles, the first step in PNF is to contract the calf muscles: A partner can provide resistance for an isometric contraction. Following a brief period of relaxation, the next step is to stretch the calf muscles by pulling the tops of the feet toward the body. A duration of 6 seconds for the contraction and 10–30 seconds for the stretch is recommended. PNF appears to allow more effective stretching, but it tends to cause more muscle stiffness and soreness than static stretching. It usually requires a partner and takes more time.

Passive and Active Stretching

Stretches can be done either passively or actively.

Passive Stretching In **passive stretching**, an outside force or resistance provided by yourself, a partner, gravity, or a weight helps your joints move through their range of motion. For example, a seated stretch of the hamstring and back muscles can be done by reaching the hands toward the feet until a "pull" is felt in those muscles. You can achieve a greater range of motion (a more intense stretch) using passive stretching. However, because the stretch is not controlled by the muscles themselves, there is a greater risk of injury. Communication between partners in passive stretching is very important so joints aren't forced outside their normal functional range of motion.

Active Stretching In **active stretching**, a muscle is stretched by a contraction of the opposing muscle (the muscle on the opposite side of the limb). For example, an active seated stretch of the calf muscles occurs when a person actively contracts the muscles on the top of the shin. The contraction of this opposing muscle produces a reflex that relaxes the muscles to be stretched. The muscle can be stretched farther with a low risk of injury.

The only disadvantage of active stretching is that a person may not be able to produce enough stress (enough stretch) to increase flexibility using only the contraction

- Do stretching exercises statically. Stretch to the point of mild discomfort, and hold the position for 10–30 seconds, rest for 30–60 seconds, and repeat, trying to stretch a bit farther.
- Do not stretch to the point of pain.
- Relax and breathe easily as you stretch. Try to relax the muscles being stretched.
- Perform all exercises on both sides of your body.

- Increase intensity and duration gradually over time. Improved flexibility takes many months to develop.
- Stretch when your muscles are warm. Do gentle warm-up exercises such as easy jogging or calisthenics before doing a pre-exercise stretching routine.
- There are large individual differences in joint flexibility. Don't feel you have to compete with others during stretching workouts.

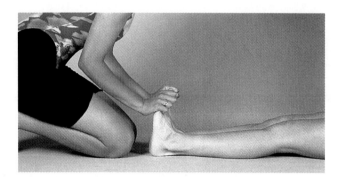 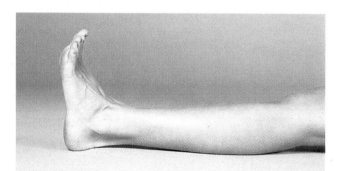

In passive stretching (left), an outside force—such as pressure exerted by another person—helps move the joint and stretch the muscles. In active stretching (right), the force to move the joint and stretch the muscles is provided by a contraction of the opposing muscles.

of opposing muscle groups. The safest and most convenient technique is active static stretching, with an occasional passive assist. For example, you might stretch your calves both by contracting the muscles on the top of your shin and by pulling your feet toward you. This way you combine the advantages of active stretching—safety and the relaxation reflex—with those of passive stretching—greater range of motion.

Intensity and Duration

For each exercise, slowly apply stretch to your muscles to the point of slight tension or mild discomfort. Hold the stretch for 10–30 seconds. As you hold the stretch, the feeling of slight tension should slowly subside; at that point, try to stretch a bit farther. Throughout the stretch, try to relax and breathe easily. Rest for about 30–60 seconds between each stretch, and do at least 4 repetitions of each stretch. A complete flexibility workout usually takes about 20–30 minutes.

Frequency

The American College of Sports Medicine recommends that stretching exercises be performed a minimum of 2–3 days a week. Many people do flexibility training more of-

ten—3–5 days a week—for even greater benefits. It's best to stretch when your muscles are warm, so try incorporating stretching into your cool-down after cardiorespiratory endurance exercise or weight training. Stretching can also be a part of your warm-up, but it's important to increase the temperature of your muscles first by doing the active part of the warm-up (for example, walking or slow jogging) for 5–10 minutes. Stretching before exercise without warming up does not prevent injury and may even cause injury.

Refer to the box "Safe Stretching" for additional tips on creating a safe and successful stretching program, and complete Lab 5-2 when you're ready to start your own program.

Exercises to Improve Flexibility

There are hundreds of exercises that can improve flexibility. Your program should include exercises that work all the major joints of the body by stretching their associated muscles. The exercises illustrated here are simple to do and pose a minimum risk of injury. Use these exercises, or substitute your favorite stretches, to create a well-rounded program for developing flexibility. Be sure to perform each stretch using the proper technique. Hold each position for 10–30 seconds, and perform at least 4 repetitions of each exercise.

FLEXIBILITY EXERCISES

EXERCISE 1

HEAD TURNS AND TILTS

Areas stretched: Neck

Instructions

Head turns: Turn your head to the right and hold the stretch. Repeat to the left.

Head tilts: Tilt your head to the left and hold the stretch. Repeat to the right.

Variation: Place your right palm on your right cheek; try to turn your head to the right as you resist with your hand. Repeat on the left side.

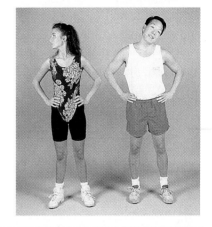

EXERCISE 2

TOWEL STRETCH

Areas stretched: Triceps, shoulders, chest

Instructions: Roll up a towel and grasp it with both hands, palms down. With your arms straight, slowly lift it back over your head as far as possible. The closer together your hands are, the greater the stretch.

Variation: Repeat the stretch with your arms down and the towel behind your back. Grasp the towel with your palms forward and thumbs pointing out. Gently raise your arms behind your back.

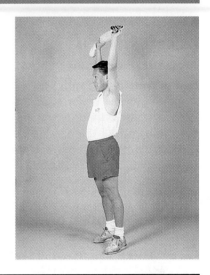

EXERCISE 3

ACROSS-THE-BODY STRETCH

Areas stretched: Shoulders, upper back

Instructions: Keeping your back straight, cross your left arm in front of your body and grasp it with your right hand. Stretch your arm, shoulders, and back by gently pulling your arm as close to your body as possible. Repeat the stretch with your right arm.

Variation: Bend your right arm over and behind your head. Grasp your right hand with your left, and gently pull your arm until you feel the stretch. Repeat for your left arm.

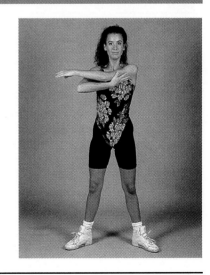

UPPER-BACK STRETCH

Areas stretched: Upper back

Instructions: Stand with your feet shoulder-width apart, knees slightly bent, and pelvis tucked under. Clasp your hands in front of your body, and press your palms forward.

Variation: In the same position, wrap your arms around your body as if you were giving yourself a hug.

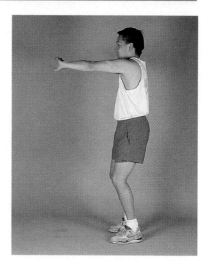

LATERAL STRETCH

Areas stretched: Trunk muscles

Instructions: Stand with your feet shoulder-width apart, knees slightly bent, and pelvis tucked under. Raise one arm over your head and bend sideways from the waist. Support your trunk by placing the hand or forearm of your other arm on your thigh or hip for support. Be sure you bend directly sideways, and don't move your body below the waist. Repeat on the other side.

Variation: Perform the same exercise in a seated position.

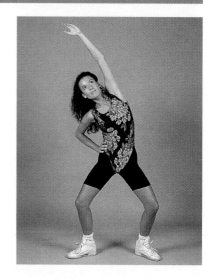

STEP STRETCH

Areas stretched: Hip, front of thigh (quadriceps)

Instructions: Step forward and flex your forward knee, keeping your knee directly above your ankle. Stretch your other leg back so that it is parallel to the floor. Press your hips forward and down to stretch. Your arms can be at your sides, on top of your knee, or on the ground for balance. Repeat on the other side.

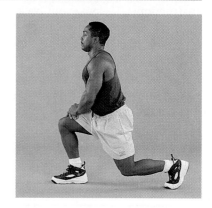

SIDE LUNGE

Areas stretched: Inner thigh, hip, calf

Instructions: Stand in a wide straddle with your legs turned out from your hip joints and your hands on your thighs. Lunge to one side by bending one knee and keeping the other leg straight. Keep your knee directly over your ankle; do not bend it more than 90 degrees. Repeat on the other side.

Variation: In the same position, lift the heel of the bent knee to provide additional stretch. The exercise may also be performed with your hands on the floor for balance.

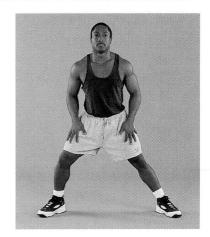

SOLE STRETCH

Areas stretched: Inner thigh, hip

Instructions: Sit with the soles of your feet together. Push your knees toward the floor using your hands or forearms.

Variation: When you first begin to push your knees toward the floor, use your legs to resist the movement. Then relax and press your knees down as far as they will go.

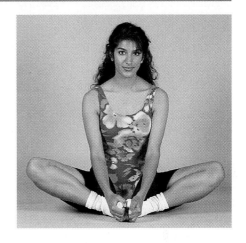

TRUNK ROTATION

Areas stretched: Trunk, outer thigh and hip, lower back

Instructions: Sit with your right leg straight, left leg bent and crossed over the right knee, and left hand on the floor next to your left hip. Turn your trunk as far as possible to the left by pushing against your left leg with your right forearm or elbow. Keep your left foot on the floor. Repeat on the other side.

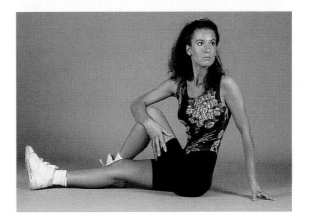

ALTERNATE LEG STRETCHER

Areas stretched: Back of the thigh (hamstring), hip, knee, ankle, buttocks

Instructions: Lie flat on your back with both legs straight. **(a)** Grasp your left leg behind the thigh, and pull in to your chest. **(b)** Hold this position, and then extend your left leg toward the ceiling. **(c)** Hold this position, and then bring your left knee back to your chest and pull your toes toward your shin with your left hand. Stretch the back of the leg by attempting to straighten your knee. Repeat for the other leg.

Variation: Perform the stretch on both legs at the same time.

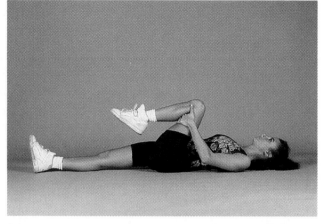

(a)

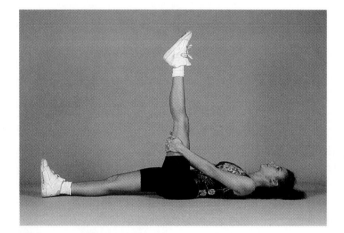

(b)

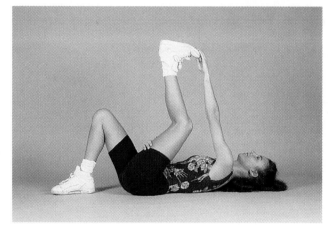

(c)

MODIFIED HURDLER STRETCH
(Seated Single-Toe Touch)

Areas stretched: Back of the thigh (hamstring), lower back

Instructions: Sit with your right leg straight and your left leg tucked close to your body. Reach toward your right foot as far as possible. Repeat for the other leg.

Variation: As you stretch forward, alternately flex and point the foot of your extended leg.

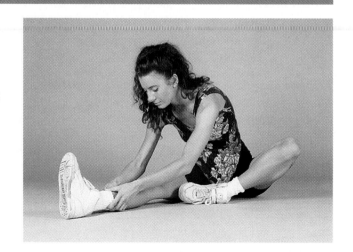

LOWER-LEG STRETCH

Areas stretched: Back of the lower leg (calf, soleus, Achilles tendon)

Instructions: Stand with one foot about 1–2 feet in front of the other, with both feet pointing forward. **(a)** Keeping your back leg straight, lunge forward by bending your front knee and pushing your rear heel backward. Hold this position. **(b)** Then pull your back foot in slightly, and bend your back knee. Shift your weight to your back leg. Hold. Repeat on the other side.

Variation: Place your hands on a wall and extend one foot back, pressing your heel down to stretch; or stand with the balls of your feet on a step or bench and allow your heels to drop below the level of your toes.

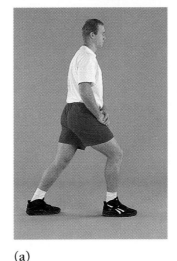

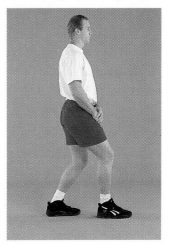

(a)　　　　　　　　　　　　　　(b)

PREVENTING AND MANAGING LOW-BACK PAIN

More than 85% of Americans experience back pain at some time in their lives. Low-back pain is the second most common ailment in the United States—headache tops the list—and the second most common reason for absences from work. Low-back pain is estimated to cost as much as $50 billion a year in lost productivity, medical and legal fees, and disability insurance and compensation.

Back pain can result from sudden traumatic injuries, but it is more often the long-term result of weak and inflexible muscles, poor posture, or poor body mechanics during activities like lifting and carrying. Any abnormal strain on the back can result in pain. Most cases of low-back pain clear up on their own within a few weeks or months, but some people have recurrences or suffer from chronic pain. Surgery for back pain is on the rise in the United States, but prevention is by far the best strategy.

Function and Structure of the Spine

The spinal column performs many important functions in the body.

- It provides structural support for the body, especially the thorax (upper-body cavity).
- It surrounds and protects the spinal cord.
- It supports much of the body's weight and transmits it to the lower body.
- It serves as an attachment site for a large number of muscles, tendons, and ligaments.
- It allows movement of the neck and back in all directions.

The spinal column is made up of bones called **vertebrae** (Figure 5-3). The spine consists of 7 cervical vertebrae in the neck, 12 thoracic vertebrae in the upper back, and 5 lumbar vertebrae in the lower back. The 9 vertebrae at the base of the spine are fused into two sections and form the sacrum and the coccyx (tailbone). The spine has four curves: the cervical, thoracic, lumbar, and sacral curves. These curves help bring the body weight supported by the spine in line with the axis of the body.

Although the structure of vertebrae depends on their location on the spine, the different types of vertebrae do share common characteristics. Each consists of a body, an arch, and several bony processes (Figure 5-4). The vertebral body is cylindrical, with flattened surfaces where **intervertebral disks** are attached. The vertebral body is designed to carry the stress of body weight and physical activity. The vertebral arch surrounds and protects the spinal cord. The bony processes serve as joints for adjacent vertebrae and attachment sites for muscles and ligaments. **Nerve roots** from the spinal cord pass through notches in the vertebral arch.

Intervertebral disks, which absorb and disperse the stresses placed on the spine, separate vertebrae from each

vertebrae Bony segments composing the spinal column that provide structural support for the body and protect the spinal cord. **TERMS**

intervertebral disk A tough, elastic disk located between adjoining vertebrae consisting of a gel- and water-filled nucleus surrounded by fibrous rings; it serves as a shock absorber for the spinal column.

nerve root The base of one of the 31 pairs of spinal nerves that branch off the spinal cord through spaces between vertebrae.

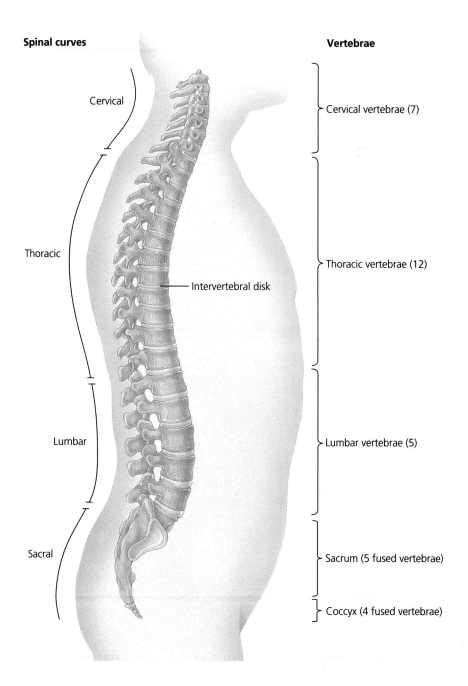

Cervical

Cervical vertebrae (7)

Thoracic

Thoracic vertebrae (12)

Intervertebral disk

Lumbar

Lumbar vertebrae (5)

Sacral

Sacrum (5 fused vertebrae)

Coccyx (4 fused vertebrae)

Figure 5-3 The spinal column.
The spine is made up of five separate
regions and has four distinct curves. An
intervertebral disk is located between
vertebrae.

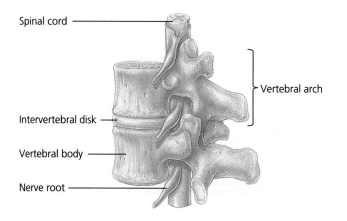

Spinal cord

Vertebral arch

Intervertebral disk

Vertebral body

Nerve root

**Figure 5-4 Vertebrae and an
intervertebral disk.**

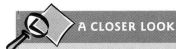

- Age greater than 34 years
- Degenerative disease (e.g., osteoporosis, arthritis)
- Family history of back pain
- History of back trauma
- Lack of physical activity
- Low job satisfaction
- Low muscular strength relative to body weight
- Low socioeconomic status
- Male sex (in some studies)
- Obesity

- Occupations or activities requiring frequent lifting, twisting, bending, or standing up
- Occupations with high concentration demands (e.g., computer programming)
- Physically hard work
- Poor posture
- Psychological depression
- Repetitive strain in forced positions over long time periods
- Smoking
- Vibration affecting the whole body (such as that experienced by truck drivers)

other. Disks are made up of a gel- and water-filled nucleus surrounded by a series of fibrous rings. The liquid nucleus can change shape when it is compressed, allowing the disk to absorb shock. The intervertebral disks also help maintain the spaces between vertebrae where the spinal nerve roots are located.

Causes of Back Pain

Back pain can occur at any point along your spine; the lumbar area, because it bears the majority of your weight, is the most common site. Any movement that causes excessive stress on the spinal column can cause injury and pain. The spine is well equipped to bear body weight and the force or stress of body movements along its long axis. However, it is less capable of bearing loads at an angle to its long axis. You do not have to carry a heavy load or participate in a vigorous contact sport to injure your back. Picking a pencil up from the floor using poor body mechanics—reaching too far out in front of you or bending over with your knees straight, for example—can also result in back pain (see the box "Risk Factors for Low-Back Pain").

Underlying causes of back pain include weak or inflexible muscles in the back, hips, abdomen, and legs; excess body weight; poor posture or body position when standing, sitting, or sleeping; and poor body mechanics when performing actions like lifting and carrying, or sports movements. Abnormal spinal loading resulting from any of these causes can have short-term or long-term direct and indirect effects on the spine. Strained muscles, tendons, or ligaments can cause pain and can, over time, lead to injuries to vertebrae or the intervertebral disks.

Stress can cause disks to break down and lose some of their ability to absorb shock. A damaged disk may bulge out between vertebrae and put pressure on a nerve root, a condition commonly referred to as a slipped disk. Painful pressure on nerves can also occur if damage to a disk narrows the space between two vertebrae. With age, you lose fluid from the disks, making them more likely to bulge and put pressure on nerve roots. Depending on the amount of pressure on a nerve, symptoms may include numbness in the back, hip, leg, or foot; radiating pain; loss of muscle function; depressed reflexes; and muscle spasm. If the pressure is severe enough, loss of function can be permanent.

Preventing Low-Back Pain

Incorrect posture when standing, sitting, lying, and lifting is responsible for many back injuries. In general, think about moving your spine as a unit, with the force directed through its long axis. Strategies for maintaining good posture during daily activities are presented in the box "Avoiding Low-Back Pain." Follow the same guidelines for posture and movement when you engage in sports or recreational activities. Maintain control over your body movements, and warm up thoroughly before you exercise. Take special care when lifting weights as part of a resistance training program. (Refer to Chapter 4 for more information on proper weight-lifting techniques.)

The role of exercise in preventing and treating back pain is still being investigated. However, many experts do recommend exercise, especially for people who have already experienced an episode of low-back pain. Regular exercise aimed at strengthening the back and abdominal muscles is often recommended to prevent back pain, as is lifestyle physical activity such as walking. When walking, stand up straight, keep your head centered over your body, and swing your arms freely. Movement helps lubricate your spinal disks and increases muscle fitness in your trunk and legs. Other lifestyle recommendations for preventing back pain include:

- Lose weight, if you are overweight, to lessen the strain on the back.

Changes in everyday behavior can help prevent and alleviate low-back pain.

- *Lying down.* When resting or sleeping, lie on your side with your knees and hips bent. If you lie on your back, place a pillow under your knees. Don't lie on your stomach. If your mattress isn't firm, place a plywood board under it.

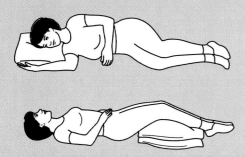

- *Sitting.* Sit with your lower back slightly rounded, knees bent, and feet flat on the floor. Alternate crossing your legs, or use a footrest to keep your knees higher than your hips. If this position is uncomfortable or if your back flattens when you sit, try using a lumbar roll pillow behind your lower back.

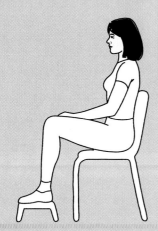

- *Lifting.* If you need to lower yourself to grasp an object, bend at the knees and hips rather than at the waist. Your feet should be about shoulder-width apart. Lift gradually, keeping your arms straight, by standing up or by pushing with your leg muscles. Keep the object close to your body. Don't twist; if you have to turn with the object, change the position of your feet.

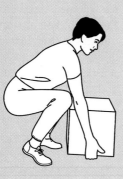

- *Standing.* When you are standing, a straight line should run from the top of your ear through the center of your shoulder, the center of your hip, the back of your kneecap, and the front of your ankle bone. Support your weight mainly on your heels, with one or both knees slightly bent. Try to keep your lower back flat by placing one foot on a stool. Don't let your pelvis tip forward or your back arch. Shift your weight back and forth from foot to foot. Avoid prolonged standing. (To check your posture, stand in a normal way with your back to a wall. Your upper back and buttocks should touch the wall; your heels may be a few inches away. Slide one hand into the space between your lower back and the wall. It should slide in easily but should almost touch both your back and the wall. Adjust your posture as needed, and try to hold this position as you walk away from the wall.)

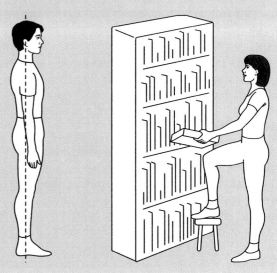

- *Walking.* Walk with your toes pointed straight ahead. Keep your back flat, head up, and chin in. Don't wear high-heeled shoes.

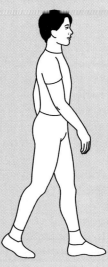

- Stop smoking, if you smoke, because smoking appears to increase degenerative changes in the spine.
- Avoid sitting, standing, or working in the same position for too long.
- Use a supportive seat while driving.
- Use a firm mattress.
- Reduce emotional stress, because stress causes muscle tension.
- Warm up thoroughly before engaging in vigorous exercise or sports.
- Progress gradually when attempting to improve strength or fitness.

The exercises that follow are designed to help you maintain a healthy back by stretching and strengthening the major muscle groups that affect the back—the abdominal muscles, the muscles along your spine and sides, and the muscles of your hips and thighs. If you have back problems, check with your physician before beginning any exercise program. Perform the exercises slowly, and progress very gradually. Stop and consult your physician if any exercise causes back pain.

LOW-BACK EXERCISES

EXERCISE 1

WALL STRETCH

Areas stretched: Back of thigh (hamstring), calf

Instructions: Sit on the floor with one leg extended and your foot flat against a wall or other immovable object. Bend the other leg and place your foot flat on the floor next to the knee of the straight leg. Clasp your hands behind your back or rest them loosely on the floor behind you. Bend forward from your hips, keeping your lower back flat and straight. Your bent knee can be moved slightly to the side to make room for your upper body as you lean forward. Repeat with the other leg.

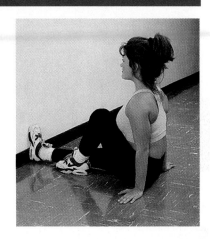

EXERCISE 2

STEP STRETCH (see Exercise 6 in the flexibility program)

EXERCISE 3

ALTERNATE LEG STRETCHER (see Exercise 10 in the flexibility program)

DOUBLE KNEE-TO-CHEST

Areas stretched: Lower back, hips

Instructions: Lie on your back with both knees bent and feet flat on the floor. **(a)** With one hand on the back of each thigh, slowly pull both knees to your chest; hold the stretch. **(b)** Then straighten your knees so that both legs are extended toward the ceiling. Return to the starting position by drawing your legs back to your chest and then placing your feet on the floor.

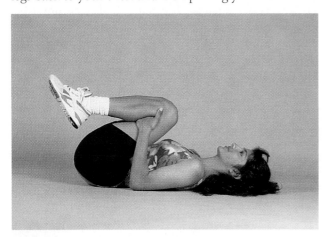

(a)

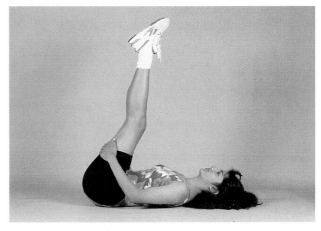

(b)

TRUNK TWIST

Area stretched: Lower back, sides

Instructions: Lie on your side with top knee bent, lower leg straight, lower arm extended out in front of you on the floor, and upper arm at your side. Push down with your upper knee while you twist your trunk backward. Try to get your shoulders and upper body flat on the floor, turning your head as well. Return to the starting position, and then repeat on the other side.

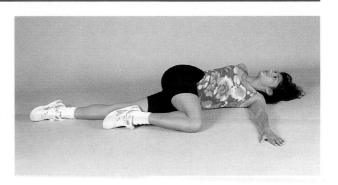

BACK BRIDGE

Areas strengthened: Hips, buttocks

Instructions: Lie on your back with knees bent and arms extended to the side. Tuck your pelvis under, and then lift your tailbone, buttocks, and lower back from the floor. Hold this position for 5–10 seconds with your weight resting on your feet, arms, and shoulders, and then return to the starting position. Work up to 10 repetitions of the exercise.

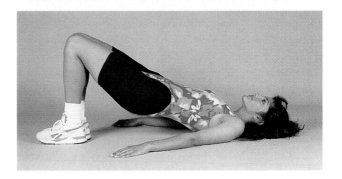

PELVIC TILT

Areas strengthened: Abdomen, buttocks

Instructions: Lie on your back with knees bent and arms extended to the side. Tilt your pelvis under, and try to flatten your lower back against the floor. Tighten your buttock and abdominal muscles while you hold this position for 5–10 seconds. Don't hold your breath. Work up to 10 repetitions of the exercise. Pelvic tilts can also be done standing or leaning against a wall.

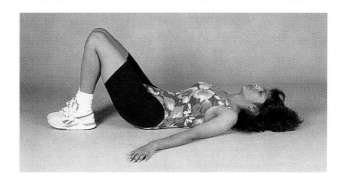

MODIFIED SIT-UP

Areas strengthened: Abdomen

Instructions: Lie on your back with knees bent and arms crossed on your chest. Tilt your pelvis under, flattening your back. Tuck your chin in and slowly curl up, one vertebra at a time as you lift your head first and then your shoulders. Stop when you can see your knees, and hold for 5–10 seconds before returning to the starting position. Do 10 repetitions.

Variation: Add a twist to develop other abdominal muscles. When you have curled up so that your shoulder blades are off the floor, twist your upper body so that one shoulder is higher than the other; reach past your knee with your upper arm. Hold, and then return to the starting position. Repeat on the opposite side.

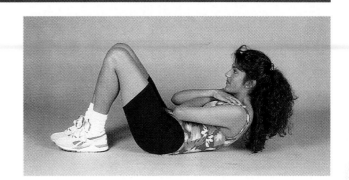

PRESS-UP

Areas stretched: Lower back, abdomen

Instructions: Lie face down with your hands under your face. Slowly push yourself up until your upper body is resting on your forearms. Relax and hold for 5–10 seconds. Gradually progress to straightening your elbows while keeping your pubic bone on the floor. (Stop if this exercise produces any pain.)

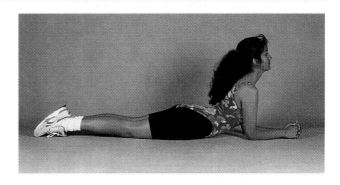

WALL SQUAT (Phantom Chair)

Areas strengthened: Lower back, thighs, abdomen

Instructions: Lean against a wall and bend your knees as though you are sitting in a chair. Support your weight with your legs. Begin by holding the position for 5–10 seconds. Build up to 1 minute or more.

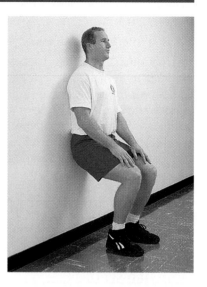

SPINE EXTENSIONS (see Exercise 9 in the free weights program in Chapter 4, p. 92)

COMMON QUESTIONS ANSWERED

Are there any stretching exercises I shouldn't do? Yes. Avoid exercises that put excessive pressure on your joints, particularly your spine and knees. Previous injuries and poor flexibility may make certain exercises dangerous for some people. Exercises that may cause problems are described in the box "Stretches to Avoid."

Is stretching the same as warming up? People often confuse stretching and pre-exercise warm-up. Although they are complementary, they are two distinct activities. A warm-up involves light exercise that increases body temperature so your metabolism works better when you're exercising at high intensity. Stretching increases the movement capability of your joints, so you can move more easily, with less risk of injury.

Whenever you stretch, first spend 5–10 minutes engaged in some form of low-intensity exercise, such as walking, jogging, or low-intensity calisthenics. When your muscles are warmed, begin your stretching routine. Warmed muscles stretch better than cold ones and are less prone to injury. Many experts recommend that people do stretching exercises at the end of the workout.

How much flexibility do I need? This question is not always easy to answer. If you're involved in a sport such as gymnas-

tics, figure skating, or ballet, you are often required to reach extreme joint motions to achieve success. However, nonathletes do not need to reach these extreme joint positions. In fact, too much flexibility may, in some cases, increase your risk of injury. As with other types of fitness, moderation is the key. You should regularly stretch your major joints and muscle groups but not aspire to reach extreme flexibility.

Can I stretch too far? Yes. As muscle tissue is progressively stretched, it reaches a point where it becomes damaged and may rupture. The greatest danger occurs during passive stretching when a partner is doing the stretching for you. It is critical that your stretching partner not force your joint outside its normal functional range of motion.

Does weight training limit flexibility? Weight training, or any physical activity, will decrease flexibility if the exercises are not performed through a full range of motion. When done properly, weight training increases flexibility.

Does jogging impair flexibility? Because of the limited range of motion used during the running stride, jogging tends to compromise flexibility. It is very important for runners to practice flexibility exercises for the hamstrings and quadriceps regularly.

Does wearing an abdominal belt at work prevent me from getting a back injury? Many employers require or encourage workers to use abdominal belts, but the benefits of these devices are far from clear. People sometimes gain a false sense of security from wearing a belt and think they can lift more weight than they really can. Although this may be true to some extent, research shows that people who are injured while wearing a belt tend to suffer more serious injuries. Wearing a belt also increases abdominal pressure and blood pressure. The best protections against back injuries are to maintain good posture and body position when standing, sitting, lifting, and sleeping; get plenty of exercise; and maintain strong, flexible back and abdominal muscles.

SUMMARY

- Flexibility, the ability of joints to move through their full range of motion, is highly adaptable and specific to each joint.
- The benefits of flexibility include preventing abnormal stresses that lead to joint deterioration and possibly reducing the risk of injuries and low-back pain.
- Range of motion can be limited by joint structure, by limited muscle elasticity, and by stretch receptor activity.
- Developing flexibility depends on stretching the elastic tissues within muscles regularly and gently until they lengthen. Overstretching can make connective tissue brittle and lead to rupture.
- Signals sent between stretch receptors and the spinal cord can enhance flexibility because contracting a muscle stimulates a relaxation response, thereby allowing a longer muscle stretch, and because stretch receptors become less sensitive after repeated stretches, initiating fewer contractions.
- The sit-and-reach test is most often used to assess flexibility; comparisons can also be made to a chart showing normal range of motion for major joints.
- Static stretching is done slowly and held to the point of mild tension; ballistic stretching consists of bouncing stretches and can lead to injury. Proprioceptive neuromuscular facilitation uses muscle receptors in contracting and relaxing a muscle.
- Passive stretching, using an outside force in moving muscles and joints, achieves a greater range of motion (and has a higher injury risk) than active stretching, which uses opposing muscles to initiate a stretch.
- Stretches should be held for 10–30 seconds; perform at least 4 repetitions. Flexibility training should be done 2 or more days a week, preferably following activity, when muscles are warm.
- The spinal column consists of vertebrae separated by intervertebral disks. It provides structure and support for the body and protects the spinal cord.
- In addition to good posture, proper body mechanics, and regular physical activity, a program for preventing low-back pain includes exercises that stretch and strengthen major muscle groups that affect the lower back.

FOR MORE INFORMATION

Books

Alter, M. J. 1996. *Science of Flexibility,* 2d ed. Champaign, Ill.: Human Kinetics. *An extremely well researched book that discusses the scientific basis of stretching exercises and flexibility.*

Anderson, B., and J. Anderson. 2000. *Stretching,* 20th anniv. ed. Bolinas, Calif.: Shelter Publications. *A best-selling exercise book, updated with more than 200 stretches for 60 sports and activities.*

Andes, K. 2000. *Fitness Stretching.* Pittsburgh, Pa.: Three Rivers Press. *Takes you through every muscle group with fully illustrated, step-by-step instructions for more than 100 yoga- and sport-inspired stretches.*

Maharam, L. 1998. *A Healthy Back: A Sports Medicine Doctor's Back-Care Program for Everybody.* New York: Henry Holt. *Lifestyle advice for preventing and eliminating back pain.*

McAtee, R. E., and J. Charland. 1999. *Facilitated Stretching,* 2d ed. Champaign, Ill.: Human Kinetics. *Provides detailed descriptions of a variety of proprioceptive neuromuscular facilitation (PNF) techniques.*

Oswald, C., and S. Bacso. 1998. *Stretching for Fitness, Health, and Performance: The Complete Handbook for All Ages and*

The safe alternatives listed here are described and illustrated on pages 121–125 as part of the complete program of safe flexibility exercises presented in this chapter.

Standing Toe Touch

Problem: Puts excessive strain on the spine

Alternatives: Alternate leg stretcher (Exercise 10), modified hurdler stretch (Exercise 11), and lower leg stretch (Exercise 12)

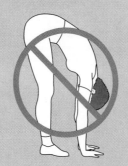

Full Squat

Problem: Puts excessive strain on the ankles, knees, and spine

Alternatives: Alternate leg stretcher (Exercise 10) and lower leg stretch (Exercise 12)

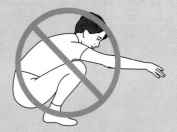

Standing Ankle-to-Buttocks Quadriceps Stretch

Problem: Puts excessive strain on the ligaments of the knee

Alternative: Step stretch (Exercise 6)

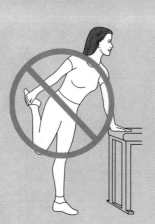

Prone Arch

Problem: Puts excessive strain on the spine, knees, and shoulders

Alternatives: Towel stretch (Exercise 2) and step stretch (Exercise 6)

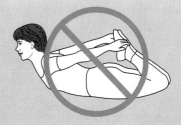

Fitness Levels. Somerset, Mass.: Sterling Publications. *A user-friendly manual providing all the basic and advanced concepts of stretching for everyone from infants to senior citizens.*

Sinel, M. S., and W. W. Deardorff. 1999. *Back Pain Remedies for Dummies.* Indianapolis, Ind.: IDG Books Worldwide. *Reviews a wide variety of self-help and professional remedies for back pain.*

St. George, F. 1997. *Stretching for Flexibility and Health.* Freedom, Calif.: Crossing Press. *A good basic book on stretching exercises.*

Web Sites

Exercise: A Guide from the National Institute on Aging and the National Aeronautics and Space Administration. Practical advice on fitness for seniors; includes animated instructions for specific flexibility exercises.

http://weboflife.arc.nasa.gov/exerciseandaging

FitnessLink/Stretching Exercises. Information on a safe, effective stretching program.

http://www.fitnesslink.com/exercise/stretch.shtml

Georgia State University: Flexibility. Provides information about the benefits of stretching and how to develop a safe and effective program; includes illustrations of stretches.

http://gsu.edu/~wwwfit/flexibility.html

NIH Back Pain Fact Sheet. Basic information on the prevention and treatment of back pain.

http://www.ninds.nih.gov/patients/disorder/back%20pain/backpain.htm

Southern California Orthopedic Institute. Provides information about a variety of orthopedic problems, including back injuries; also has illustrations of spinal anatomy.

http://www.scoi.com

Stretching and Flexibility. Provides information about the physiology of stretching and different types of stretching exercises.

http://www.taiko.com/history/stretching/stretching_toc.html

Workout.Com: Exercise Zone. Includes illustrated sample programs for developing flexibility and balance.

http://www.workout.com/exercises/exercises.asp?nav=1

See also the listings for Chapters 2 and 4.

The safe alternatives listed here are described and illustrated on pages 121–125 as part of the complete program of safe flexibility exercises presented in this chapter.

Standing Hamstring Stretch

Problem: Puts excessive strain on the knee and lower back

Alternatives: Alternate leg stretcher (Exercise 10) and modified hurdler stretch (Exercise 11)

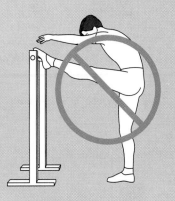

Yoga Plow

Problem: Puts excessive strain on the neck, shoulders, and back

Alternatives: Head turns and tilts (Exercise 1), across-the-body stretch (Exercise 3), and upper-back stretch (Exercise 4)

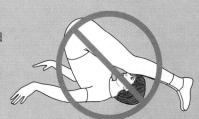

Hurdler Stretch

Problem: Turning out the bent leg can put excessive strain on the ligaments of the knee

Alternative: Modified hurdler stretch (Exercise 11)

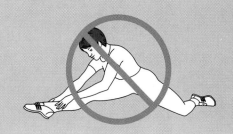

SELECTED BIBLIOGRAPHY

Abenheim, L., et al. 2000. The role of activity in the therapeutic management of back pain. *Spine* 25 (4 Suppl.): 1S–33S.

American College of Sports Medicine. 1998. *ACSM's Resource Manual for Guidelines for Exercise Testing and Prescription*, 3d ed. Baltimore, Md.: Williams & Wilkins.

Anderson, G. B., et al. 1999. Epidemiological features of chronic low-back pain. *Lancet*, 354:581–585.

Better than your bed. New therapy for sciatic pain, 1999. *Prevention*, 8:37.

Bobo, M., and M. Yarbrough. 1999. The effects of long-term aerobic dance on agility and flexibility. *Journal of Sports Medicine and Physical Fitness* 39:165–168.

Carpenter, D. M., and B. W. Nelson. 1999. Low back strengthening for the prevention and treatment of low back pain. *Medicine and Science in Sports and Exercise* 31:18–24.

Evanoff, A., and W. P. Newton. 1999. An alternative treatment for low back pain. *Journal of Family Practice* 48: 416–417.

Fischer, J. S. 1999. News you can use: your achin' back. *U.S. News and World Report,* 11 October, 64–70.

Glascoe, W. M. et al. 1999. Weight-bearing immobilization and early exercise treatment following a grade 2 lateral ankle sprain. *Journal of Orthopaedic and Sports Physical Therapy* 29: 394–399.

Hartigan, C., et al. 2000. Long-term exercise adherence after intensive rehabilitation for chronic low back pain. *Medicine and Science in Sports and Exercise* 32(3): 551–557.

Jones, C. J., et al. 1998. The reliability and validity of a chair sit-and-reach test as a measure of hamstring flexibility in older adults. *Research Quarterly for Exercise and Sport* 29:338–343.

Keen, S., et al. 1999. Individuals with low back pain: How do they view physical activity? *Family Practice* 16:39–45.

Lauerman, W. and N. White. 1999. Toward optimal health: The experts respond to 'my achin' back,' *Journal of Women's Health* 8:27–31.

Leggett, S., et al. 1999. Restorative exercise for clinical low back pain: A prospective two-center study with 1-year follow-up. *Spine* 24:889–898.

Lieber, R. L., and J. Friden. 2000. Mechanisms of muscle injury after eccentric contraction. *Journal of Science and Medicine in Sport* 2(3): 253–265.

Lonn, J. H., et al. 1999. Active back school: Prophylactic management for low back pain. A randomized, controlled, 1-year follow-up study. *Spine* 24:865–871.

Moffett, J. K., et al. 1999. Randomised controlled trial of exercise for low back pain: Clinical outcomes, costs, and preferences. *British Medical Journal* 319:279–283.

Nieman, D. C. 1999. *Exercise Testing and Prescription: A Health-Related Approach,* 4th ed. Mountain View, Calif.: Mayfield.

Novy, D. M., et al. 1999. Physical performance: Differences in men and women with and without low back pain. *Archives of Physical Medicine and Rehabilitation* 80:195–298.

Parente, D. 2000. Influence of aerobic and stretching exercise on anxiety and sensation-seeking mood state. *Perceptual and Motor Skills* 90(1): 347–348.

Patel, A. T., and A. A. Ogle. 2000. Diagnosis and management of acute low back pain. *American Family Physician* 61(6): 1779–1786, 1789–1790.

Pope, R. P., et al. 2000. A randomized trial of preexercise stretching for prevention of lower limb injury. *Medicine and Science in Sports and Exercise* 32 (2): 271–277.

Roberts, J. M., and K. Wilson. 1999. Effect of stretching duration on active and passive range of motion in the lower extremity. *British Journal of Sports Medicine* 33:259–263.

Samanta, A. and J. Beardsley. 1999. Low back pain: Which is the best way forward? *British Medical Journal* 318: 1122–1123.

Suni, J. H., et al. 1999. Health-related fitness test battery for middle-aged adults: Associations with physical activity patterns. *International Journal of Sports Medicine* 20:183–191.

Tyler, T. F., et al. 1999. Reliability and validity of a new method of measuring posterior shoulder tightness. *Journal of Orthopaedic and Sports Physical Therapy* 29:262–274.

Name _____ Section _____ Date _____

LAB 5-1 *Assessing Your Current Level of Flexibility*

Part I Sit-and-Reach Test

Equipment

A flexibility box or measuring device (see photograph). If you make your own measuring device, use two pieces of wood 12 inches high attached at right angles to each other. Use a ruler or yardstick to measure the extent of reach. With the low numbers of the ruler toward the person being tested, set the 6-inch mark of the ruler at the footline of the box. (Individuals who cannot reach as far as the footline will have scores below 6 inches; those who can reach past their feet will have scores above 6 inches.)

Preparation

Warm up your muscles with some low-intensity activity such as walking or easy jogging.

Instructions

1. Remove your shoes, and sit facing the flexibility box with your knees fully extended and your feet about 4 inches apart. Your feet should be flat against the box.

2. Reach as far forward as you can, with palms down and one hand placed on top of the other. Hold the position of maximum reach for 1–2 seconds. Keep your knees locked at all times.

3. Repeat the stretch two times. Your score is the most distant point reached with the fingertips of both hands on the third trial, measured to the nearest quarter of an inch.

   Footline of your box: _____ in.   Score of third trial: _____ in.

The sit-and-reach test.

Rating Your Flexibility

Find your score in the table below to determine your flexibility rating.

Rating: _____

Ratings for Sit-and-Reach Test

| | Rating/Score (in.)* | | | | |
Men	*Very Poor*	*Poor*	*Moderate*	*High*	*Very High*
Age: 15–19	Below 5.25	5.25–6.75	7.00–8.75	9.00–10.75	Above 10.75
20–29	Below 5.50	5.50–7.00	7.25–8.75	9.00–11.00	Above 11.00
30–39	Below 4.75	4.75–6.50	6.75–8.50	8.75–10.25	Above 10.25
40–49	Below 2.75	2.75–5.00	5.25–6.75	7.00–9.25	Above 9.25
50–59	Below 2.00	2.00–5.00	5.25–6.50	6.75–9.25	Above 9.25
60 and over	Below 1.75	1.75–3.25	3.50–5.25	5.50–8.50	Above 8.50
Women					
Age: 15–19	Below 7.25	7.25–8.75	9.00–10.50	10.75–12.25	Above 12.25
20–29	Below 6.75	6.75–8.50	8.75–10.00	10.25–11.50	Above 11.50
30–39	Below 6.50	6.50–8.00	8.25–9.50	9.75–11.50	Above 11.50
40–49	Below 5.50	5.50–7.25	7.50–8.75	9.00–10.50	Above 10.50
50–59	Below 5.50	5.50–7.25	7.50–8.50	8.75–10.75	Above 10.75
60 and over	Below 4.75	4.75–6.00	6.25–7.75	8.00–9.25	Above 9.25

*Footline is set at 6 inches.

SOURCE: Published in the *Canadian Standardized Test of Fitness Operations Manual,* 3rd edition, 1986. Reprinted by permission from the Canadian Society for Exercise Physiology.

Part II Range-of-Motion Assessment

This portion of the lab can be completed by doing visual comparisons or by measuring joint range of motion with a goniometer or other instrument.

Equipment

1. A partner to do visual comparisons or to measure the range of motion of your joints. (You can also use a mirror to perform your own visual comparisons.)
2. For the measurement method, you need a goniometer, flexometer, or other instrument to measure range of motion.

Preparation

None

Instructions

A. *Visual comparison method:* On the following pages, the average range of motion is illustrated for some of the major joints. Compare the range of motion in your joints to that shown in the illustrations. For each joint, note (with a check mark) whether your range of motion is average or greater or needs improvement.

B. *Measurement method:* Measure the appropriate range of motion with a goniometer, flexometer, or other instrument. Record your range of motion in degrees, and find your rating in the appropriate table. (Ratings are taken from several published sources.)

For both methods, record your scores on the following pages and on the chart on the final page of this lab.

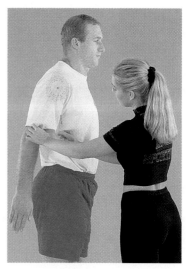

Assessment of range of motion using a goniometer.

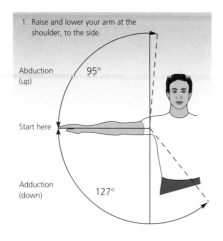

1. Raise and lower your arm at the shoulder, to the side.

Abduction (up) 95°

Start here

Adduction (down) 127°

A. Comparison Method (✓)

    Abduction: Average or above _____ Needs improvement _____

    Adduction: Average or above _____ Needs improvement _____

B. Measurement Method

    Abduction: _____ ° Rating: _____

    Adduction: _____ ° Rating: _____

Ratings

	Abduction	Adduction
Below average	<92°	<124°
Average	92°–95°	124°–127°
Above average	96°–99°	128°–130°
Excellent	>99°	>130°

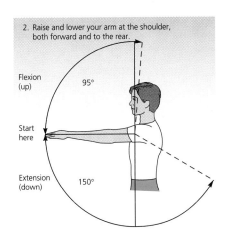

2. Raise and lower your arm at the shoulder, both forward and to the rear.

Flexion (up) 95°

Start here

Extension (down) 150°

A. Comparison Method (✓)

Flexion: Average or above _____ Needs improvement _____

Extension: Average or above _____ Needs improvement _____

B. Measurement Method

Flexion: _____ °   Rating: _____

Extension: _____ °   Rating: _____

Ratings

	Flexion	Extension
Below average	<92°	<145°
Average	92°–95°	145°–150°
Above average	96°–99°	151°–156°
Excellent	>99°	>156°

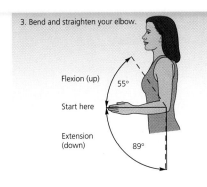

3. Bend and straighten your elbow.

Flexion (up) 55°

Start here

Extension (down) 89°

A. Comparison Method (✓)

Flexion: Average or above _____ Needs improvement _____

Extension: Average or above _____ Needs improvement _____

B. Measurement Method

Flexion: _____ °   Rating: _____

Extension: _____ °   Rating: _____

Ratings

	Flexion	Extension
Below average	<51°	<88°
Average	51°–55°	88°–89°
Above average	56°–60°	90°–91°
Excellent	>60°	>91°

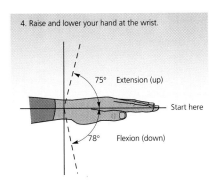

4. Raise and lower your hand at the wrist.

75° Extension (up)

Start here

78° Flexion (down)

A. Comparison Method (✓)

Extension: Average or above _____ Needs improvement _____

Flexion: Average or above _____ Needs improvement _____

B. Measurement Method

Extension: _____ °   Rating: _____

Flexion: _____ °   Rating: _____

Ratings

	Extension	Flexion
Below average	<70°	<73°
Average	70°–75°	73°–78°
Above average	76°–81°	79°–84°
Excellent	>81°	>84°

ACTIVITIES

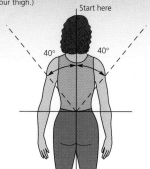

Bend directly sideways at your waist. (To prevent injury, keep your knees slightly bent, and support your trunk by placing your hand or forearm on your thigh.)

Start here

40° 40°

A. Comparison Method (✓)

Right lateral flexion: Average or above _____ Needs improvement _____

Left lateral flexion: Average or above _____ Needs improvement _____

B. Measurement Method:

Right lateral flexion: _____ ° Rating: _____

Left lateral flexion: _____ ° Rating: _____

Ratings

	Right or Left Lateral Flexion
Below average	<36°
Average	36°–40°
Above average	41°–45°
Excellent	>45

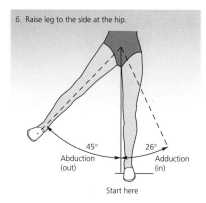

6. Raise leg to the side at the hip.

45°
Abduction
(out)

26°
Adduction
(in)

Start here

A. Comparison Method (✓)

Abduction: Average or above _____ Needs improvement _____

Adduction: Average or above _____ Needs improvement _____

B. Measurement Method

Abduction: _____ ° Rating: _____

Adduction: _____ ° Rating: _____

Ratings

	Abduction	Adduction
Below average	<40°	<23°
Average	40°–45°	23°–26°
Above average	46°–51°	27°–30°
Excellent	>51°	>30°

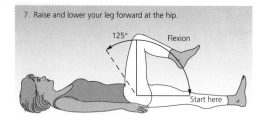

7. Raise and lower your leg forward at the hip.

125° Flexion

Start here

A. Comparison Method (✓)

Average or above _____ Needs improvement _____

B. Measurement Method

Flexion: _____ ° Rating: _____

Ratings

	Flexion
Below average	<121°
Average	121°–125°
Above average	126°–130°
Excellent	>130°

LABORATORY ACTI

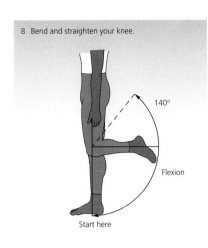

8. Bend and straighten your knee.

140°

Flexion

Start here

A. Comparison Method (✓)

Average or above _____ Needs improvement _____

B. Measurement Method

Flexion: _____° Rating: _____

Ratings

	Flexion
Below average	<136°
Average	136°–140°
Above average	141°–145°
Excellent	>145°

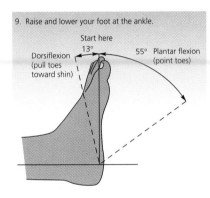

9. Raise and lower your foot at the ankle.

Start here

13°

Dorsiflexion (pull toes toward shin)

55° Plantar flexion (point toes)

A. Comparison Method (✓)

Dorsiflexion: Average or above _____ Needs improvement _____

Plantar flexion: Average or above _____ Needs improvement _____

B. Measurement Method

Dorsiflexion: _____° Rating: _____

Plantar flexion: _____° Rating: _____

Ratings

	Dorsiflexion	Plantar flexion
Below average	<9°	<50°
Average	9°–13°	50°–55°
Above average	14°–17°	56°–60°
Excellent	>17°	>60°

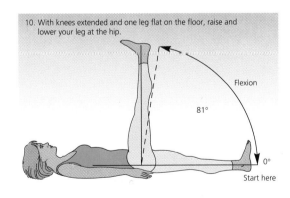

10. With knees extended and one leg flat on the floor, raise and lower your leg at the hip.

Flexion

81°

0°

Start here

A. Comparison Method (✓)

Average or above _____ Needs improvement _____

B. Measurement Method

Flexion: _____° Rating: _____

Ratings

	Flexion
Below average	<79°
Average	79°–81°
Above average	82°–84°
Excellent	>84°

Rating Your Flexibility

Sit-and-Reach Test

Score: _____ in.　Rating: _____

Range of Motion Assessment

			Comparison Method (✓)		Measurement Method	
Joint		*Average ROM*	*Average or above*	*Needs improvement*	*Current range of motion (°)*	*Rating*
Shoulder (side-to-side)	Abduction	95°				
	Adduction	127°				
Shoulder (front-to-back)	Flexion	95°				
	Extension	150°				
Elbow (up-and-down)	Flexion	55°				
	Extension	89°				
Wrist (up-and-down)	Extension	75°				
	Flexion	78°				
Low back (side-to-side)	Right flexion	40°				
	Left flexion	40°				
Hip (side-to-side)	Abduction	45°				
	Adduction	26°				
Hip (bent knee)	Flexion	125°				
Knee	Flexion	140°				
Ankle	Dorsiflexion	13°				
	Plantar flexion	55°				
Hip (straight knee)	Flexion	81°				

To monitor your progress toward your goal, enter the results of this lab in the Preprogram Assessment column of Appendix D. After following the stretching program for several weeks, do this lab again, and enter the results in the Postprogram Assessment column of Appendix D. How do the results compare?

Name _____ Section _____ Date _____

 LAB 5-2 *Creating a Personalized Program for Developing Flexibility*

Complete the program plan below, and start on your flexibility program.

Exercises: The exercises contained in the program plan below are those from the general stretching program presented in Chapter 5. You can add or delete exercises depending on your needs, goals, and preferences. For any exercises you add, fill in the areas of the body affected.

Frequency: A minimum frequency of 2–3 days per week is recommended. You may want to do your stretching exercises the same days you plan to do cardiorespiratory endurance exercise or weight training, because muscles stretch better following exercise, when they are warm.

Intensity: All stretches should be done to the point of mild discomfort, not pain.

Duration: All stretches should be held for 10–30 seconds. (PNF techniques should include a 6-second contraction followed by a 10–30-second assisted stretch.)

Repetitions: All stretches should be performed at least 4 times.

Program Plan for Flexibility

Exercise	Areas Stretched	Frequency (check ✔)						
		M	T	W	Th	F	Sa	Su
Head turns and tilts	Neck							
Towel stretch	Triceps, shoulders, chest							
Across-the-body stretch	Shoulders, upper back							
Upper-back stretch	Upper back							
Lateral stretch	Trunk muscles							
Step stretch	Hip, front of thigh (quadriceps)							
Side lunge	Inner thigh, hip, calf							
Sole stretch	Inner thigh, hip							
Trunk rotation	Trunk, outer thigh and hip, lower back							
Alternate leg stretcher	Back of the thigh (hamstring), hip, knee, ankle, buttocks							
Modified hurdler stretch	Back of the thigh (hamstring), lower back							
Lower-leg stretch	Back of the lower leg (calf, soleus, Achilles tendon)							

You can monitor your program using a chart like the one on the next page.

Flexibility Program Chart

Fill in the dates you perform each stretch, the number of seconds you hold each stretch (should be 10–30), and the number of repetitions of each (should be at least 4). For an easy check on the duration of your stretches, count "one thousand one, one thousand two," and so on. You will probably find that over time you'll be able to hold each stretch longer (in addition to being able to stretch farther).

Exercise/Date																						
	Duration																					
	Reps																					
	Duration																					
	Reps																					
	Duration																					
	Reps																					
	Duration																					
	Reps																					
	Duration																					
	Reps																					
	Duration																					
	Reps																					
	Duration																					
	Reps																					
	Duration																					
	Reps																					
	Duration																					
	Reps																					
	Duration																					
	Reps																					
	Duration																					
	Reps																					
	Duration																					
	Reps																					
	Duration																					
	Reps																					
	Duration																					
	Reps																					
	Duration																					
	Reps																					
	Duration																					
	Reps																					

Body Composition

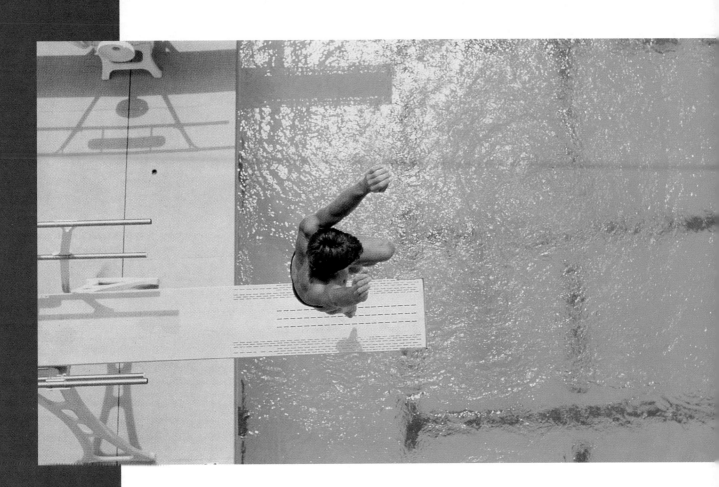

LOOKING AHEAD

After reading this chapter, you should be able to answer these questions about body composition:

- What are fat-free mass, essential fat, and nonessential fat, and what are their functions in the body?

- How does body composition affect wellness?

- How are body composition and body fat distribution measured?

- What is recommended body weight, and how is it determined?

145

ody composition, the body's relative amount of fat and fat-free mass, is an important component of fitness for wellness. People whose body composition is optimal tend to be healthier, to move more efficiently, and to feel better about themselves. To reach wellness, you must determine what body composition is right for you and then work to achieve and maintain it.

Although people pay lip service to the idea of exercising for health, a more immediate goal for many is to look fit and healthy. Unfortunately, many people don't succeed in their efforts to obtain a fit and healthy body because they emphasize short-term weight loss rather than the permanent changes in lifestyle that lead to fat loss and a healthy body composition. Successful management of body composition requires the coordination of many aspects of a wellness program, including proper nutrition, adequate exercise, and stress management.

This chapter focuses on defining and measuring body composition and determining recommended body weight; Chapter 9 provides specific strategies for changing your lifestyle to reach your body composition goal.

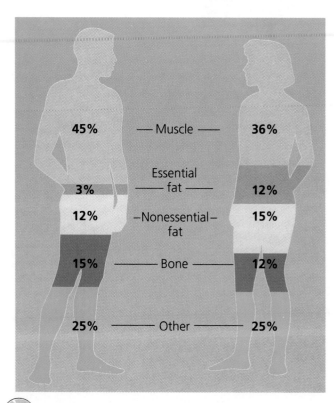

Figure 6-1　Body composition of a typical man and woman, 20–24 years old. SOURCE: Adapted from Brooks, G. A., et al. 2000. *Exercise Physiology: Human Bioenergetics and Its Applications,* 3d ed. Mountain View, Calif.: Mayfield.

WHAT IS BODY COMPOSITION, AND WHY IS IT IMPORTANT?

The human body can be divided into fat-free mass and body fat. Fat-free mass is composed of all the body's nonfat tissues: bone, water, muscle, connective tissue, organ tissues, and teeth. Body fat includes both essential and nonessential body fats (Figure 6-1). **Essential fat** includes lipids incorporated into the nerves, brain, heart, lungs, liver, and mammary glands. These fat deposits, crucial for normal body functioning, make up approximately 3% of total body weight in men and 12% in women. (The larger percentage in women is due to fat deposits in the breasts, uterus, and other sites specific to females.) **Nonessential (storage) fat** exists primarily within fat cells, or **adipose tissue,** often located just below the skin and around major organs. The amount of storage fat varies from individual to individual based on many factors, including gender, age, heredity, metabolism, diet, and activity level. Excess storage fat is usually the result of consuming more energy (as food) than is expended (in metabolism and physical activity).

How much body fat is too much? In the past, many people relied on height-weight tables based on insurance company mortality statistics to answer this question. Unfortunately, these tables can be highly inaccurate for some people; at best, they provide only an indirect measure of fatness. Because, as explained in Chapter 4, muscle tissue is denser and heavier than fat, a fit person can easily weigh more and an unfit person weigh less than recommended weights on a height-weight table.

The most important consideration when a person is looking at body composition is the proportion of the body's total weight that is fat—the **percent body fat.** For example, two women may both be 5 feet, 5 inches tall and weigh 130 pounds. But one woman, a runner, may have only 15% of her body weight as fat, whereas the second, sedentary woman could have 33% body fat. Although neither woman is overweight by most standards, the second woman is overfat. Too much body fat (not total weight) has a negative effect on health and well-being.

Some of the most commonly used methods to assess and classify body composition are described later in the chapter. Although less accurate than standards based on body fat, some methods are based on total body weight because it is easier to measure. **Overweight** is usually defined as total body weight above the recommended range for good health (as determined by large-scale population surveys). **Obesity** is defined as a more serious degree of overweight; the cutoff point for obesity may be set in terms of percent body fat, as in Table 6-1, or in terms of some measure of total body weight.

By any measure, Americans are getting fatter. Since 1991, the number of Americans having a body composition categorized as obese has nearly doubled (from 12.0% in 1991 to 17.9 in 1998), and more than 50% of Ameri-

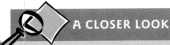

Negative Health Consequences of Obesity

An obese person is at increased risk for the following:

Early death

Death from CVD, including sudden death

Hypertension

Diabetes and insulin resistance

Gallbladder disease

Cancer of the colon, prostate, esophagus, gallbladder, ovary, endometrium, breast, and cervix

Arthritis and gout

Back pain

Complications during pregnancy

Menstrual abnormalities

Shortness of breath

Sleep apnea (intermittent cessation of breathing while sleeping)

Obesity is also associated with the following:

Increased LDL and triglyceride concentrations

Decreased HDL concentration

Impaired heart function (ventricles)

Impaired immune function

---

can adults are now overweight. The increased incidence of obesity between 1991 and 1998 was 67.2% in the South Atlantic states. The reason for increased body fat in the population is not totally clear, but it is related to decreased physical activity and increased caloric consumption. As discussed in Chapter 2, more than half of all Americans do not meet the minimum recommendation of 30 minutes per day of moderate physical activity. More people are working in white-collar and service professions than in jobs involving physical activity. And increased access to items such as home computers and cable television has also contributed to more sedentary lifestyles. In addition to exercising less, Americans are eating more. The Centers for Disease Control and Prevention has estimated that caloric intake has increased by 100–300 calories a day during the past decade. (For more on the causes of obesity, see Chapter 9.)

Though not as prevalent a problem, having too little body fat is also dangerous (see Table 6-1). Too much or too little body fat can have negative effects on health, performance, and self-image.

Health

Obesity is associated with a wide variety of health problems, many of which are listed in the box "Negative Health Consequences of Obesity." Obese people have an overall mortality rate almost twice that of nonobese people. They are more than five times as likely to develop diabetes (see the box "Diabetes"). In 1998, the American Heart Association classified obesity as one of the major risk factors for heart disease. It is estimated that if all Americans had a healthy body composition, the incidence of coronary heart disease would drop by 25%.

The distribution of fat is also an important indicator of future health. Although fat distribution is a controversial topic among scientists, studies suggest that people who tend to gain weight in the abdominal area ("apples") have

TABLE 6-1	*Percent Body Fat Standards for Men and Women*	
	Men	**Women**
At risk[a]	≤5%	≤8%
Below average	6–14%	9–22%
Average	15%	23%
Above Average	16–24%	24–31%
At risk[b]	≥25%	≥32%

[a]At risk for diseases and disorders associated with malnutrition
[b]At risk for diseases associated with obesity

Note: These percentages represent approximate standards for body composition; the healthy range varies, depending on health status and risk factors for disease. For example, a man with high blood pressure and high cholesterol levels might want to reduce his percentage of body fat, even if it is within the acceptable range for the general population.

SOURCE: Heyward, V. H. 1998. *Advanced Fitness Assessment and Exercise Prescription.* Champaign, Ill.: Human Kinetics.

TERMS

essential fat   The fat in the body necessary for normal body functioning.

nonessential (storage) fat   Extra fat or fat reserves stored in the body.

adipose tissue   Connective tissue in which fat is stored.

percent body fat   The percentage of total body weight that is composed of fat.

overweight   Characterized by a body weight above a recommended range for good health; ranges are set through large-scale population surveys.

obese   Severely overweight, characterized by an excessive accumulation of body fat: 25% of body weight or more as fat in men, and 32% or more as fat in women. Obesity may also be defined in terms of some measure of total body weight.

Diabetes mellitus is a disease that causes a disruption of normal metabolism. The pancreas, a long, thin organ located behind the stomach, normally secretes the hormone insulin, which stimulates cells to take up glucose to produce energy. In a person with diabetes, this process is disrupted, causing a buildup of glucose in the bloodstream. Over the long term, diabetes is associated with kidney failure; nerve damage; circulation problems; retinal damage and blindness; and increased rates of heart attack, stroke, and hypertension. The rate of diabetes has increased steadily over the past 40 years, and it is currently the seventh leading cause of death in the United States.

Types of Diabetes

Approximately 16 million Americans—nearly 6% of the population—have one of two major forms of diabetes. About 5–10% of people with diabetes have the more serious form, known as Type 1 diabetes. In this type of diabetes, the pancreas produces little or no insulin, so daily doses of insulin are required. (Without insulin, a person with Type 1 can lapse into a coma.) Type 1 diabetes usually strikes before age 30.

The remaining 15 million Americans with diabetes have Type 2 diabetes. This condition can develop slowly, and about half of affected individuals are unaware of their condition. In Type 2 diabetes, the pancreas doesn't produce enough insulin, the cells don't respond to the hormone, or both. This condition is usually diagnosed in people over age 40. About one-third of people with Type 2 diabetes must inject insulin; others may take medications that increase insulin production or stimulate cells to take up glucose.

A third type of diabetes occurs in about 2–3% of women during pregnancy. So-called gestational diabetes usually disappears after pregnancy, but more than half of women who experience it eventually develop Type 2 diabetes.

The major factors involved in the development of diabetes are age, obesity, physical inactivity, a family history of diabetes, and lifestyle. Excess body fat reduces cell sensitivity to insulin, and it is a major risk factor for Type 2 diabetes. Ethnic background also plays a role. African Americans and people of Hispanic background are 55% more likely than non-Hispanic whites to develop Type 2 diabetes; more than 20% of Hispanics over age 65 have diabetes. Native Americans also have a higher-than-average incidence of diabetes.

Treatment

There is no cure for diabetes, but it can be successfully managed. Treatment involves keeping blood sugar levels within safe limits through diet, exercise, and, if necessary, medication. Blood sugar levels can be monitored using a home test. Recent research indicates that close monitoring and control of glucose levels can significantly reduce the rate of serious complications among people with diabetes. Nearly 90% of people with Type 2 diabetes are overweight when diagnosed, and an important step in treatment is to lose weight. Even a small amount of weight loss can be beneficial. People with diabetes should eat regular meals with an emphasis on complex carbohydrates and ample dietary fiber; a dietitian can help design a healthy eating plan. Regular exercise and a healthy diet are often sufficient to control Type 2 diabetes.

Prevention

Recent studies have shown that exercise can help prevent the development of Type 2 diabetes, a benefit especially important in individuals with one or more risk factors for the disease. Exercise burns excess sugar and makes cells more sensitive to insulin. Exercise also helps keep body fat at healthy levels.

Eating a moderate diet to help control body fat is perhaps the most important dietary recommendation for the prevention of diabetes. However, there is some evidence that the composition of the diet may also be important. In a long-term study of more than 65,000 nurses, a diet low in fiber and high in sugar and refined carbohydrates was found to increase risk for Type 2 diabetes. The foods most closely linked to higher diabetes risk were regular (non-diet) cola beverages, white bread, white rice, french fries, and potatoes; consumption of cereal fibers such as those found in cold breakfast cereals was associated with lower risk. (See chapter 8 for more information on different types of carbohydrates and specific strategies for increasing fiber intake.)

Warning Signs and Testing

A wellness lifestyle that includes a healthy diet and regular exercise is the best strategy for preventing diabetes. If you do develop diabetes, the best way to avoid complications is to recognize the symptoms and get early diagnosis and treatment. Be alert for the following warning signs:

- Frequent urination
- Extreme hunger or thirst
- Unexplained weight loss
- Extreme fatigue
- Blurred vision
- Frequent infections, especially of the bladder, gums, skin, or vagina
- Cuts and bruises that are slow to heal
- Tingling or numbness in the hands and feet
- Generalized itching, with no rash

Type 2 diabetes is often asymptomatic in the early stages, and major health organizations now recommend routine screening for people over age 45 and anyone younger who is at high risk, including anyone who is obese. (The Web site for the American Diabetes Association, listed in the For More Information section at the end of the chapter, includes an interactive diabetes risk assessment.) Screening involves a blood test to check glucose levels after either a period of fasting or the administration of a set dose of glucose. If you are concerned about your risk for diabetes, talk with your physician about being tested.

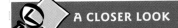
While obesity is at epidemic levels in the United States, many girls and women strive for unrealistic thinness in response to pressure from peers and a society obsessed with appearance. This quest for thinness has led to an increasingly common, underreported condition called the **female athlete triad.**

The triad consists of three interrelated disorders: abnormal eating patterns (and excessive exercising), followed by lack of menstrual periods (amenorrhea), followed by decreased bone density (premature osteoporosis). Left untreated, the triad can lead to decreased physical performance, increased incidence of bone fractures, disturbances of heart rhythm and metabolism, and even death.

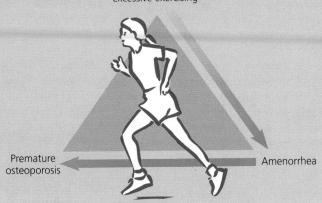

Abnormal eating patterns and excessive exercising

Premature osteoporosis

Amenorrhea

Abnormal eating is the event from which the other two components of the triad flow. Abnormal eating ranges from moderately restricting food intake, to binge eating and purging (bulimia), to severely restricting food intake (anorexia nervosa). Whether serious or relatively mild, eating disorders prevent women from consuming enough calories to meet their bodies' needs.

Eating disorders, combined with intense exercise and emotional stress, can suppress the hormones that control the menstrual cycle. If the menstrual cycle stops for three consecutive months, the condition is called amenorrhea. Prolonged amenorrhea can lead to osteoporosis; bone density may erode to the point that a woman in her 20s will have the bone density of a woman in her 60s. Women with osteoporosis have fragile, easily fractured bones.

All physically active women and girls have the potential to develop one or more components of the female athlete triad; for example, it is estimated that 5–20% of women who exercise regularly and vigorously may develop amenorrhea. But the triad is most prevalent among athletes who participate in certain sports: those in which appearance is highly important, those that emphasize a prepubertal body shape, those that require contour-revealing clothing for competition, those that require endurance, and those that use weight categories for participation. Such sports include gymnastics, figure skating, swimming, distance running, cycling, cross-country skiing, track, volleyball, rowing, horse racing, and cheerleading.

The female athlete triad can be life-threatening, and health professionals are taking it seriously. Typical signs of the eating disorders that trigger the condition are extreme weight loss, dry skin, loss of hair, brittle fingernails, cold hands and feet, low blood pressure and heart rate, swelling around the ankles and hands, and weakening of the bones. Female athletes who have repeated stress fractures may be suffering from the condition. Early intervention is the key to stopping this series of interrelated conditions. Unfortunately, once the condition has progressed, long-term consequences, especially bone loss, are unavoidable. Teenagers may need only to learn about good eating habits; college-age women with a long-standing problem may require psychological counseling.

SOURCES: Otis, C. 1998. Too slim, amenorrheic, fracture-prone: The female athlete triad. *ACSM's Health and Fitness Journal* 2(1): 20–25. Smith, A. 1996. The female athlete triad: Causes, diagnosis, and treatment. *Physician and Sportsmedicine* 24(7). Art: Adapted from Yeager, K. K., et al. The female athlete triad: Disordered eating, amenorrhea, osteoporosis. *Medicine and Science in Sports and Exercise* 25: 775–777. Reprinted by permission of Lipincott, Williams & Wilkins.

a risk of coronary heart disease, high blood pressure, diabetes, and stroke twice as high as that of people who tend to gain weight in the hip area ("pears"). The reason for this increased risk is not entirely clear, but it appears that fat in the abdomen is more easily mobilized and sent into the bloodstream, increasing disease-related blood fat levels. In general, men tend to gain weight in the abdominal area and women in the hip area, but women who exhibit the male pattern of fat distribution face the increased health risks associated with it. Researchers have also found ethnic differences in the relative significance of increased abdominal fat, but more studies are needed to clarify the relationships among fat distribution, ethnicity, and disease.

Body fat distribution is usually assessed by measuring waist circumference or by calculating waist-to-hip ratio (the relative circumference of the waist and hips). A person doesn't have to be technically overfat to have fat distribution be a risk factor, nor do all overfat people face this increased risk. However, individuals in the obese range should not be complacent about their body composition regardless of their fat distribution—all obesity has serious health consequences.

TERMS

female athlete triad A condition consisting of three interrelated disorders: abnormal eating patterns (and excessive exercising) followed by lack of menstrual periods (amenorrhea) and decreased bone density (premature osteoporosis).

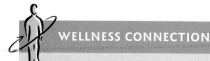

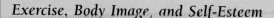

If you gaze into the mirror and wish you could change the way your body looks, consider getting some exercise—not to re-shape your contours but to firm up your body image and enhance your self-esteem. In a recent study, 82 adults completed a 12-week aerobic exercise program (using cycle ergometry) and had 12 months of follow-up. Compared with the control group, the participants improved their fitness and also benefited psychologically in tests of mood, anxiety, and self-concept. These same physical and psychological benefits were still significant at the 1-year follow-up.

One reason for the findings may be that people who exercise regularly often gain a sense of mastery and competence that enhances their self-esteem and body image. In addition, exercise contributes to a more toned look, which many adults prefer. Research suggests that physically active people are more comfortable with their bodies and their image than sedentary people are. In one workplace study, 60 employees were asked to complete a 36-session stretching program whose main purpose was to prevent muscle strains at work. At the end of the program, besides the significant increase by all participants in measurements of flexibility, their perceptions of their bodies improved and so did their overall sense of self-worth.

Similar results were obtained in a Norwegian study, in which 219 middle-aged people at risk for heart disease were randomly assigned to one of four groups: diet, diet plus exercise, exercise, and no intervention. The greater the participation of individuals in the exercise component of the program, the higher were their scores in perceived competence/self-esteem and coping.

SOURCES: DiLorenzo, T. M., et al. 1999. Long-term effects of aerobic exercise on psychological outcomes. *Preventive Medicine* 28(1): 75–85. Sorensen, M., et al. 1999. The effect of exercise and diet on mental health and quality of life in middle-aged individuals with elevated risk factors for cardiovascular disease. *Journal of Sports Science* 17(5): 369–377. Moore, T. M. 1998. A workplace stretching program. *AAOHN Journal* 46(12): 563–568.

Is it possible to be too lean? Health experts have generally viewed too little body fat—less than 8% for women and 5% for men—as a threat to health and well-being. Extreme leanness has been linked with reproductive, circulatory, and immune system disorders. Extremely lean people may experience muscle wasting and fatigue; they are also more likely to suffer from a dangerous eating disorder. For women, an extremely low percentage of body fat is associated with **amenorrhea** and loss of bone mass. (see the box "The Female Athlete Triad"). However, a study from Harvard Medical School found that among nonsmoking women who did not suffer from eating disorders, the leanest lived longer than women of "normal" weight. The authors of this study concluded that even mild to moderate overweight is associated with a substantial increase in the risk of premature death. Additional research is needed to determine all the effects of extremely low body fat levels on health.

Performance of Physical Activities

Too much body fat makes all types of physical activity more difficult because just moving the body through everyday activities means working harder and using more energy. In general, overfat people are less fit than others and don't have the muscular strength, endurance, and flexibility that make normal activity easy. Because exercise is more difficult, they do less of it, depriving themselves of an effective way to improve body composition.

Self-Image

The "fashionable" body image has changed dramatically during the past 50 years, varying from slightly plump to an almost unhealthy thinness. Today a fit and healthy-looking body, developed through a healthy lifestyle, is the goal for most people (see the box "Exercise, Body Image and Self-Esteem."). The key to this "look" is a balance of proper nutrition and exercise—in short, a lifestyle that emphasizes wellness.

Goals for body composition should be realistic, however; a person's ability to change body composition through diet and exercise depends not only on a wellness program, but also on heredity. Unrealistic expectations about body composition can have a negative impact on self-image and can lead to the development of eating disorders. (For more information on eating disorders, see Chapter 9.)

For most people, body fat percentage falls somewhere between ideal and a level that is significantly unhealthy. If they consistently maintain a wellness lifestyle that includes a healthy diet and regular exercise, the right body composition will naturally develop.

Wellness for Life

A healthy body composition is vital for wellness throughout life. Strong scientific evidence suggests that controlling your weight will increase your life span; reduce the risk of heart disease, cancer, diabetes, insulin resistance, and back pain; increase your energy level; and improve your self-esteem.

ASSESSING BODY COMPOSITION

The morning weighing ritual on the bathroom scale can't reveal whether a fluctuation in weight is due to a change in muscle, body water, or fat and can't differentiate be-

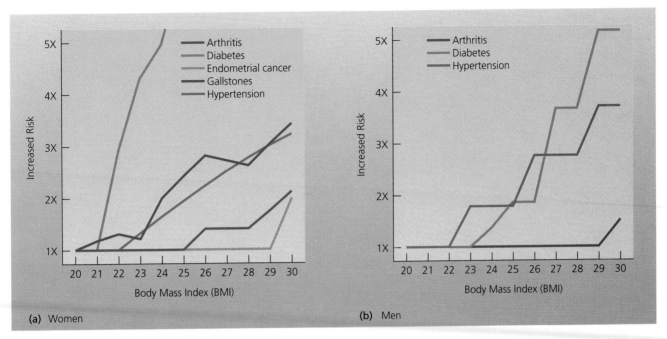

Figure 6-2   BMI and risk of health problems.   SOURCE: How's your weight? 1997. *Nutrition Action Healthletter,* December. Copyright © 1999 CSPI. Adapted from Nutrition Action Healthletter (1875 Connecticut Avenue, N.W., Suite 300, Washington, D.C. 20009-5728. $24.00 for 10 issues).

tween overweight and overfat. A 260-pound football player may be overweight according to population height-weight standards yet actually have much less body fat than average. Likewise, a 40-year-old woman may weigh the same as she did 20 years earlier yet have a considerably different body composition.

There are a number of simple, inexpensive ways to estimate body composition that are superior to the bathroom scale. These methods include body mass index and skinfold measurements.

Body Mass Index

Body mass index (BMI) is a rough measure of body composition that is useful if you don't have access to sophisticated equipment. Though more accurate than height-weight tables, body mass index is also based on the concept that a person's weight should be proportional to height. The measurement is fairly accurate for people who do not have an unusual amount of muscle mass and who are not very short. BMI is calculated by dividing your body weight (expressed in kilograms) by the square of your height (expressed in meters). For example, a person who weighs 130 pounds (59 kilograms) and is 5 feet, 3 inches tall (1.6 meters) would have a BMI of 59 kg ÷ $(1.6 \text{ m})^2$, or 23 kg/m². (Refer to Lab 6-1 for instructions on how to calculate your BMI.)

The relative risk for several health problems associated with different values of BMI is shown in Figure 6-2. At high values of BMI, the risk of arthritis, diabetes, hypertension, endometrial cancer, and other disorders increases substantially. The increased risk of diabetes at

even fairly low values of BMI, especially among women, is of particular concern.

In June 1998, new federal guidelines for classifying overweight and obesity on the basis of BMI were released by the National Heart, Lung, and Blood Institute (NHLBI), a division of the National Institutes of Health. Under these guidelines, a person is classified as overweight if he or she has a BMI of 25 or above and obese if he or she has a BMI of 30 or above (Table 6-2). Previously, the cutoff point for defining overweight was higher; the new guidelines reflect standards used in other countries as well as those used by the World Health Organization. Nearly 55% of American adults have a BMI of 25 or above.

In classifying the health risks associated with overweight and obesity, the NHLBI guidelines consider body fat distribution and other disease risk factors in addition to BMI. As described earlier, excess fat in the abdomen is of greater concern than excess fat in other areas. Methods of assessing body fat distribution are discussed later in the chapter; the NHLBI guidelines use measurement of waist circumference (see Table 6-2). At a given level of overweight, people with a large waist circumference and/or

amenorrhea   Absent or infrequent menstruation, sometimes **TERMS** related to low levels of body fat and excessive quantity or intensity of exercise.

body mass index (BMI)   A measure of relative body weight correlating highly with more direct measures of body fat, calculated by dividing total body weight (in kilograms) by the square of body height (in meters).

TABLE 6-2 *Body Mass Index (BMI) Classification and Disease Risk*

Classification	BMI (kg/m²)	Obesity Class	Disease Risk Relative to Normal Weight and Waist Circumferenceª	
			Men ≤ 40 in. (102 cm) Women ≤ 35 in. (88 cm)	> 40 in. (102 cm) > 35 in. (88 cm)
Underweightᵇ	<18.5		—	—
Normalᶜ	18.5–24.9		—	—
Overweight	25.0–29.9		Increased	High
Obesity	30.0–34.9	I	High	Very high
	35.0–39.9	II	Very high	Very high
Extreme obesity	≥ 40.0	III	Extremely high	Extremely high

ªDisease risk for Type 2 diabetes, hypertension, and cardiovascular disease. The waist circumference cutoff points for increased risk are 40 inches (102 cm) for men and 35 inches (88 cm) for women.

ᵇResearch suggests that a low BMI can be healthy in some cases, as long as it is not the result of smoking, an eating disorder, or an underlying disease process.

ᶜIncreased waist circumference can also be a marker for increased risk, even in persons of normal weight.

SOURCE: Adapted from National Heart, Lung, and Blood Institute. 1998. *Clinical Guidelines on the Identification, Evaluation, and Treatment of Overweight and Obesity in Adults: The Evidence Report.* Bethesda, Md.: National Institutes of Health.

additional disease risk factors are at greater risk for health problems. For example, a man with a BMI of 27, a waist circumference of more than 40 inches, and high blood pressure is at greater risk for health problems than another man who has a BMI of 27 but has a smaller waist circumference and no other risk factors. Thus, optimal BMI for good health depends on many factors; if your BMI is 25 or above, consult a physician for help in determining a healthy BMI for you. (Weight loss recommendations based on the NHLBI guidelines are discussed further in Chapter 9.) Despite its widespread use, BMI does have limitations. Although it is good for large population studies, it is less useful for measuring changes in body composition in individuals.

Skinfold Measurements

Skinfold measurement is a simple, inexpensive, and practical way to assess body composition. Skinfold measurements can be used to assess body composition because equations can link the thickness of skinfolds at various sites to percent body fat calculations from more precise laboratory techniques.

Skinfolds are measured with a device called a **caliper**, which consists of a pair of spring-loaded, calibrated jaws. High-quality calipers are made of metal and have parallel jaw surfaces and constant spring tension. Inexpensive

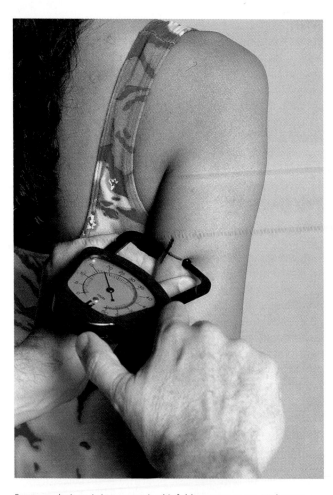

Proper technique is important in skinfold measurement. It's best to take several measurements at each site to ensure accuracy.

TERMS **caliper** A pressure-sensitive measuring instrument with two jaws that can be adjusted to determine thickness.

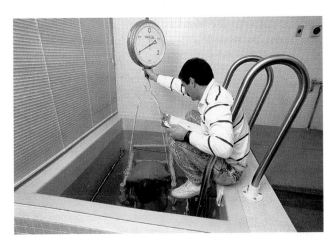

This man is having his body composition assessed in an underwater weighing tank. Muscle has a higher density than water, so people with more lean body mass weigh more under water.

plastic calipers are also available; to ensure accuracy, plastic calipers should be spring-loaded and have metal jaws. Refer to Lab 6-1 for the procedure for taking skinfold measurements. Taking accurate measurements with calipers requires patience, experience, and considerable practice. It's best to take several measurements at each site (or have several different people take each measurement) to help ensure accuracy. Be sure to take the measurements in the exact location called for in the procedure. Because the amount of water in your body changes during the day, skinfold measurements taken in the morning and evening often differ. If you repeat the measurements in the future to track changes in your body composition, measure skinfolds at approximately the same time of day.

Other Methods of Measuring Body Composition

Most of the many other methods for determining body composition are very sophisticated and require expensive equipment. For example, the DXA (dual energy X-ray absorptiometry) technique lets scientists measure body fat by splitting an X-ray beam into two levels. The TOBEC (total body electrical conductivity) technique lets scientists estimate lean body mass by passing a body through a magnetic field. Less expensive methods are available in many health clubs and sports medicine clinics, including underwater weighing, the Bod Pod, and bioelectrical impedance analysis.

Underwater Weighing   Hydrostatic (underwater) weighing is considered one of the most accurate indirect ways to measure body composition. It is the standard used for other techniques, including skinfold measurements. For this method, an individual is submerged and weighed under water. The percentages of fat and fat-free weight are calculated from body density. Muscle has a higher density and fat a lower density than water (1.1 grams per cubic

centimeter for fat-free mass, 0.91 gram per cubic centimeter for fat, and 1 gram per cubic centimeter for water). Therefore, fat people tend to float and weigh less under water, and lean people tend to sink and weigh more under water.

Although somewhat cumbersome and expensive, this method is not beyond limited budgets. A harness and a spring-loaded scale can be connected to a diving board, and the school pool can be used as the underwater weighing tank. Most university exercise physiology departments or sports medicine laboratories have an underwater weighing facility. If you want an accurate assessment of your body composition, find a place that does underwater weighing.

The Bod Pod   The Bod Pod, a small chamber containing computerized sensors, measures body composition by air displacement rather than water displacement. It determines the percentage of fat by calculating how much air is displaced by the person sitting inside the chamber. Many people prefer this short, 5-minute test over underwater weighing because it takes the place of the difficult "dunking" process and is just as accurate.

Bioelectrical Impedance Analysis (BIA)   The BIA technique works by sending a small electrical current through the body and measuring the body's resistance to it. Fat-free tissues, where most body water is located, are good conductors of electrical current, whereas fat is not. Thus, the amount of resistance to electrical current is related to the amount of fat-free tissue in the body (the lower the resistance, the greater the fat-free mass) and can be used to estimate percent body fat. Bioelectrical impedance analysis is fairly accurate for most people (about the same as skinfold measurements). To avoid error, it is important to follow the manufacturer's instructions carefully and to avoid overhydration or underhydration (more or less body water than normal). Because measurement varies with the type of BIA analyzer, use the same instrument to compare measurements over time.

Assessing Body Fat Distribution

Researchers have studied many different methods for determining the risk associated with body fat distribution. Two of the simplest to perform are waist circumference measurement and waist-to-hip ratio calculation. In the first method, you measure your waist circumference; in the second, you divide your waist circumference by your hip circumference. Waist circumference has been found to be a better indicator of abdominal fat than waist-to-hip ratio. More research is needed to determine the precise degree of risk associated with specific values for these two assessments of body fat distribution. However, a total waist measurement of more than 40 inches (102 cm) for men and 35 inches (88 cm) for women and a waist-to-hip ratio above 0.94 for young men and 0.82 for young women are associated with a significantly increased risk of disease. Follow the instructions in Lab 6-1 to measure and rate your body fat distribution.

DETERMINING RECOMMENDED BODY WEIGHT

If the assessment tests indicate that fat loss would be beneficial for you, your first step is to establish a goal. Use the ratings in Table 6-1 or Table 6-2 to choose a target value for percent body fat or BMI (depending on which type of assessment you completed). Select a goal that is realistic for you and will ensure good health. Genetics may limit your capacity to change your body composition. Few people can expect to develop the body of a fashion model or competitive bodybuilder. However, you can improve your body composition through a regular program of exercise and a healthy diet. If you have known risk factors for disease, such as high blood pressure or high levels of blood cholesterol, consult your physician to determine the ideal body composition for your individual risk profile.

Once you've established your goal, you can calculate a target body weight. (Though body weight is not an accurate means of assessing body composition, it's a useful method for tracking progress in a program to change body composition. If you're losing a small or moderate amount of weight and exercising, you're probably losing fat while building muscle mass.) Follow the instructions

in Lab 6-2 to put the results of all the assessment tests together, get an overview of your body composition, and determine a range for recommended body weight.

Using percent body fat or BMI will generate a fairly accurate target body weight for most people. However, it's best not to stick rigidly to a recommended body weight calculated from any formula; individual genetic, cultural, and lifestyle factors are also important. Decide whether the body weight that the formulas generate for you is realistic, meets all your goals, is healthy, *and* is reasonable for you to maintain.

After selecting your overall goal, set realistic intermediate goals. For example, if you want to lose a total of 10 pounds, you might set short-term goals of losing 2 pounds during the first month of your program and 2 more pounds during the second month. To help ensure success, reevaluate your program and your goals frequently.

Track your progress toward your target body composition by checking your body weight periodically. To get a more accurate idea of your progress, especially when weight loss is large, you should directly reassess your body composition occasionally during your program: Body composition changes as weight changes. Losing a lot of weight usually includes losing some muscle mass no matter how hard a person exercises, partly because carrying less weight requires the muscular system to bear a smaller burden. (Conversely, a large gain in weight without exercise still causes some gain in muscle mass because muscles are working harder to carry the extra weight.)

See Chapter 9 for specific strategies for losing or gaining weight and improving body composition.

COMMON QUESTIONS ANSWERED

Is spot reducing effective? No. Spot reducing refers to attempts to lose body fat in specific parts of the body by doing exercises for those parts. For example, a person might try to spot reduce in the legs by doing leg lifts. Spot-reducing exercises contribute to fat loss only to the extent that they burn calories. The only way you can reduce fat in any specific area is to create an overall negative energy balance: Take in less energy (food) than you use up through exercise and metabolism.

How does exercise affect body composition? Cardiorespiratory endurance exercise burns calories, thereby helping create a negative energy balance. Weight training does not use many calories and therefore is of little use in creating a negative energy balance. However, weight training increases muscle mass, which maintains a high metabolic rate (the body's energy level) and helps improve body composition. To minimize body fat and increase muscle mass, thereby improving body composition, combine cardiorespiratory endurance exercise and weight training (Figure 6-3).

How do I develop a toned, healthy-looking body? The development of a healthy-looking body requires regular exercise, proper diet, and other good health habits. However, it helps to have heredity on your side. Some people put on or take off fat more easily than others just as some people are taller than others. Be realistic in your goals, and be satisfied with the improvements in body composition you can make by observing the principles of a wellness lifestyle.

Are people who have a desirable body composition physically fit? Having a healthy body composition is not necessarily associated with overall fitness. For example, many bodybuilders have very little body fat but have poor cardiorespiratory capacity and flexibility. To be fit, you must rate high on all the components of fitness.

What is liposuction, and will it help me lose body fat? Suction lipectomy, popularly known as liposuction, has become the most popular type of elective surgery in the United States. The procedure involves removing limited amounts of fat from specific areas. Typically, no more than 2.5 kg (5.5 lb) of adipose tissue is removed at a time. The procedure is usually successful if the amount of excess fat is limited and skin elasticity is good. The procedure is most effective if integrated into a program of dietary restriction and exercise. Side effects include infection, dimpling, and wavy skin contours. Liposuction has a death rate of 1 in 5000 patients, primarily from pulmonary thromboembolism (a blood clot in the lungs) or fat embolism (circulatory blockage caused by a dislodged piece of fat). Other serious complications include shock, bleeding, and impaired blood flow to vital organs.

What is cellulite, and how do I get rid of it? Cellulite is the name commonly given to ripply, wavy fat deposits that collect just under the skin. However, these rippling fat deposits are really the same as fat deposited anywhere else in the body. The only way to control them is to create a negative energy balance—burn up more calories than are taken in. There are no creams or lotions that will rub away surface (subcutaneous) fat deposits, and spot reducing is also ineffective. The solution is sensible eating habits and exercise.

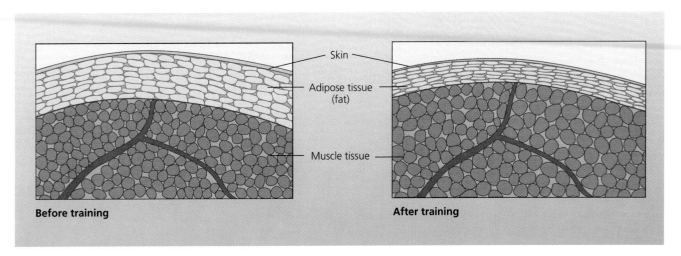

Figure 6-3 Effects of exercise on body composition. Endurance exercise and strength training reduce body fat and increase muscle mass.

SUMMARY

- The human body is composed of fat-free mass (which includes bone, muscle, organ tissues, and connective tissues) and body fat (essential and nonessential).

- Having too much body fat has negative health consequences, especially in terms of cardiovascular disease. Distribution of fat is also a significant factor in health.

- A fit and healthy-looking body, with the right body composition for a particular person, develops from habits of proper nutrition and exercise.

- Measuring body weight is not an accurate way to assess body composition because it does not differentiate between muscle weight and fat weight.

- Two measurements of body composition are body mass index (formulated through weight and height measurements) and percent body fat (formulated through skinfold measurements).

- Hydrostatic weighing is based on body density; muscle has a higher density and fat a lower density than water. The Bod Pod measures the air displaced by a person in a chamber and then calculates the body's density. Bioelectrical impedance analysis estimates the amount of body water (and thereby fat-free tissue) by measuring the body's resistance to a small electrical current.

- Body fat distribution can be assessed through the total waist measurement or the waist-to-hip ratio.

- Recommended body weight can be determined by choosing a target BMI or target body fat percentage. Keep heredity in mind when setting a goal.

Underwater weighing, the Bod Pod, and bioelectrical impedance analysis are often available through campus adult fitness
programs, and health clubs may also provide tests for percent
body fat.

Books

American Diabetes Association. 2000. *American Diabetes Association Complete Guide to Diabetes*, 2d ed. Alexandria, Va.:
American Diabetes Association. *Explains the causes, symptoms, diagnosis, treatment, and self-care of diabetes.*

Brooks, G. A., et al. 2000. *Exercise Physiology: Human Bioenergetics and Its Applications*, 3d ed. Mountain View, Calif.: Mayfield.
*A basic exercise physiology textbook that describes principles of
metabolism and body composition.*

Gaesser, G. A. 1999. *Big Fat Lies: The Truth About Your Weight and
Your Health*. New York: Ballantine Books. *Emphasizes the importance of diet and exercise in maintaining metabolic health.*

Heyward, V. H., and L. M. Stolarczyk. 1996. *Applied Body Composition Assessment*. Champaign, Ill.: Human Kinetics. *Describes different methods of measuring and assessing body composition.*

Kopelman, P. G., and M. J. Stock, eds. 1998. *Clinical Obesity*.
London: Blackwell Science. *An anthology by international experts on current knowledge about obesity; for people who want in-
depth information.*

Otis, C. L., and R. Goldingay. 2000. *The Athletic Woman's Survival Guide*. Champaign, Ill.: Human Kinetics. *Information on
the female athlete triad and suggestions for changing attitudes toward weight, self-esteem, and body image.*

Organizations and Web Sites

American Diabetes Association. Provides information, a free
newsletter, and referrals to local support groups; the Web site
includes an online diabetes risk assessment.
    800-342-2383
    http://www.diabetes.org
National Heart, Lung, and Blood Institute. Provides information
on the latest federal obesity standards and a BMI calculator.
    http://www.nhlbi.nih.gov/guidelines/obesity/ob_home.htm
*National Institute of Diabetes and Digestive and Kidney Diseases
Health Information/Nutrition and Obesity*. Provides information
about adult obesity: how it is defined and assessed, the risk factors associated with it, and its causes.
    800-WIN-8098
    http://www.niddk.nih.gov/health/nutrit/nutrit.htm
Shape Up America. A site devoted to promoting healthy weight
management; calculates and rates BMI and looks at why BMI is
an important measure of health.
    http://shapeup.org
See also the listings for Chapters 2 and 9.

American College of Sports Medicine. 1998. *ACSM's Resource
Manual for Guidelines for Exercise Testing and Prescription*, 3d
ed. Baltimore, Md.: Williams & Wilkins.

American lifestyle leading to diabetes at younger and younger
ages. 1999. *Tufts University Health and Nutrition Letter*, January, 6.

Borghouts, L. B., and H. A. Keizer. 2000. Exercise and insulin
sensitivity: A review. *International Journal of Sports Medicine*
21(1): 1–12.

Brochu, M., et al. 2000. Coronary risk profiles in men with
coronary artery disease: Effects of body composition, fat
distribution, age and fitness. *Coronary Artery Disease* 11(2):
137–144.

Bussolotto, M., et al. 1999. Assessment of body composition in
elderly: Accuracy of bioelectrical impedance analysis. *Gerontology* 45:39–43.

Clark, C. M., Jr. 2000. Combating sloth as well as gluttony: The
role of physical fitness in mortality among men with type 2
diabetes. *Annals of Internal Medicine* 132(8): 669–670.

Elia, M., and L. C. Ward. 1999. New techniques in nutritional
assessment: Body composition methods. *Proceedings of the
Nutrition Society* 58:33–38.

Epstein, L. H., et al. 2000. Decreasing sedentary behaviors in
treating pediatric obesity. *Archives of Pediatrics and Adolescent
Medicine* 154(3): 220–226.

Forbes, G. B. 1999. Body composition: Overview. *Journal of Nutrition* 129(Suppl.): 270S–272S.

Grazer, F. M., and R. H. de Jong. 2000. Fatal outcomes from liposuction: Census survey of cosmetic surgeons. *Plastic and
Reconstructive Surgery* 105(1): 436.

Kriska, A. 2000. Physical activity and the prevention of type 2
diabetes mellitus: How much for how long? *Sports Medicine*
29(3): 147–151.

Managing Type 2 diabetes. 2000. *Journal of the American Medical
Association* 283(2): 288.

McCrory, M. A., et al. 1999. Overeating in America: Association
between restaurant food consumption and body fatness in
healthy adult men and women ages 19 to 80. *Obesity Research* 7(6): 564–571.

Megnien, J. L., et al. 1999. Predictive value of waist-to-hip ratio
on cardiovascular risk events. *International Journal of Obesity
and Related Metabolic Disorders* 23:90–97.

National Heart, Lung, and Blood Institute. 1998. *Clinical Guidelines on the Identification, Evaluation, and Treatment of Overweight and Obesity in Adults: The Evidence Report*. Bethesda,
Md.: National Institutes of Health.

Ross, R., I. Janssen, and A. Tremblay. 2000. Obesity reduction
through lifestyle modification. *Canadian Journal of Applied
Physiology* 25(1): 1–18.

Samaras, K., et al. 1998. Genes versus environment: The relationship between dietary fat and total and central abdominal
fat. *Diabetes Care* 21:2069–2076.

Scully, D., et al. 1998. Physical exercise and psychological well
being: A critical review. *British Journal of Sports Medicine*
32(2): 111–120.

To, W. W., M. W. Wong, and K. M. Chan. 1997. Association between body composition and menstrual dysfunction in col-
legiate dance students. *Journal of Obstetrics and Gynecology
Research* 23:529–535.

Utter, A. C., et al. 2000. Effects of exercise training on gallbladder function in an obese female population. *Medicine and Science in Sports and Exercise* 32(1): 41–45.

LAB 6-1 *Assessing Body Composition*

Body Mass Index

Equipment

1. Weight scale
2. Tape measure or other means of measuring height

Preparation

None

Instructions

Measure your height and weight, and record the results. Be sure to record the unit of measurement.

Height: _____   Weight: _____

Calculating BMI

1. Convert your body weight to kilograms by dividing your weight in pounds by 2.2.

    Body weight _____ lb ÷ 2.2 lb/kg = body weight _____ kg

2. Convert your height measurement to meters by multiplying your height in inches by 0.0254.

    Height _____ in. × 0.0254 m/in. = height _____ m

3. Square your height measurement.

    Height _____ m × height _____ m = height _____ m^2

4. BMI equals body weight in kilograms divided by height in meters squared (kg/m^2).

    Body weight _____ kg ÷ height _____ m^2 = BMI _____ kg/m^2
             (from step 1)   (from step 3)

Rating Your BMI

Refer to Table 6-2 (p. 152) for a rating of your BMI. Record the results below and in the chart on the final page of this lab.

BMI _____ kg/m^2

Classification (from Table 6-2) _____

Skinfold Measurements

Equipment

1. Skinfold calipers
2. Partner to take measurements
3. Marking pen (optional)

Preparation

None

Instructions

1. *Select and locate the correct sites for measurement.* All measurements should be taken on the right side of the body with the subject standing. Skinfolds are normally measured on the natural fold line of the skin, either vertically or at a slight angle. The skinfold measurement sites for males are chest, abdomen, and thigh; for females, triceps, suprailium, and thigh. If the person taking skinfold measurements is inexperienced, it may be helpful to mark the correct sites with a marking pen.

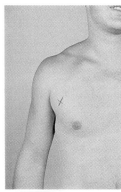 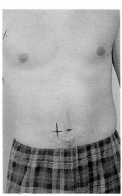 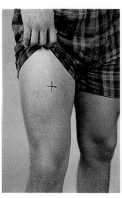 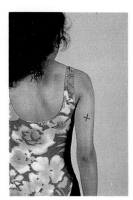 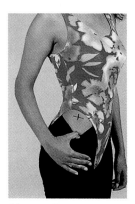

(a) Chest   (b) Abdomen   (c) Thigh   (d) Triceps   (e) Suprailium

(a) Chest. Pinch a diagonal fold halfway between the nipple and the shoulder crease. *(b) Abdomen.* Pinch a vertical fold about 1 inch to the right of the umbilicus (navel). *(c) Thigh.* Pinch a vertical fold midway between the top of the hipbone and the kneecap. *(d) Triceps.* Pinch a vertical skinfold on the back of the right arm midway between the shoulder and elbow. The arm should be straight and should hang naturally. *(e) Suprailium.* Pinch a fold at the top front of the right hipbone. The skinfold here is taken slightly diagonally according to the natural fold tendency of the skin.

2. *Measure the appropriate skinfolds.* Pinch a fold of skin between your thumb and forefinger. Pull the fold up so that no muscular tissue is included; don't pinch the skinfold too hard. Hold the calipers perpendicular to the fold, and measure the skinfold about 0.25 inch away from your fingers. Allow the tips of the calipers to close on the skinfold, and let the reading settle before marking it down. Take readings to the nearest half-millimeter. Continue to repeat the measurements until two consecutive measurements match, releasing and repinching the skinfold between each measurement. Make a note of the final measurement for each site.

Time of day of measurements: _____

Men	Women
Chest: _____ mm	Triceps: _____ mm
Abdomen: _____ mm	Suprailium: _____ mm
Thigh: _____ mm	Thigh: _____ mm

Determining Percent Body Fat

Add the measurements of your three skinfolds, and then find the percent body fat that corresponds to your total in the appropriate table. For example, a 19-year-old female with measurements of 16 mm, 19 mm, and 22 mm would have a skinfold sum of 57 mm; according to the table on page 160, her percent body fat is 22.7.

Sum of three skinfolds: _____ mm

Percent body fat: _____ %

Rating Your Body Composition

Refer to the table on page 161 to rate your percent body fat. Record it below and in the chart at the end of this lab.

Rating: _____

Percent Body Fat Estimate for Men: Sum of Chest, Abdomen, and Thigh Skinfolds

Sum of Skinfolds (mm)	Age								
	Under 22	23–27	28–32	33–37	38–42	43–47	48–52	53–57	Over 57
8–10	1.3	1.8	2.3	2.9	3.4	3.9	4.5	5.0	5.5
11–13	2.2	2.8	3.3	3.9	4.4	4.9	5.5	6.0	6.5
14–16	3.2	3.8	4.3	4.8	5.4	5.9	6.4	7.0	7.5
17–19	4.2	4.7	5.3	5.8	6.3	6.9	7.4	8.0	8.5
20–22	5.1	5.7	6.2	6.8	7.3	7.9	8.4	8.9	9.5
23–25	6.1	6.6	7.2	7.7	8.3	8.8	9.4	9.9	10.5
26–28	7.0	7.6	8.1	8.7	9.2	9.8	10.3	10.9	11.4
29–31	8.0	8.5	9.1	9.6	10.2	10.7	11.3	11.8	12.4
32–34	8.9	9.4	10.0	10.5	11.1	11.6	12.2	12.8	13.3
35–37	9.8	10.4	10.9	11.5	12.0	12.6	13.1	13.7	14.3
38–40	10.7	11.3	11.8	12.4	12.9	13.5	14.1	14.6	15.2
41–43	11.6	12.2	12.7	13.3	13.8	14.4	15.0	15.5	16.1
44–46	12.5	13.1	13.6	14.2	14.7	15.3	15.9	16.4	17.0
47–49	13.4	13.9	14.5	15.1	15.6	16.2	16.8	17.3	17.9
50–52	14.3	14.8	15.4	15.9	16.5	17.1	17.6	18.2	18.8
53–55	15.1	15.7	16.2	16.8	17.4	17.9	18.5	19.1	19.7
56–58	16.0	16.5	17.1	17.7	18.2	18.8	19.4	20.0	20.5
59–61	16.9	17.4	17.9	18.5	19.1	19.7	20.2	20.8	21.4
62–64	17.6	18.2	18.8	19.4	19.9	20.5	21.1	21.7	22.2
65–67	18.5	19.0	19.6	20.2	20.8	21.3	21.9	22.5	23.1
68–70	19.3	19.9	20.4	21.0	21.6	22.2	22.7	23.3	23.9
71–73	20.1	20.7	21.2	21.8	22.4	23.0	23.6	24.1	24.7
74–76	20.9	21.5	22.0	22.6	23.2	23.8	24.4	25.0	25.5
77–79	21.7	22.2	22.8	23.4	24.0	24.6	25.2	25.8	26.3
80–82	22.4	23.0	23.6	24.2	24.8	25.4	25.9	26.5	27.1
83–85	23.2	23.8	24.4	25.0	25.5	26.1	26.7	27.3	27.9
86–88	24.0	24.5	25.1	25.7	26.3	26.9	27.5	28.1	28.7
89–91	24.7	25.3	25.9	26.5	27.1	27.6	28.2	28.8	29.4
92–94	25.4	26.0	26.6	27.2	27.8	28.4	29.0	29.6	30.2
95–97	26.1	26.7	27.3	27.9	28.5	29.1	29.7	30.3	30.9
98–100	26.9	27.4	28.0	28.6	29.2	29.8	30.4	31.0	31.6
101–103	27.5	28.1	28.7	29.3	29.9	30.5	31.1	31.7	32.3
104–106	28.2	28.8	29.4	30.0	30.6	31.2	31.8	32.4	33.0
107–109	28.9	29.5	30.1	30.7	31.3	31.9	32.5	33.1	33.7
110–112	29.6	30.2	30.8	31.4	32.0	32.6	33.2	33.8	34.4
113–115	30.2	30.8	31.4	32.0	32.6	33.2	33.8	34.5	35.1
116–118	30.9	31.5	32.1	32.7	33.3	33.9	34.5	35.1	35.7
119–121	31.5	32.1	32.7	33.3	33.9	34.5	35.1	35.7	36.4
122–124	32.1	32.7	33.3	33.9	34.5	35.1	35.8	36.4	37.0
125–127	32.7	33.3	33.9	34.5	35.1	35.8	36.4	37.0	37.6

SOURCE: Jackson, A. S., and M. L. Pollock. 1985. Practical assessment of body composition. *Physician and Sportsmedicine* 13(5): 76–90. Reproduced by permission of McGraw-Hill, Inc.

Percent Body Fat Estimate for Women: Sum of Triceps, Suprailium, and Thigh Skinfolds

Sum of Skinfolds (mm)	Under 22	23–27	28–32	33–37	38–42	43–47	48–52	53–57	Over 57
23–25	9.7	9.9	10.2	10.4	10.7	10.9	11.2	11.4	11.7
26–28	11.0	11.2	11.5	11.7	12.0	12.3	12.5	12.7	13.0
29–31	12.3	12.5	12.8	13.0	13.3	13.5	13.8	14.0	14.3
32–34	13.6	13.8	14.0	14.3	14.5	14.8	15.0	15.3	15.5
35–37	14.8	15.0	15.3	15.5	15.8	16.0	16.3	16.5	16.8
38–40	16.0	16.3	16.5	16.7	17.0	17.2	17.5	17.7	18.0
41–43	17.2	17.4	17.7	17.9	18.2	18.4	18.7	18.9	19.2
44–46	18.3	18.6	18.8	19.1	19.3	19.6	19.8	20.1	20.3
47–49	19.5	19.7	20.0	20.2	20.5	20.7	21.0	21.2	21.5
50–52	20.6	20.8	21.1	21.3	21.6	21.8	22.1	22.3	22.6
53–55	21.7	21.9	22.1	22.4	22.6	22.9	23.1	23.4	23.6
56–58	22.7	23.0	23.2	23.4	23.7	23.9	24.2	24.4	24.7
59–61	23.7	24.0	24.2	24.5	24.7	25.0	25.2	25.5	25.7
62–64	24.7	25.0	25.2	25.5	25.7	26.0	26.7	26.4	26.7
65–67	25.7	25.9	26.2	26.4	26.7	26.9	27.2	27.4	27.7
68–70	26.6	26.9	27.1	27.4	27.6	27.9	28.1	28.4	28.6
71–73	27.5	27.8	28.0	28.3	28.5	28.8	29.0	29.3	29.5
74–76	28.4	28.7	28.9	29.2	29.4	29.7	29.9	30.2	30.4
77–79	29.3	29.5	29.8	30.0	30.3	30.5	30.8	31.0	31.3
80–82	30.1	30.4	30.6	30.9	31.1	31.4	31.6	31.9	32.1
83–85	30.9	31.2	31.4	31.7	31.9	32.2	32.4	32.7	32.9
86–88	31.7	32.0	32.2	32.5	32.7	32.9	33.2	33.4	33.7
89–91	32.5	32.7	33.0	33.2	33.5	33.7	33.9	34.2	34.4
92–94	33.2	33.4	33.7	33.9	34.2	34.4	34.7	34.9	35.2
95–97	33.9	34.1	34.4	34.6	34.9	35.1	35.4	35.6	35.9
98–100	34.6	34.8	35.1	35.3	35.5	35.8	36.0	36.3	36.5
101–103	35.3	35.4	35.7	35.9	36.2	36.4	36.7	36.9	37.2
104–106	35.8	36.1	36.3	36.6	36.8	37.1	37.3	37.5	37.8
107–109	36.4	36.7	36.9	37.1	37.4	37.6	37.9	38.1	38.4
110–112	37.0	37.2	37.5	37.7	38.0	38.2	38.5	38.7	38.9
113–115	37.5	37.8	38.0	38.2	38.5	38.7	39.0	39.2	39.5
116–118	38.0	38.3	38.5	38.8	39.0	39.3	39.5	39.7	40.0
119–121	38.5	38.7	39.0	39.2	39.5	39.7	40.0	40.2	40.5
122–124	39.0	39.2	39.4	39.7	39.9	40.2	40.4	40.7	40.9
125–127	39.4	39.6	39.9	40.1	40.4	40.6	40.9	41.1	41.4
128–130	39.8	40.0	40.3	40.5	40.8	41.0	41.3	41.5	41.8

SOURCE: Jackson, A. S., and M. L. Pollock. 1985. Practical assessment of body composition. *Physician and Sportsmedicine* 13(5): 76–90. Reproduced by permission of McGraw-Hill, Inc.

LABORATORY ACTIVITIES

Body Composition Ratings

Percent Body Fat

Men	Very Lean	Excellent	Good	Fair	Poor	Very Poor
Age: 18–29	Below 5.3	5.3–9.4	9.5–14.1	14.2–17.4	17.5–22.4	Above 22.4
30–39	Below 9.2	9.2–13.9	14.0–17.5	17.6–20.5	20.6–24.2	Above 24.2
40–49	Below 11.5	11.5–16.3	16.4–19.6	19.7–22.5	22.6–26.1	Above 26.1
50–59	Below 13.0	13.0–17.9	18.0–21.3	21.4–24.1	24.2–27.5	Above 27.5
60 and over	Below 13.2	13.2–18.4	18.5–22.0	22.1–25.0	25.1–28.5	Above 28.5
Women						
Age: 18–29	Below 10.9	10.9–17.1	17.2–20.6	20.7–23.7	23.8–27.7	Above 27.7
30–39	Below 13.5	13.5–18.0	18.1–21.6	21.7–24.9	25.0–29.3	Above 29.3
40–49	Below 16.2	16.2–21.3	21.4–24.9	25.0–28.1	28.2–32.1	Above 32.1
50–59	Below 18.9	18.9–25.0	25.1–28.5	28.6–31.6	31.7–35.6	Above 35.6
60 and over	Below 16.9	16.9–25.1	25.2–29.3	29.4–32.5	32.6–36.6	Above 36.6

*These ratings are derived from norms based on the measurement of thousands of individuals. In evaluating your body composition, also consider the health-related recommendations for body fat given in Table 6-1 (p. 147). Obesity is defined as having 25% of body weight or more as fat for men and 32% of body weight or more as fat for women. Norms reflect the status of the population, whereas recommendations represent a healthier and more desirable status.

SOURCE: Based on norms from the Cooper Institute for Aerobics Research, Dallas, Tex.; used with permission.

Other Methods of Assessing Percent Body Fat

Other methods of assessing percent body fat, including underwater weighing, the Bod Pod, and bioelectrical impedance analysis, may be available on your campus or in your community. If you use one of these alternative methods, record the name of the method and the result below and in the chart at the end of this lab. Find your body composition rating on the table above.

Method used: _____

Percent body fat: _____ %

Rating (from table above): _____

Waist Circumference and Waist-to-Hip Ratio

Equipment

1. Tape measure
2. Partner to take measurements

Preparation

Wear clothes that will not add significantly to your measurements.

Instructions

Stand with your feet together and your arms at your sides. Raise your arms only high enough to allow for taking the measurements. Your partner should make sure the tape is horizontal around the entire circumference and pulled snugly against your skin. The tape shouldn't be pulled so tight that it causes indentations in your skin. Record measurements to the nearest millimeter or one-sixteenth of an inch.

Waist. Measure at the smallest waist circumference. If you don't have a natural waist, measure at the level of your navel.

Waist measurement: _____

Hip. Measure at the largest hip circumference.

Hip measurement: _____

Waist-to-Hip Ratio: You can use any unit of measurement (for example, inches or centimeters), as long as you're consistent. Waist-to-hip ratio equals waist measurement divided by hip measurement.

Waist-to-hip ratio: _____ ÷ _____ = _____
  (waist measurement)   (hip measurement)

Determining Your Risk

The table below indicates values for waist circumference and waist-to-hip ratio above which the risk of health problems increases significantly. If your measurement or ratio is above either cutoff point, put a check on the appropriate line below and in the chart on the final page of this lab.

Waist circumference: _____ (✔ high risk)

Waist-to-hip ratio: _____ (✔ high risk)

Body Fat Distribution

Cutoff Points for High Risk

	Waist Circumference	Waist-to-Hip Ratio
Men	more than 40 in. (102 cm)	more than 0.94
Women	more than 35 in. (88 cm)	more than 0.82

SOURCES: National Heart, Lung, and Blood Institute. 1998. *Clinical Guidelines on the Identification, Evaluation, and Treatment of Overweight and Obesity in Adults: The Evidence Report.* Bethesda, Md.: National Institutes of Health. American College of Sports Medicine. 1998. *ACSM's Resource Manual for Guidelines for Exercise Testing and Prescription,* 3d ed. Baltimore, Md.: Williams & Wilkins.

Rating Your Body Composition

Assessment	Value	Classification
BMI	_____ kg/m²	_____
Skinfold measurements or alternative method of determining percent body fat Specify method: _____	_____ % body fat	_____
Waist circumference Waist-to-hip ratio	_____ in. or cm _____ (ratio)	_____ (✔ high risk) _____ (✔ high risk)

Enter the results of this lab in the Preprogram Assessment column of Appendix D. After several weeks of a program to improve body composition, do this lab again, and enter the results in the Postprogram Assessment column of Appendix D. How do the results compare?

LAB 6-2 *Determining Desirable Body Weight*

Complete this lab if assessment tests indicate that a change in your body composition is appropriate.

Equipment

Calculator (or pencil and paper for calculations)

Preparation

Determine percent body fat and/or calculate BMI as described in Lab 6-1. Keep track of height and weight as measured for these calculations.

Height: _____

Weight: _____

Calculations for desirable body weight can be based on target values for BMI and/or percent body fat. The instructions given below contain formulas for both methods; depending on which assessments you performed in Lab 6-1, you may complete the calculations for one or both methods. Choose a target BMI from Table 6-2, and/or choose a target percent body fat from Table 6-1. For example, a 190-pound male who is 5 feet, 7 inches tall and has a BMI of 29.9 and a percent body fat of 26 might set goals of 26 for BMI and 18 for percent body fat.

Instructions

1. To calculate desirable weight from target BMI:

   a. Convert your height measurement to meters by multiplying your height in inches by 0.0254.

   b. Square your height measurement.

   c. Multiply your target BMI by your height in meters, squared, to get your target weight in kilograms.

   d. Multiply your target weight in kilograms by 2.2 to get your desirable body weight in pounds.

   a. Height _____ in. × 0.0254 m/in. = height _____ m

   b. Height _____ m × height _____ m = height _____ m²

   c. Target BMI _____ × height _____ m² = target weight _____ kg

   d. Target weight _____ kg × 2.2 lb/kg = desirable body weight _____ lb

2. To calculate desirable body weight from actual and target body fat percentages:

   a. To determine the fat weight in your body, multiply your current weight by percent body fat (determined through skinfold measurements and expressed as a decimal).

   b. Subtract the fat weight from your current weight to get your current fat-free weight.

   c. Subtract your target percent body fat from 1 to get target percent fat-free weight.

Example (see above)

1. Desirable weight from target BMI:

   67 in. × 0.0254 m/in. = 1.70 m

   1.70 m × 1.70 m = 2.89 m²

   26 kg/m² × 2.89 m² = 75.1 kg

   75.1 kg × 2.2 lb/kg = 165 lb

2. Desirable weight from actual and target body fat percentages:

   190 lb × 0.26 = 49.4 lb

   190 lb − 49.4 lb = 140.6 lb

   1 − 0.18 = 0.82

d. To get your desirable body weight, divide your
fat-free weight by your target percent fat-free weight.   140.6 lb ÷ 0.82 = 171 lb

Note: Weight can be expressed in either pounds or kilograms, as long as the unit of measurement is used consistently.

a. Current body weight _____ × percent body fat _____ = fat weight _____

b. Current body weight _____ − fat weight _____ = fat-free weight _____

c. 1 − target percent body fat _____ = target percent fat-free weight _____

d. Fat-free weight _____ ÷ target percent fat-free weight _____ =

    desirable body weight _____

Based on these calculations and other factors (including heredity, individual preference, and current health status), select a target weight or range of weights for yourself.

Target body weight: _____

Putting Together a Complete Fitness Program

7

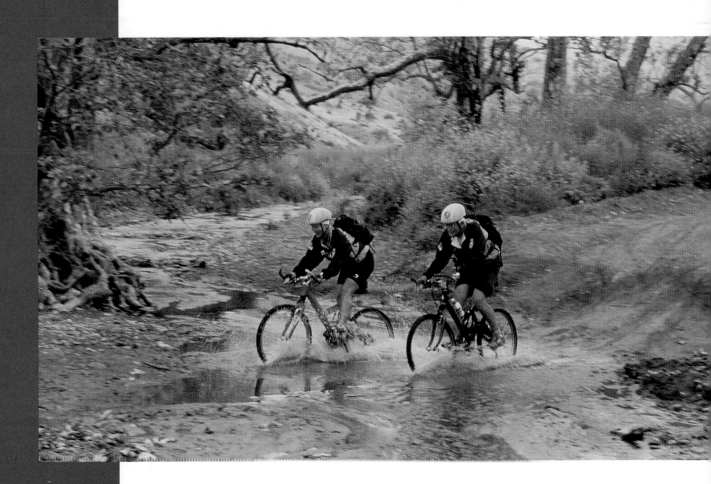

LOOKING AHEAD

After reading this chapter, you should be able to answer these questions about putting together a complete personalized exercise program:

- What are the steps for putting together a successful personal fitness program?

- What strategies can help maintain a fitness program over the long term?

- How can a fitness program be tailored to accommodate special health concerns?

Understanding the physiological basis and wellness benefits of health related physical fitness, as explained in Chapters 1–6, is the first step toward creating a well-rounded exercise program. The next challenge is to combine activities into a program that develops all the fitness components and maintains motivation.

This chapter presents a step-by-step procedure for creating and maintaining a well-rounded program. Following the chapter, you'll find sample programs based on popular activities. The structure these programs provide can be helpful if you're beginning an exercise program for the first time.

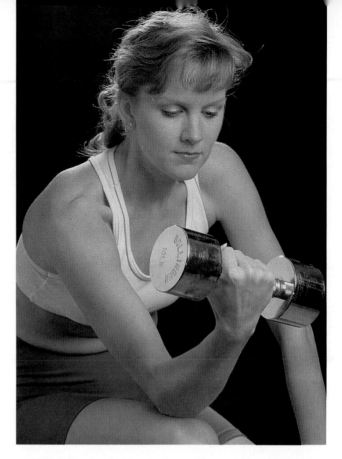

Weight training does little to develop cardiorespiratory endurance but is excellent for developing muscular strength and endurance. An overall fitness program includes exercises to develop all the components of physical fitness.

DEVELOPING A PERSONAL FITNESS PLAN

If you're ready to create a complete fitness program based around the activities you enjoy most, begin by preparing the program plan and contract in Lab 7-1. By carefully developing your plan and signing a contract, you'll increase your chances of success. The step-by-step procedure outlined here (adapted from *Your Guide to Getting Fit,* by Ivan Kusinitz and Morton Fine) will guide you through the steps of Lab 7-1 to the creation of an exercise program that's right for you. Refer to Figure 7-1 for a sample personal fitness program plan and contract.

If you'd like additional help in setting up your program, choose one of the sample programs at the end of this chapter (pp. 179–188). Sample programs are provided for walking/jogging/running, cycling, swimming, and in-line skating; they include detailed instructions for starting a program and developing and maintaining fitness.

1. Set Goals

Setting goals to reach through exercise is a crucial first step. Ask yourself, "What do I want from my fitness program?" Develop different types of goals—general and specific, long term and short term. General or long-term goals might include things like lowering your risk for chronic disease, improving posture, and having more energy. It's a good idea to also develop some specific, short-term goals based on measurable factors. Specific goals might be raising $\dot{V}O_{2max}$ by 10%, reducing the time it takes you to jog 2 miles from 22 minutes to 19 minutes, increasing the number of push-ups you can do from 15 to 25, and lowering BMI from 26 to 24. Having specific goals will allow you to track your progress and enjoy the measurable changes brought about by your fitness program.

Physical fitness assessment tests are essential to determining your goals. They help you decide which types of exercise you should emphasize, and they help you understand the relative difficulty of attaining specific goals. If you have health problems, such as high blood pressure, heart disease, obesity, or serious joint or muscle disabil-

ities, see your physician before taking assessment tests. Measure your progress by taking these tests every 3 months.

You'll find it easier to stick with your program if you choose goals that are both important to you and realistic. Remember that heredity, your current fitness level, and other individual factors influence the amount of improvement and the ultimate level of fitness you can expect to obtain through physical training. Fitness improves most quickly during the first 6 months of an exercise program. After that, gains come more slowly and usually require a higher-intensity program. So don't expect to improve indefinitely. Improve your fitness to a reasonable target level, and then train consistently to maintain it.

Think carefully about your reasons for exercising, and then fill in the goals portion of your program plan in Lab 7-1.

2. Select Activities

If you have already chosen activities and created separate program plans for different fitness components in Chapters 3, 4, and 5, you can put those plans together into a single program. It's usually best to include exercises to develop each of the health-related components of physical fitness.

A. I ___Tracie Kaufman___ am contracting with myself to follow a physical
   (name)
fitness program to work toward the following goals:

Specific or short-term goals
1. Improving cardiorespiratory fitness by raising my $\dot{V}O_{2max}$ to 37 ml/kg/min
2. Improving upper body muscular strength and endurance
3. Improving body composition (from 30% to 25% body fat)
4. Improving my tennis game (hitting 20 playable shots in a row against the ball machine)

General or long-term goals
1. Developing a more positive attitude about myself
2. Reducing my risk for diabetes and heart disease
3. Building and maintaining bone mass to reduce my risk of osteoporosis
4. Increasing my life expectancy

B. My program plan is as follows:

Activities	Components (Check ✓)					Intensity*	Duration	Frequency (Check ✓)						
	CRE	MS	ME	F	BC			M	Tu	W	Th	F	Sa	Su
Swimming	✓	✓	✓	✓	✓	140-150 bpm	35min	✓		✓		✓		
Tennis	✓	✓	✓	✓	✓	RPE=14	90min						✓	
Weight training		✓	✓	✓	✓	see Lab 4-3	30min		✓		✓	✓		
Stretching				✓		—	25min	✓		✓		✓	✓	

*List your target heart rate range or an RPE value if appropriate.

C. My program will begin on Sept. 21. My program includes the following schedule
of mini-goals. For each step in my program, I will give myself the reward listed.

Completing 2 full weeks of program (mini-goal 1)	Oct 5 (date)	movie with friends (reward)
$\dot{V}O_{2max}$ of 34 ml/kg/min (mini-goal 2)	Nov 2 (date)	new CD (reward)
Completing 10 full weeks of program (mini-goal 3)	Nov 30 (date)	new sweater (reward)
Percent body fat of 28% (mini-goal 4)	Dec 22 (date)	weekend away (reward)
$\dot{V}O_{2max}$ of 36 ml/kg/min (mini-goal 5)	Jan 18 (date)	new CD (reward)

D. My program will include the addition of physical activity to my daily routine (such
as climbing stairs or walking to class):
1. Walking to and from campus job
2. Taking the stairs to dorm room instead of elevator
3. Bicycling to the library instead of driving
4. _____
5. _____

E. I will use the following tools to monitor my program and my progress toward
my goals: I'll use a chart that lists the number of laps and minutes I swim and the
charts for strength and flexibility from Labs 4-3 & 5-2.

I sign this contract as an indication of my personal commitment to reach my goal.

___Tracie Kaufman___   ___Sept 10___
(your signature)   (date)

I have recruited a helper who will witness my contract and
swim with me three days per week
(list any way your helper will participate in your program)

___Russell Walker___   ___Sept 10___
(witness's signature)   (date)

Figure 7-1 A sample personal fitness program plan and contract.

TABLE 7-1 *A Summary of Sports and Fitness Activities*

This table classifies sports and activities as high (H), moderate (M), or low (L) in terms of their ability to develop each of the five components of physical fitness: cardiorespiratory endurance (CRE), muscular strength (MS), muscular endurance (ME), flexibility (F), and body composition (BC). The skill level needed to obtain fitness benefits is noted: Low (L) means little or no skill is required to obtain fitness benefits; moderate (M) means average skill is needed to obtain fitness benefits; and high (H) means much skill is required to obtain fitness benefits. The fitness prerequisite, or conditioning needs of a beginner, is also noted: Low (L) means no fitness prerequisite is required, moderate (M) means some preconditioning is required, and high (H) means substantial fitness is required. The last two columns list the calorie cost of each activity when performed moderately and vigorously. To determine how many calories you burn, multiply the value in the appropriate column by your body weight and then by the number of minutes you exercise. Work up to using 300 or more calories per workout.

| Sports and Activities | Components | | | | | Skill Level | Fitness Prerequisite | Approximate Calorie Cost (cal/lb/min) | |
	CRE	MS*	ME*	F*	BC			Moderate	Vigorous
Aerobic dance	H	M	H	H	H	L	L	.046	.062
Backpacking	H	M	H	M	H	L	M	.032	.078
Badminton, skilled, singles	H	M	M	M	H	M	M	—	.071
Ballet (floor combinations)	M	M	H	H	M	M	L	—	.058
Ballroom dancing	M	L	M	L	M	M	L	.034	.049
Baseball (pitcher and catcher)	M	M	H	M	M	H	M	.039	—
Basketball, half court	H	M	H	M	H	M	M	.045	.071
Bicycling	H	M	H	M	H	M	L	.049	.071
Bowling	L	L	L	L	L	L	L	—	—
Calisthenic circuit training	H	M	H	M	H	L	L	—	.060
Canoeing and kayaking (flat water)	M	M	H	M	M	M	M	.045	—
Cheerleading	M	M	M	M	M	M	L	.033	.049
Fencing	M	M	H	H	M	M	L	.032	.078
Field hockey	H	M	H	M	H	M	M	.052	.078
Folk and square dancing	M	L	M	L	M	L	L	.039	.049
Football, touch	M	M	M	M	M	M	M	.049	.078
Frisbee, ultimate	H	M	H	M	H	M	M	.049	.078
Golf (riding cart)	L	L	L	M	L	L	L	—	—
Handball, skilled, singles	H	M	H	M	H	M	M	—	.078
Hiking	H	M	H	L	H	L	M	.051	.073
Hockey, ice and roller	H	M	H	M	H	M	M	.052	.078
Horseback riding	M	M	M	L	M	M	M	.052	.065
Interval circuit training	H	H	H	M	H	L	L	—	.062
Jogging and running	H	M	H	L	H	L	L	.060	.104

*Ratings are for the muscle groups involved.

- Cardiorespiratory endurance is developed by activities such as walking, cycling, and aerobic dance that involve continuous rhythmic movements of large-muscle groups like those in the legs (see Chapter 3).

- Muscular strength and endurance are developed by training against resistance (see Chapter 4).

- Flexibility is developed by stretching the major muscle groups (see Chapter 5).

- Healthy body composition can be developed by

combining a sensible diet and a program of regular exercise, including cardiorespiratory endurance exercise to burn calories and resistance training to build muscle mass (see Chapter 6).

Table 7-1 rates many popular activities for their ability to develop each of the health-related components of fitness. Check the ratings of the activities you're considering to make sure the program you put together will develop all fitness components and help you achieve your goals. One strategy is to select one activity for each component of fitness—bicycling, weight training, and stretching, for example. Another strategy applies the principle of **cross-training**, using several different activities to develop a

TERMS **cross-training** Alternating two or more activities to improve a single component of fitness.

TABLE 7-1   *A Summary of Sports and Fitness Activities*

Sports and Activities	CRE	MS*	ME*	F*	BC	Skill Level	Fitness Prerequisite	Approximate Calorie Cost (cal/lb/min) Moderate	Vigorous
Judo	M	H	H	M	M	M	L	.049	.090
Karate	H	M	H	H	H	L	M	.049	.090
Lacrosse	H	M	H	M	H	H	M	.052	.078
Modern dance (moving combinations)	M	M	H	H	M	L	L	—	.058
Orienteering	H	M	H	L	H	L	M	.049	.078
Outdoor fitness trails	H	M	H	M	H	L	L	—	.060
Popular dancing	M	L	M	M	M	M	L	—	.049
Racquetball, skilled, singles	H	M	M	M	H	M	M	.049	.078
Rock climbing	M	H	H	H	M	H	M	.033	.033
Rope skipping	H	M	H	L	H	M	M	.071	.095
Rowing	H	H	H	H	H	L	L	.032	.097
Rugby	H	M	H	M	H	M	M	.052	.097
Sailing	L	L	M	L	L	M	L	—	—
Skating, ice, roller, and in-line	M	M	H	M	M	H	M	.049	.095
Skiing, alpine	M	H	H	M	M	H	M	.039	.078
Skiing, cross-country	H	M	H	M	H	M	M	.049	.104
Soccer	H	M	H	M	H	M	M	.052	.097
Squash, skilled, singles	H	M	M	M	H	M	M	.049	.078
Stretching	L	L	L	H	L	L	L	—	—
Surfing (including swimming)	M	M	M	M	M	H	M	—	.078
Swimming	H	M	H	M	H	M	L	.032	.088
Synchronized swimming	M	M	H	H	M	M	M	.032	.052
Table tennis	M	L	M	M	M	M	L	—	.045
Tennis, skilled, singles	H	M	M	M	H	M	M	—	.071
Volleyball	M	L	M	M	M	M	M	—	.065
Walking	H	L	M	L	H	L	L	.029	.048
Water polo	H	M	H	M	H	H	M	—	.078
Water skiing	M	M	H	M	M	H	M	.039	.055
Weight training	L	H	H	H	M	L	L	—	—
Wrestling	H	H	H	H	H	H	H	.065	.094
Yoga	L	L	M	H	L	H	L	—	—

*Ratings are for the muscle groups involved.

SOURCE: Kusinitz, I., and M. Fine. 1995. *Your Guide to Getting Fit*, 3d ed. Mountain View, Calif.: Mayfield.

particular fitness component—aerobics classes, swimming, and volleyball for cardiorespiratory endurance, for example. Cross-training is discussed in the next section.

If you select activities that support your commitment rather than activities that turn exercise into a chore, the right program will be its own incentive for continuing. Consider the following factors in making your choices.

- *Fun and interest.* Your fitness program is much more likely to be successful if you choose activities that you enjoy doing. Start by considering any activities you currently engage in and enjoy. Often you can modify your current activities to fit your fitness program. As you consider new activities, ask yourself, "Is this activity fun?" "Will it hold my interest over time?" For new activities, it is a good idea to undertake a trial period before making a final choice. Figure 7-2 shows popular fitness activities among Americans.

- *Your current skill and fitness level.* Although many activities are appropriate for beginners, some sports and activities require participants to have a moderate level of skill to obtain fitness benefits. For example, a beginning tennis player will probably not be able to sustain rallies long enough to develop cardiorespiratory endurance. Refer to the skill level column in Table 7-1 to determine the level of skill needed for full participation in the activities you're considering. If your current skill level doesn't

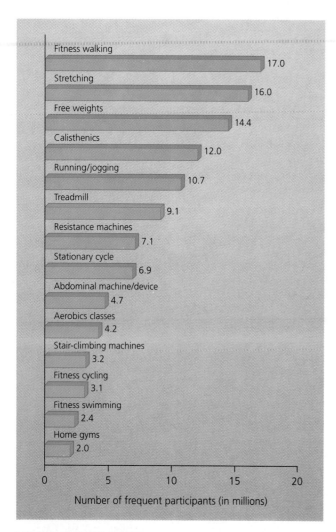

Figure 7-2 Popular fitness activities among Americans.
Frequent participants in the activities shown here are those age 6 and over who engage in the activity at least 100 days per year. DATA SOURCE: Fitness Products Council/American Sports Data, Inc. 1999. Frequent participation in Fitness Activities, 1998. Press release dated April 8 (http://www.sportlink.com/press_room/1999_releases/fitness99-002.html).

meet the requirement, you may want to begin your program with a different activity. For example, a beginning tennis player may be better off with a walking program while improving his or her tennis game. To build skill for a particular activity, consider taking a class or getting some instruction from a coach or fellow participant.

Your current fitness level may also limit the activities that are appropriate for your program. For example, if you have been inactive, a walking program would be more appropriate than a jogging program. Activities in which participants control the intensity of effort—walking, cycling, and swimming, for example—are more appropriate for a beginning fitness program than sports and activities that are primarily "other paced"—soccer,

basketball, and tennis, for example. Refer to the fitness prerequisite column of Table 7-1 to determine the minimum level of fitness required for participation in the activities you're considering.

• *Time and convenience.* Unless exercise fits easily into your daily schedule, you are unlikely to maintain your program over the long term. As you consider activities, think about whether a special location or facility is required. Can you participate in the activity close to your residence, school, or job? Are the necessary facilities open and available at times convenient to you? Do you need a partner or a team to play? Can you participate in the activity year-round, or will you need to find an alternative during the summer or winter?

• *Cost.* Some sports and activities require equipment, fees, or some type of membership investment. If you are on a tight budget, limit your choices to activities that are inexpensive or free. Investigate the facilities on your campus, which you may be able to use at little or no cost. Many activities require no equipment beyond an appropriate pair of shoes (see the box "Choosing Exercise Footwear" for more information). Refer back to Chapters 2 and 3 for consumer guidelines for evaluating exercise equipment and facilities.

• *Special health needs.* If you have special exercise needs due to a particular health problem, choose activities that will conform to your needs and enhance your ability to cope. If necessary, consult your physician about how best to tailor an exercise program to your particular needs and goals. Guidelines and safety tips for exercisers with common chronic conditions are provided later in the chapter.

3. Set a Target Intensity, Duration, and Frequency for Each Activity

The next step in planning your fitness program is to set a target intensity, duration, and frequency for each activity you've chosen (see the sample in Figure 7-1). Refer to the calculations and plans you completed in Chapters 3, 4, and 5.

Cardiorespiratory Endurance Exercise For intensity, note your target heart rate zone or RPE value. Your target total duration should be about 20–60 minutes, depending on the intensity of the activity (shorter durations are appropriate for high-intensity activities, longer durations for activities of more moderate intensity). You can exercise in a single session or in multiple sessions of 10 or more minutes. One way to check whether the total duration you've set is appropriate is to use the **calorie costs** (calories per minute per pound of body weight) given in Table 7-1. Your goal should be to work up to burning about 300 calories per workout; beginners should start with a calorie cost of about 100–150 calories per workout. You can calculate the calorie cost of your activities by

Name Tracie Kaufman

Enter duration, distance, or other factor to track your progress.

Activity/Date	M	Tu	W	Th	F	S	S	Weekly Total	M	Tu	W	Th	F	S	S	Weekly Total
1 Swimming	800 yd		725 yd		800 yd			2325 yd	800 yd		800 yd		850 yd			2450 yd
2 Tennis					90 min			90 min							95 min	95 min
3 Weight Training		✓		✓		✓				✓		✓		✓	✓	
4 Stretching	✓		✓		✓	✓			✓			✓	✓	✓	✓	
5																
6																

Figure 7-3   A sample program log.

multiplying the appropriate factor from Table 7-1 by your body weight and the duration of your workout. For example, walking at a moderate pace burns about 0.029 calorie per minute per pound of body weight. A person weighing 150 pounds could begin her exercise program by walking for 30 minutes, burning about 130 calories. Once her fitness improves, she might choose to start cycling for her cardiorespiratory endurance workouts. Cycling at a moderate pace has a higher calorie cost than walking (0.049 calorie per minute per pound), and if she cycled for 40 minutes, she would burn the target 300 calories during her workout.

An appropriate frequency for cardiorespiratory endurance exercise is 3–5 times per week.

Muscular Strength and Endurance Training   As described in Chapter 4, a general fitness strength training program includes 1 or more sets of 8–12 repetitions of 8–10 exercises that work all major muscle groups. For intensity, choose a weight that is heavy enough to fatigue your muscles but not so heavy that you cannot complete the full number of repetitions with proper form. A frequency of 2–3 days per week is recommended.

Flexibility Training   Stretches should be performed for all major muscle groups. For each exercise, stretch to the point of slight tension or mild discomfort and hold the stretch for 10–30 seconds; do at least 4 repetitions of each exercise. Stretches should be performed at least 2–3 days per week, preferably when muscles are warm.

4. Set Up a System of Mini-Goals and Rewards

To keep your program on track, it is important to set up a system of goals and rewards. Break your specific goals into several steps, and set a target date for each step. For example, if one of the goals of an 18-year-old male stu-dent's program is to improve upper-body strength and endurance, he could use the push-up test in Lab 4-2 to set intermediate goals. If he can currently perform 15 push-ups (for a rating of "very poor"), he might set intermediate goals of 20, 25, and 30 push-ups (for a final rating of "fair"). By allowing 4–6 weeks between mini-goals and specifying rewards, he'll be able to track his progress and reward himself as he moves toward his final goal. For more on choosing appropriate rewards, refer to p. 11 in Chapter 1 and Activity 4 in the Behavior Change Workbook at the end of the text.

5. Include Lifestyle Physical Activity in Your Program

As described in Chapter 2, daily physical activity is an important part of a fit and well lifestyle. As part of your fitness program plan, specify ways that you will be more active during your daily routine. You may find it helpful to first use your health journal to track your activities for several days. Review the records in your journal, identify routine opportunities to be more active, and add these to your program plan in Lab 7-1.

6. Develop Tools for Monitoring Your Progress

A record that tracks your daily progress will help remind you of your ongoing commitment to your program and give you a sense of accomplishment. Figure 7-3 shows you how to create a general program log and record the activity type, frequency, and durations. Or if you wish, complete specific activity logs like those in Labs 3-2, 4-3, and 5-2 in addition to, or instead of, a general log. Post your log in a place where you'll see it often as a reminder

calorie cost   The amount of energy used to perform a particular activity, usually expressed in calories per minute per pound of body weight.   **TERMS**

Footwear is perhaps the most important item of equipment for almost any activity. Shoes protect and support your feet and improve your traction. When you jump or run, you place as much as six times more force on your feet than when you stand still. Shoes can help cushion against the stress that this additional force places on your lower legs and thus prevent injuries. Some athletic shoes are also designed to help prevent ankle rollover, another common source of injury.

Shoe Terminology

Understanding the structural features of athletic shoes can help you make sound choices.

Outsole: The bottom of the shoe that touches the ground and provides traction. The shape and composition of an outsole depend on the activity for which the shoe is designed.

Midsole: The layer of shock-absorbing material located between the insole and the outsole; typically composed of polyurethane, ethyl vinyl acetate (EVA), or another cushioning material. For improved durability, some shoe midsoles include encapsulated air or gel.

Insole: The insert or sock lining that the foot rests on inside the shoe, usually contoured to fit the foot and containing additional cushioning and arch and heel support.

Collar: The opening of the shoe where the foot goes in.

Upper: The top part of the shoe, usually made of nylon, canvas, or leather.

Toe box: The front part of the upper, which surrounds the toes.

Heel counter: The stiff cup in the back of the inside of the shoe that provides support and stability.

Notched heel: Some shoes have raised heel padding to support the Achilles tendon.

Stabilizers: Bars or strips of rubber, polyurethane, or nylon near the heel or forefoot area of some shoes; they provide additional stability.

Wedge: The thick portion of the midsole that makes the heel higher than the ball of the foot in some shoes.

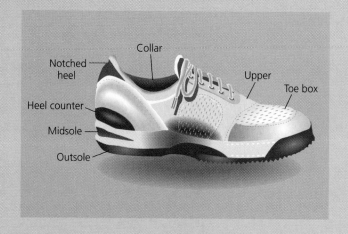

General Guidelines

When choosing athletic shoes, first consider the activity you've chosen for your exercise program. Shoes appropriate for different activities have very different characteristics. For example, running shoes typically have highly cushioned midsoles, rubber outsoles with elevated heels, and a great deal of flexibility in the forefoot. The heels of walking shoes tend to be lower, less padded, and more beveled than those designed for running. For aerobic dance, shoes must be flexible in the forefoot and have straight, nonflared heels to allow for safe and easy lateral movements. Court shoes also provide substantial support for lateral movements; they typically have outsoles made from white rubber that will not damage court surfaces.

Also consider the location and intensity of your workouts. If you plan to walk or run on trails, you should choose shoes with water-resistant, highly durable uppers and more outsole traction. If you work out intensely or have a relatively high body weight, you'll need thick, firm midsoles to avoid bottoming-out the cushioning system of your shoes.

Foot type is another important consideration. If your feet tend to roll in excessively (overpronate), you may need shoes with additional stability features on the inner side of the shoe to counteract this movement. If your feet tend to roll outward excessively (oversupinate), you may need highly flexible and cushioned shoes that promote foot motion. For aerobic dancers

and as an incentive for improvement. If you have specific, measurable goals, you can also graph your weekly or monthly progress toward your goal (Figure 7-4).

7. Make a Commitment

Your final step in planning your program is to make a commitment by signing a contract. Find a witness for your contract—preferably one who will be actively involved in your program. Keep your contract in a visible spot to remind you of your commitment.

PUTTING YOUR PLAN INTO ACTION

Once you've developed a detailed plan and signed your contract, you are ready to begin your fitness program. Refer to the specific training suggestions provided in Chapters 2–5 for advice on beginning and maintaining your program. Some key guidelines are summarized below.

• *Start slowly and increase intensity and duration gradually.* Overzealous exercising can result in discouraging discomforts and injuries. Your program is meant to last a

with feet that tend to pronate or supinate, mid-cut to high-cut shoes may be more appropriate than low-cut aerobic shoes or cross-trainers (shoes designed to be worn for several different activities). Compared with men, women have narrower feet overall and narrower heels relative to the forefoot. Most women will get a better fit if they choose shoes that are specifically designed for women's feet rather than those that are downsized versions of men's shoes.

For successful shoe shopping, keep these strategies in mind:

- Shop at an athletic shoe or specialty store that has personnel trained to fit athletic shoes and a large selection of styles and sizes.

- Shop late in the day or, ideally, following a workout. Your foot size increases over the course of the day and as a result of exercise.

- Wear socks like those you plan to wear during exercise. If you have an old pair of athletic shoes, bring them with you. The wear pattern on your old shoes can help you select a pair with extra support or cushioning in the places you need it the most.

- Ask for help. Trained salespeople know which shoes are designed for your foot type and your level of activity. They can also help fit your shoes properly.

- Don't insist on buying shoes in what you consider to be your typical shoe size. Sizes vary from shoe to shoe. In addition, foot sizes change over time, and many people have one foot that is larger or wider than the other. Try

several sizes in several widths if necessary. Don't buy shoes that are too small.

- Try on both shoes, and wear them around for at least 10 minutes. Try walking on a noncarpeted surface. Approximate the movements of your activity: walk, jog, run, jump, and so on.

- Check the fit and style carefully.

   Is the toe box roomy enough? Your toes will spread out when your foot hits the ground or you push off. There should be at least one thumb's width of space from the longest toe to the end of the toe box.

   Do they have enough cushioning? Do your feet feel cushioned and supported when you bounce up and down? Try bouncing on your toes and on your heels.

   Do your heels fit snugly into the shoe? Do they stay put when you walk, or do they rise up?

   Are the arches of your feet right on top of the shoes' arch supports?

   Do the shoes feel stable when you twist and turn on the balls of your feet? Try twisting from side to side while standing on one foot.

   Do you feel any pressure points?

- If the shoe isn't comfortable in the store, don't buy it. Don't expect athletic shoes to stretch over time in order to fit your feet properly.

lifetime. The important first step is to break your established pattern of inactivity. Be patient and realistic. Once your body has adjusted to your starting level of exercise, slowly increase the amount of overload. Small increases are the key—achieving a large number of small improvements will eventually result in substantial gains in fitness. It's usually best to increase duration and frequency before increasing intensity.

- *Find an exercise buddy.* The social side of exercise is an important factor for many regular exercisers. Working out with a friend will make exercise more enjoyable and increase your chances of sticking with your program. Find an exercise partner who shares your goals and general fitness level.

- *Vary your program.* You can make your program more fun over the long term if you participate in a variety of different activities that you enjoy. You can also add interest by strategies such as varying the routes you take when walking, running, biking, or in-line skating; finding a new tennis or racquetball partner; changing your music for aerobic dance; or switching to a new volleyball or basketball court.

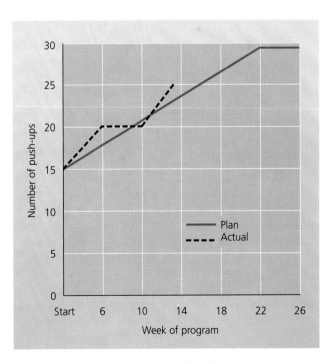

Figure 7-4 A sample program progress chart.

Engaging in any program of exercise requires a generous amount of common sense to minimize risk and prevent injury. Here are ten precautions to take into account as you begin an exercise program:

1. **Be smart.** Minimize risk. If you are over 45 years old or in a high-risk group, see a physician and have an EKG stress test before you begin an exercise program.

2. **Keep your muscles in balance.** Combine aerobic exercise with a sound strength training program. When your muscles are strong in proportion to each other, they are less likely to be injured.

3. **Take care of your feet.** Select shoes that provide adequate support and cushioning. Promptly take care of any exercise-related problem that plagues your feet (blisters, bone bruises, blackened toenails, and the like).

4. **Train by stressing your body to its limits and then just a little bit more.** Allow your body to adapt to a relatively small increase in stress. Don't overstress.

5. **Use proper techniques while exercising.** Keep your body in proper alignment when you're exercising. This will decrease the likelihood of your being injured.

6. **Respect signals from your body that something may be wrong.** Stop exercising if you experience abnormal heart beats, pain or pressure in your chest, dizziness, light-headedness, nausea during or after exercise, prolonged fatigue, or insomnia.

7. **Get adequate rest.** Without adequate rest, you can not achieve the maximum benefits from your exercise regimen.

8. **Keep an exercise diary.** If you get injured, a diary may help you learn how and why the injury occurred. A diary can also help your health care provider to diagnose and treat you most successfully.

9. **Keep in mind that exercise by itself cannot produce good health.** Exercise is only one factor conducive to basic wellness. Combine it with other elements of wellness—nutritional, emotional, social/interpersonal, intellectual, spiritual, and environmental—to be truly healthy.

10. **Minimize the constant stress on your joints.** If you prefer high-impact exercise, be sure to include low- or nonimpact forms of exercise on a regular basis (preferably on an alternating basis).

SOURCE: Adapted from Peterson, J. 1999. Ten common-sense precautions for exercisers. *ACSM's Health and Fitness Journal* 3(3): 48.

Varying your activities, a strategy known as cross-training, has other benefits. It can help you develop balanced, total body fitness. For example, by alternating running with swimming, you build both upper- and lower-body strength. Cross-training can thus prepare you for a wider range of activities and physical challenges. It can also reduce the risk of injury and overtraining because the same muscles, bones, and joints are not continuously subjected to the stresses of the same activity. Cross training can be done either by choosing different activities on different days or by alternating activities within a single workout.

• *Expect fluctuations and lapses.* On some days, your progress will be excellent, but on others, you'll barely be able to drag yourself through your scheduled activities. Don't let off-days or lapses discourage you or make you feel guilty. Instead, feel a renewed commitment for your fitness program. Focus on the improvements you obtain from your program and how good you feel after exercise. Reward yourself often for sticking with your program. Visualize what it will be like to reach your goals, and keep these pictures in your mind as an incentive to stick with your program.

If you notice you're slacking off, use your health journal to identify the negative thoughts and behaviors that are causing noncompliance. Devise a strategy to decrease the frequency of these negative thoughts and behaviors. Make changes in your program plan and reward system to help renew your enthusiasm and commitment to your program. Expect to make many adjustments in your program along the way.

See the box "Exercising Common Sense" for additional suggestions on how to keep your program on track.

EXERCISE GUIDELINES FOR PEOPLE WITH SPECIAL HEALTH CONCERNS

Regular, appropriate exercise is safe and beneficial for many people with chronic conditions or other special health concerns. For example, people with heart disease or hypertension who exercise may lower their blood pressure and improve their cholesterol levels. For people with diabetes, exercise can improve insulin sensitivity and body composition. For people with asthma, regular exercise may reduce the risk of acute attacks during exertion. For many people with special health concerns, the risks associated with *not* exercising are far greater than those associated with a moderate program of regular exercise.

The fitness recommendations for the general population presented in this text can serve as a general guideline

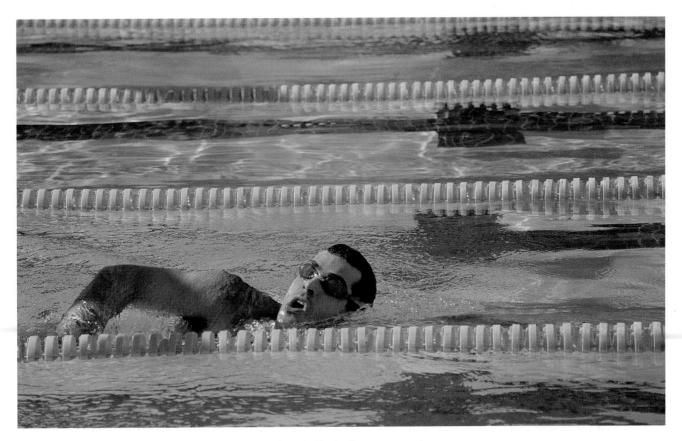

An individual with special health concerns can develop a safe and effective fitness program by choosing activities carefully and making appropriate modifications in the program. Swimming is an excellent activity choice for this man with asthma because breathing warm, moist air reduces the risk of asthma attacks during exercise.

for any exercise program. However, for people with special health concerns, certain precautions and monitoring may be required. Anyone with special health concerns should consult a physician before beginning an exercise program. Guidelines and cautions for some common conditions are described below.

Arthritis

- Begin an exercise program as early as possible in the course of the disease.
- Warm up thoroughly before each exercise session to loosen stiff muscles and lower the risk of injury.
- For cardiorespiratory endurance exercise, avoid high-impact activities that may damage arthritic joints; consider a swimming program or another type of exercise in a warm pool.
- Perform strength training exercises for the whole body; pay special attention to muscles that support and protect affected joints (for example, build quadriceps, hamstring, and calf strength for the knee). Start with small loads and build intensity gradually.

- Perform flexibility exercises regularly to maintain joint mobility.

Asthma

- Exercise regularly. Acute attacks are more likely if you exercise only occasionally.
- Carry medication during workouts, and avoid exercising alone.
- Warm up and cool down slowly to reduce the risk of acute attacks.
- When starting an exercise program, choose self-paced endurance activities, especially those involving **interval training** (short bouts of exercise followed by a rest period). Increase the intensity of cardiorespiratory endurance exercise gradually.
- Cold, dry air can trigger or worsen an attack. Drink water before, during, and after a workout to moisten

interval training A training technique that alternates exercise intervals with rest intervals or intense exercise intervals with low to moderate intervals.   **TERMS**

your airways. In cold weather, cover your mouth with a mask or scarf to warm and humidify the air you breathe. Swimming in a heated pool is an excellent activity choice for people with asthma.

- Avoid outdoor activities during pollen season or when the air is polluted. Avoid exercise in dry or dusty indoor environments.

Diabetes

- Don't begin an exercise program unless your diabetes is under control and you have checked about exercise safety with your physician. Because people with diabetes have an increased risk for heart disease, an exercise stress test may be recommended.

- Don't exercise alone. Wear a bracelet identifying yourself as having diabetes.

- If you are taking insulin or another medication, you may need to adjust the timing and amount of each dose. Work with your physician and check your blood sugar levels regularly so you can learn to balance your energy intake and output and your medication dosage.

- To prevent abnormally rapid absorption of injected insulin, inject it over a muscle that won't be exercised, and wait at least an hour before exercising.

- Check blood sugar levels before, during, and after exercise, and adjust your diet or insulin dosage if needed. Carry high-carbohydrate foods during a workout.

- Don't lift heavy weights. Straining can damage blood vessels.

- If you have poor circulation or numbness in your extremities, check your skin regularly for blisters and abrasions, especially on your feet. Avoid high-impact activities, and wear comfortable shoes.

- For maximum benefit and minimum risk, choose low-to-moderate-intensity activities

Heart Disease and Hypertension

- Check with your physician about exercise safety before increasing your activity level.

- Exercise at a moderate rather than a high intensity. Keep your heart rate below the level at which abnormalities appear on an exercise stress test.

- Warm-up and cool-down sessions should be gradual and last at least 10 minutes.

- Monitor your heart rate during exercise, and stop if you experience dizziness or chest pain.

- If your physician has prescribed it, carry nitroglycerin with you during exercise. If you are taking beta-blockers for hypertension, use RPE rather than heart rate to monitor exercise intensity (beta-blockers

reduce heart rate). Exercise at an RPE level of "somewhat hard"; your breathing should be unlabored, and you should be able to talk.

- Don't hold your breath when exercising. Doing so can cause sudden, steep increases in blood pressure. Take special care during weight training; don't lift extremely heavy loads.

- Increase exercise intensity, duration, and frequency very gradually.

Obesity

- For maximum benefit and minimum risk, choose low-to-moderate-intensity activities.

- Choose non- or low-weight-bearing activities such as swimming, water exercises, cycling, or walking. Low-impact activities are less likely to lead to joint problems or injuries.

- Stay alert for symptoms of heat-related problems during exercise (see Chapter 3). People who are obese are particularly vulnerable to problems with heat intolerance.

- Ease into an exercise program, and increase overload gradually. Increase duration and frequency of exercise before increasing intensity.

- Include strength training in your fitness program to build or maintain fat-free mass.

Osteoporosis

- For cardiorespiratory endurance activities, exercise at the maximum intensity that causes no significant discomfort. If possible, choose low-impact weight-bearing activities to help safely maintain bone density (see Chapter 8 for more strategies for building and maintaining bone density).

- To prevent fractures, avoid any activity or movement that stresses the back or carries a risk of falling.

- Include weight training in your exercise program to improve strength and balance and reduce the risk of falls and fractures. Avoid lifting heavy loads.

Pregnancy

Exercise is important during pregnancy, but women should be cautious because some types of exercise can pose increased risk to the mother and the unborn child. The following guidelines are consistent with the recommendations of the American College of Obstetrics and Gynecology.

- See your physician about possible modifications needed for your particular pregnancy.

- Continue mild-to-moderate exercise routines at least three times a week. Avoid exercising vigorously or to exhaustion, especially in the third trimester. Monitor exercise intensity by assessing how you feel rather than by monitoring your heart rate.

- Favor non- or low-weight-bearing exercises such as swimming or cycling over weight-bearing exercises, which can carry increased risk of injury.

- Avoid exercise in a supine position—lying on your back—after the first trimester. Research indicates that this position restricts blood flow to the uterus. Also avoid prolonged periods of motionless standing.

- Avoid exercise that could cause loss of balance, especially in the third trimester, and exercise that might injure the abdomen, stress the joints, or carry a risk of falling (such as contact sports, vigorous racquet sports, skiing, and in-line skating).

- Avoid activities involving extremes in altitude—for example, scuba diving and mountain climbing.

- Especially during the first trimester, drink plenty of fluids and exercise in well-ventilated areas to avoid heat stress.

- After giving birth, resume prepregnancy exercise routines gradually, based on how you feel.

Exercise for Older Adults

Older people readily adapt and respond to endurance exercise and strength training. Exercise principles are the same as for younger people, but some specific guidelines apply:

- Include the three basic types of exercise—resistance, endurance, and flexibility.

- Drink plenty of water, and avoid exercising in excessively hot or cold environments. (Older people sometimes have a decreased ability to regulate body temperature during exercise.) Wear clothes that speed heat loss in warm environments and that prevent heat loss in cold environments.

- Warm up slowly and carefully. Increase intensity and duration of exercise gradually.

- Cool down slowly, continuing very light exercise until the heart rate is below 100.

- To help prevent soft tissue pain, do static stretching.

Exercise for Children and Adolescents

Only about half of all young people age 12–21 in the United States participate regularly in vigorous activity, and 25% report no vigorous activity at all. Inactivity is higher in females than in males. This lack of physical activity has led to alarming increases in overweight and obesity in children and adolescents. If you have children or are in a position to influence children, keep these guidelines in mind:

- Provide opportunities for children and adolescents to exercise every day. Minimize sedentary activities, such as watching television and playing video games. Children and adolescents should aim for 60 minutes of moderate physical activity most, but preferably all, days.

- During family outings, choose dynamic activities. For example, go for a walk, park away from a mall and then walk to the stores, take the stairs instead of the escalator.

- In children under 12 years, emphasize skill development and fitness rather than excellence in competitive sports. In adolescents, combine participation and training in lifetime sports with traditional, competitive sports.

- Make sure children are developmentally capable of participating in an activity. For example, catching skills are difficult for young children because their nervous system is not developed enough to fully master the skill. When teaching a child to catch a ball, start with a large ball, and throw it from a short range. Gradually increase the complexity of the skill once the child has mastered the simpler skill.

- Make sure children get plenty of water when exercising in the heat. Make sure they are dressed properly when doing sports in the cold.

Exercise guidelines for people with disabilities are discussed in Chapter 2 and for people with low-back pain, in Chapter 5.

COMMON QUESTIONS ANSWERED

Should I exercise every day?   Some daily exercise is beneficial, and health experts recommend that you engage in at least 30 minutes of moderate physical activity over the course of every day. However, if you train intensely every day without giving yourself a rest, you will likely get injured or become overtrained. When strength training, for example, rest at least 1 day between workouts before exercising the same muscle group. For cardiorespiratory endurance exercise, rest or exercise lightly the day after an intense or long-duration workout. Balancing the proper amount of rest and exercise will help you feel better and improve your fitness faster.

(continued)

I'm just starting an exercise program. How much activity should I do at first? Be conservative. Walking is a good way to begin almost any fitness program. At first, walk for approximately 10 minutes, and then increase the distance and pace. After several weeks, you can progress to something more vigorous. Let your body be your guide. If the intensity and duration of a workout seem easy, increase them a little the next time. The key is to be progressive; don't try to achieve physical fitness in one or two workouts. Build your fitness gradually.

What are kickboxing and Tae Bo? Are they effective forms of exercise? Kickboxing and Tae Bo are group fitness workouts that combine martial arts maneuvers, boxing moves, and traditional group exercise activities. Participants in martial arts workouts repetitively execute a variety of punches and kicks, building movement combinations that involve the entire body. Workouts are often choreographed to moderately paced popular music and are continuous in nature. Although more research is needed to clarify the actual training effects, the workouts certainly develop cardiovascular endurance, muscular endurance, and flexibility. Because of the potential for injury, classes should be led either by a certified fitness professional who has had ancillary training in teaching martial arts skills or a martial artist with qualifications as a fitness instructor. Other key safety elements include precise skill modeling and verbal instruction, moderate pacing, and an emphasis on health-related fitness development.

I'm concerned about my safety when I go for a jog or walk. What can I do to make sure that my training sessions are safe and enjoyable? A person exercising alone in the park can be a tempting target for criminals. Don't exercise alone. You are much less likely to be a crime victim if you are training in a group or with a partner. Another alternative is to take an exercise class. Classes are fun and much safer than exercising by yourself. If you must train alone, try to exercise where there are plenty of people. A good bet is the local high school or college track.

Make sure you're wearing proper safety equipment. If you're riding a bike, wear a helmet. If you're playing racquetball or handball, wear eye protectors. Don't go in-line skating unless you're wearing the proper pads and protective equipment. If you are jogging at night, wear reflective clothing that can be seen easily.

Refer to Appendix A for more information on personal safety.

SUMMARY

- Steps for putting together a complete fitness program include (1) setting realistic goals; (2) selecting activities to develop all the health-related components of fitness; (3) setting a target intensity, duration, and frequency for each activity; (4) setting up a system of mini-goals and rewards; (5) making lifestyle physical activity a part of the daily routine; (6) developing tools for monitoring progress; and (7) making a commitment.

- In selecting activities, consider fun and interest, your current skill and fitness levels, time and convenience, cost, and any special health concerns.

- Keys to putting a successful plan into action are starting slowly, increasing intensity and duration gradually, finding a buddy, varying the program, and expecting fluctuations and lapses.

- Regular exercise is appropriate and highly beneficial for people with special health concerns; program modifications may be necessary to maximize safety.

FOR MORE INFORMATION

See the listings for Chapters 2–6.

SELECTED BIBLIOGRAPHY

American College of Sports Medicine. 2000. *ACSM's Guidelines for Exercise Testing and Prescription*, 6th ed. Baltimore, Md.: Lippincott Williams & Wilkins.

American College of Sports Medicine. 1998. ACSM position stand: Exercise and physical activity for older adults. *Medicine and Science in Sports and Exercise* 30(6): 992–1008.

American College of Sports Medicine. 1998. ACSM position stand: The recommended quantity and quality of exercise for developing and maintaining cardiorespiratory and muscular fitness, and flexibility in healthy adults. *Medicine and Science in Sports and Exercise* 30(6): 975–991.

American College of Sports Medicine. 1998. *ACSM's Resource Manual for Guidelines for Exercise Testing and Prescription*, 3rd ed. Baltimore, Md.: Williams & Wilkins.

American College of Sports Medicine and American Diabetes Association. 1997. Joint position statement: Diabetes mellitus and exercise. *Medicine and Science in Sports and Exercise* 29(12): I–VI.

Butler, R. N. 2000. Fighting frailty: Prescription for healthier aging includes exercise, nutrition, safety, and research. *Geriatrics* 55(2): 20.

Carpenter, M. W. 2000. The role of exercise in pregnant women with diabetes mellitus. *Clinical Obstetrics and Gynecology* 43(1): 56–64.

Casperson, C. J., P. A. Nixon, and R. H. DuRant. 1998. Physical activity epidemiology applied to children and adolescents. *Exercise and Sport Sciences Reviews* 26:341–403.

Daley, M. J., and W. L. Spinks. 2000. Exercise, mobility, and aging. *Sports Medicine* 29(1): 1–12.

DePalo, V. A., and F. D. McCool. 2000. Exercise-induced asthma. *Medicine and Health, Rhode Island* 83(2): 52–55.

Eriksson J. G. 1999. Exercise and the treatment of Type 2 diabetes mellitus: An update. *Sports Medicine* 27(6): 381–391.

Galloway, M. T., and P. Jokl. 2000. Aging successfully: The importance of physical activity in maintaining health and function. *Journal of the American Academy of Orthopaedic Surgeons* 8(1): 37–44.

Goran, M. I., K. D. Reynolds, and C. H. Lindquist. 1999. Role of physical activity in the prevention of obesity in children. *International Journal of Obesity and Related Metabolic Disorders* 23(Suppl. 3): S18–S33.

Hartmann, S., and P. Bung. 1999. Physical exercise during pregnancy—Physiological considerations and recommendations. *Journal of Perinatal Medicine* 27(3): 204–215.

International Inline Skating Association. Health benefits: Burn, baby, burn (http://www.iisa.org/numbers/health.htm; retrieved December 4, 1999).

Manek, N. J., and N. E. Lane. 2000. Osteoarthritis: Current concepts in diagnosis and management. *American Family Physician* 61(6): 1795–1804.

Martin, D. R. 1997. Athletic shoes: Finding a good match. *Physician and Sports medicine* 25(9): 138–144.

Morrow, J. R., Jr., et al. 1999. A one-year follow-up to Physical Activity and Health: A Report of the Surgeon General. *American Journal of Preventive Medicine* 17(1): 24–30.

Olson, M. D., and H. N. Williford. 1999. Martial arts exercise. *ACSM's Health and Fitness Journal* 3(6): 6–14.

Rowland, T., et al. 2000. Cardiac responses to progressive exercise in normal children: A synthesis. *Medicine and Science in Sports and Exercise* 32(2): 253–259.

Shephard, R. J. 2000. Exercise and training in women, part II: Influence of menstrual cycle and pregnancy. *Canadian Journal of Applied Physiology* 25(1): 35–54.

Sothern, M. S., et al. 1999. The health benefits of physical activity in children and adolescents: Implications for chronic disease prevention. *European Journal of Pediatrics* 158(4): 271–274.

Wei, M., et al. 1999. Relationship between low cardiorespiratory fitness and mortality in normal-weight, overweight, and obese men. *Journal of the American Medical Association* 282(16): 1547–1553.

Workouts for special disorders. 2000. *Consumer Reports on Health,* January, 9.

SAMPLE PROGRAMS FOR POPULAR ACTIVITIES

Sample programs based on four different types of cardiorespiratory activities—walking/jogging/running, bicycling, swimming, and in-line skating—are presented below. Each sample program includes regular cardiorespiratory endurance exercise, resistance training, and stretching. To choose a sample program, first compare your fitness goals with the benefits of the different types of endurance exercise featured in the sample programs (see Table 7-1). Identify the programs that meet your fitness needs. Next, read through the descriptions of the programs you're considering, and decide which will work best for you based on your present routine, the potential for enjoyment, and adaptability to your lifestyle. If you choose one of these programs, complete the personal fitness program plan in Lab 7-1, just as if you had created a program from scratch.

No program will bring about enormous changes in your fitness level in the first few weeks. Give your program a good chance. Follow the specifics of the program for 3–4 weeks. Then if the exercise program doesn't seem suitable, make adjustments to adapt it to your particular needs. But retain the basic elements of the program that make it effective for developing fitness.

General Guidelines

The following guidelines can help make the activity programs more effective for you.

- *Intensity.* To work effectively for cardiorespiratory endurance training or to improve body composition, you must raise your heart rate into its target zone. Monitor your pulse, or use rates of perceived exertion to monitor your intensity.

If you've been sedentary, begin very slowly. Give your muscles a chance to adjust to their increased workload. It's probably best to keep your heart rate below target until your body has had time to adjust to new demands. At first you may not need to work very hard to keep your heart rate in its target zone, but as your cardiorespiratory endurance improves, you will probably need to increase intensity.

- *Duration and frequency.* To experience training effects, you should exercise for 20–60 minutes at least three times a week.

- *Interval training.* Some of the sample programs involve continuous activity. Others rely on interval training, which calls for alternating a relief interval with exercise (walking after jogging, for example, or coasting after biking uphill). Interval training is an effective way to achieve progressive overload: When your heart rate gets too high, slow down to lower your pulse rate until you're at the low end of your target zone. Interval training can also prolong the total time you spend in exercise and delay the onset of fatigue.

- *Warm-up and cool-down.* Begin each exercise session with a 10-minute warm-up. Begin your activity at a slow pace, and work up gradually to your target heart rate. Always slow down gradually at the end of your exercise session to bring your system back to its normal state. It's a good idea to do stretching exercises to increase your flexibility after cardiorespiratory exercise or strength training because your muscles will be warm and ready to stretch.

- *Record keeping.* After each exercise session, record your daily distance or time on a progress chart.

Walking, jogging, and running are the most popular forms of training for people who want to improve cardiorespiratory endurance; they also improve body composition and muscular endurance of the legs. It's not always easy to distinguish among these three endurance activities. For clarity and consistency, we'll consider walking to be any on-foot exercise of less than 5 miles per hour, jogging any pace between 5 and 7.5 miles per hour, and running any pace faster than that. Table 1 divides walking, jogging, and running into nine categories, with rates of speed (in both miles per hour and minutes per mile) and calorie costs for each. The faster your pace or the longer you exercise, the more calories you burn. The greater the number of calories burned, the higher the potential training effects of these activities. Tables 2 and 3 contain sample walking/jogging programs by time and distance.

Equipment and Technique

These activities require no special skills, expensive equipment, or unusual facilities. Comfortable clothing, well-fitted walking or running shoes, and a stopwatch or ordinary watch with a second hand are all you need.

Developing Cardiorespiratory Endurance

The four variations of the basic walking/jogging/running sample program that follow are designed to help you regulate the intensity, duration, and frequency of your program. Use the following guidelines to choose the variation that is right for you.

- *Variation 1: Walking (Starting).* Choose this program if you have medical restrictions, are recovering from illness or surgery, tire easily after short walks, are obese, or have a sedentary lifestyle, and if you want to prepare for the advanced walking program to improve cardiorespiratory endurance, body composition, and muscular endurance.

- *Variation 2: Advanced Walking.* Choose this program if you already can walk comfortably for 30 minutes and if you want to develop and maintain cardiorespiratory fitness, a lean body, and muscular endurance.

- *Variation 3: Preparing for a Jogging Program.* Choose this program if you already can walk comfortably for 30 minutes and if you want to prepare for the jogging/running program to improve cardiorespiratory endurance, body composition, and muscular endurance.

- *Variation 4: Jogging/Running.* Choose this program if you already can jog comfortably without muscular discomfort, if you already can jog for 15 minutes without stopping or 30 minutes with brief walking intervals within your target heart rate range, and if you want to develop and maintain a high level of cardiorespiratory fitness, a lean body, and muscular endurance.

Variation 1: Walking (Starting)

Intensity, duration, and frequency: Walk at first for 15 minutes at a pace that keeps your heart rate below your target zone. Gradually increase to 30-minute sessions. The distance you travel will probably be 1–2 miles. At the beginning, walk every other day. You can gradually increase to daily walking if you want to burn more calories (helpful if you want to change body composition).

Calorie cost: Work up to using 90–135 calories in each session (see Table 1). To increase calorie costs to the target level, walk for a longer time or for a longer distance rather than sharply increasing speed.

At the beginning: Start at whatever level is most comfortable. Maintain a normal, easy pace, and stop to rest as often as you need to. Never prolong a walk past the point of comfort. When walking with a friend (a good motivation), let a comfortable conversation be your guide to pace.

As you progress: Once your muscles have become adjusted to the exercise program, increase the duration of your sessions—but by no more than 10% each week. Increase your intensity only enough to keep your heart rate just below your target. When you're able to walk 1.5 miles in 30 minutes, using 90–135 calories per session, you should consider moving on to Variation 2 or 3. Don't be discouraged by lack of immediate progress, and don't try to speed things up by overdoing. Remember that pace and heart rate can vary with the terrain, the weather, and other factors.

Variation 2: Advanced Walking

Intensity, duration, and frequency: Start at a pace at the lower end of your target heart rate zone, and begin soon afterward to increase your pace. This might boost your heart rate into the upper levels of your target zone, which is fine for brief periods. But don't overdo the intervals of fast walking. Slow down after a short time to drop your pulse rate. Vary your pattern to allow for intervals of slow, medium, and fast walking. Walk at first for 30 minutes and gradually increase your walking time until eventually you reach 60 minutes, all the while maintaining your target heart rate. The distance you walk will probably be 2–4 miles. Walk at least every other day.

Calorie cost: Work up to using about 200–350 calories in each session (see Table 1).

At the beginning: Begin by walking somewhat faster than you did in Variation 1. Check your pulse to make sure you keep your heart rate within your target zone. Slow down when necessary to lower your heart rate when going up hills or when extending the duration of your walks.

As you progress: As your heart rate adjusts to the increased workload, gradually increase your pace and your total walking time. Gradually lengthen the periods of fast walking and shorten the relief intervals of slow walking, always maintaining target heart rate. Eventually, you will reach the fitness level you would like to maintain. And to maintain that level of fitness, continue to burn the same amount of calories in each session.

Vary your program by changing the pace and distance walked, or by walking routes with different terrains and views. Gauge your progress toward whatever calorie goal you've set by using Table 1.

Variation 3: Preparing for a Jogging Program

Intensity, duration, and frequency: Start by walking at a moderate pace (3–4 miles per hour or 15–20 minutes per mile).

SAMPLE PROGRAM TABLE I
Calorie Costs for Walking/Jogging/Running

This table gives the calorie costs of walking, jogging, and running for slow, moderate, and fast paces. Calculations for calorie costs are approximate and assume a level terrain. A hilly terrain would result in higher calorie costs. To get an estimate of the number of calories you burn, multiply your weight by the calories per minute per pound for the speed at which you're doing the activity (listed in the right-hand column), and then multiply that by the number of minutes you exercise.

Activity	Speed		Calories per Minute per Pound
	Miles per Hour	Minutes: Seconds per Mile	
Walking			
Slow	2.0	30:00	.020
	2.5	24:00	.023
Moderate	3.0	20:00	.026
	3.5	17:08	.029
Fast	4.0	15:00	.037
	4.5	13:20	.048
Jogging			
Slow	5.0	12:00	.060
	5.5	11:00	.074
Moderate	6.0	10:00	.081
	6.5	9:00	.088
Fast	7.0	8:35	.092
	7.5	8:00	.099
Running			
Slow	8.5	7:00	.111
Moderate	9.0	6:40	.116
Fast	10.0	6:00	.129
	11.0	5:30	.141

SOURCE: Kusinitz, I., and M. Fine. 1995. *Your Guide to Getting Fit,* 3d ed. Mountain View, Calif.: Mayfield.

Staying within your target heart rate zone, begin to add brief intervals of slow jogging (5–6 miles per hour or 10–12 minutes per mile). Keep the walking intervals constant at 60 seconds or at 110 yards, but gradually increase the jogging intervals until eventually you jog 4 minutes for each minute of walking. You'll probably cover between 1.5 and 2.5 miles. Each exercise session should last 15–30 minutes. Exercise every other day. If your goals include changing body composition and you want to exercise more frequently, walk on days you're not jogging.

Calorie cost: Work up to using 200–350 calories in each session (see Table 1).

At the beginning: Start slowly. Until your muscles adjust to jogging, you may need to exercise at less than your target heart rate. At the outset, expect to do two to four times as much walking as jogging, even more if you're relatively inexperienced. Be guided by how comfortable you feel—and by your heart rate—in setting the pace for your progress. Follow the guidelines presented in Chapter 3 for exercising in hot or cold weather. Drink enough liquids to stay adequately hydrated, particularly in hot weather. In addition, use the proper running technique, described below.

- Run with your back straight and your head up. Look straight ahead, not at your feet. Shift your pelvis forward, and tuck your buttocks in.

- Hold your arms slightly away from your body. Your elbows should be bent so that your forearms are parallel to the ground. You may cup your hands, but do not clench your fists. Allow your arms to swing loosely and rhythmically with each stride.

- Your heel should hit the ground first in each stride. Then roll forward onto the ball of your foot and push off for the next stride. If you find this difficult, you can try a more flat-footed style, but don't land on the balls of your feet.

- Keep your steps short by allowing your foot to strike the ground in line with your knee. Keep your knees bent at all times.

- Breathe deeply through your mouth. Try to use your abdominal muscles rather than just your chest muscles to take deep breaths.

- Stay relaxed.

As you progress: Adjust your ratio of walking to jogging to keep within your target heart rate zone as much as possible. When you have progressed to the point where most of your 30-minute session is spent jogging, consider moving on to Variation 4. To find a walking/jogging progression that suits you, refer to Tables 2 and 3 (one uses time, the other distance). Which one you choose will depend, to some extent, on where you work out. If you have access to a track or can use a measured distance with easily visible landmarks to indicate yardage covered, you may find it convenient to use distance as your organizing principle. If you'll be using parks, streets, or woods, time intervals (measured with a watch) would probably work better. The progressions in Tables 2 and 3 are not meant to be rigid; they are guidelines to help you develop your own rate of progress. Let your progress be guided by your heart rate, and increase your intensity and duration only to achieve your target zone.

Variation 4: Jogging/Running

Intensity, duration, and frequency: The key is to exercise within your target heart rate zone. Most people who sustain a continuous jog/run program will find that they can stay within their target heart rate zone with a speed of 5.5–7.5 miles per hour (8–11 minutes per mile). Start by jogging steadily for 15 minutes. Gradually increase your jog/run session to a regular 30–60 minutes (or about 2.5–7 miles). Exercise at least every other day. Increasing frequency by doing other activities on alternate days will place less stress on the weight-bearing parts of your lower body than will a daily program of jogging/running.

Calorie cost: Use about 300–750 calories in each session (see Table 1).

At the beginning: The greater number of calories you burn per minute makes this program less time-consuming for altering body composition than the three other variations in the walking/jogging/running program.

SAMPLE PROGRAM TABLE 2 *Walking/Jogging Progression by Time*

This table is based on a walking interval of 3.75 miles per hour, measured in seconds, and a jogging interval of 5.5 miles per hour, measured in minutes:seconds. The combination of the two intervals equals a single set. In the Number of Sets column, the higher figure represents the maximum number of sets to be completed.

	Walk Interval (sec)	Jog Interval (min:sec)	Number of Sets	Total Distance (mi)	Total Time (min:sec)
Stage 1	:60	:30	10–15	1.0–1.7	15:00–22:30
Stage 2	:60	:60	8–13	1.2–2.0	16:00–26:00
Stage 3	:60	2:00	5–19	1.3–2.3	15:00–27:00
Stage 4	:60	3:00	5–7	1.6–2.4	16:00–28:00
Stage 5	:60	4:00	3–6	1.5–2.7	15:00–30:00

SOURCE: Kusinitz, I., and M. Fine. 1995. *Your Guide to Getting Fit*, 3d ed. Mountain View, Calif.: Mayfield.

SAMPLE PROGRAM TABLE 3 *Walking/Jogging Progression by Distance*

This table is based on a walking interval of 3.75 miles per hour, measured in yards, and a jogging interval of 5.5 miles per hour, also measured in yards. The combination of the two intervals equals a single set. (One lap around a typical track is 440 yards.)

	Walk Interval (yd)	Jog Interval (yd)	Number of Sets	Total Distance (mi)	Total Time (min:sec)
Stage 1	110	55	11–21	1.0–2.0	15:00–28:12
Stage 2	110	110	16	2.0	26:56
Stage 3	110	220	11	2.0	26:02
Stage 4	110	330	8	2.0	24:24
Stage 5	110	440	7	2.2	26:05
Stage 6	110	440	8	2.5	29:49

SOURCE: Kusinitz, I., and M. Fine. 1995. *Your Guide to Getting Fit*, 3d ed. Mountain View, Calif.: Mayfield.

As you progress: If you choose this variation, you probably already have a moderate-to-high level of cardiorespiratory fitness. To stay within your target heart rate zone, increase your distance or both pace and distance as needed. Add variety to your workouts by varying your route, intensity, and duration. Alternate short runs with long ones. If you run for 60 minutes one day, try running for 30 minutes the next session. Or try doing sets that alternate hard and easy intervals—even walking, if you feel like it. You can also try a road race now and then, but be careful not to do too much too soon.

Developing Muscular Strength and Endurance

Walking, jogging, and running provide muscular endurance workouts for your lower body; they also develop muscular strength of the lower body to a lesser degree. To develop muscular strength and endurance of the upper body, and to make greater and more rapid gains in lower-body strength, you need to include resistance training in your fitness program. Use the general wellness weight training program from Chapter 4, or tailor one to fit your personal fitness goals. If you'd like to increase your running speed and performance, you might want to focus your program on lower-body exercises. (Don't neglect upper-body strength, however; it is important for overall well-

ness.) Regardless of what strength training exercises you choose, follow the guidelines for successful training:

- Train 2–3 days per week.
- Perform 1 or more sets of 8–12 repetitions of 8–10 exercises.
- Include exercises that work all the major muscle groups: neck, shoulders, chest, arms, upper and lower back, abdomen, thighs, and calves.

Depending on the amount of time you are able to set aside for exercise, you may find it more convenient to alternate between your cardiorespiratory endurance workouts and your muscular strength and endurance workouts. In other words, walk or jog one day and strength train the next day.

Developing Flexibility

To round out your fitness program, you also need to include exercises that develop flexibility. The best time for a flexibility workout is when your muscles are warm, as they are immediately following cardiorespiratory endurance exercise or strength training. Perform the stretching routine presented in Chapter 5 or one that you have created to meet your own goals and preferences. Be sure to pay special attention to the hamstrings and quadriceps, which are not worked through their complete range of motion during walking or jogging. As you put your program together, remember the basic structure of a successful flexibility program:

- Stretch at least 2–3 days per week, preferably when muscles are warm.

- Stretch all the major muscle groups.
- Stretch to the point of mild discomfort, and hold for 10–30 seconds.
- Repeat each stretch at least 4 times.

BICYCLING SAMPLE PROGRAM

Bicycling can also lead to large gains in physical fitness. For many people, cycling is a pleasant and economical alternative to driving and a convenient way to build fitness.

Equipment and Technique

Cycling has its own special array of equipment, including headgear, lighting, safety pennants, and special shoes. The bike is the most expensive item, ranging from about $100 to well over $1000. Avoid making a large investment until you're sure you'll use your bike regularly. While investigating what the marketplace has to offer, rent or borrow a bike. Consider your intended use of the bike. Most cyclists who are interested primarily in fitness are best served by a sturdy 10-speed rather than a mountain bike or sport bike. Stationary cycles are good for rainy days and areas that have harsh winters.

Clothing for bike riding shouldn't be restrictive or binding, nor should it be so loose-fitting or so long that it might get caught in the chain. Clothing worn on the upper body should be comfortable but not so loose that it catches the wind and slows you down. Always wear a helmet to help prevent injury in case of a fall or crash. Wearing glasses or goggles can protect the eyes from dirt, small objects, and irritation from wind.

To avoid saddle soreness and injury, choose a soft or padded saddle, and adjust it to a height that allows your legs to almost reach full extension while pedaling. Wear a pair of well-padded gloves if your hands tend to become numb while riding or if you begin to develop blisters or calluses. To prevent backache and neck strain, warm up thoroughly, and periodically shift the position of your hands on the handlebars and your body in the saddle. Keep your arms relaxed, and don't lock your elbows. To protect your knees from strain, pedal with your feet pointed straight ahead or very slightly inward, and don't pedal in high gear for long periods.

Bike riding requires a number of precise skills that practice makes automatic. If you've never ridden before, consider taking a course. In fact, many courses are not just for beginners. They'll help you develop skills in braking, shifting, and handling emergencies, as well as teach you ways of caring for and repairing your bike.

The National Injury Information Clearinghouse classifies bicycle riding as the nation's most dangerous sport. Many injuries are the result of carelessness. For safe cycling, follow these rules:

- Always wear a helmet.
- Keep on the correct side of the road. Bicycling against traffic is usually illegal and always dangerous.
- Obey all traffic signs and signals.
- On public roads, ride in single file, except in low-traffic areas (if the law permits). Ride in a straight line; don't swerve or weave in traffic.

- Be alert; anticipate the movements of other traffic and pedestrians. Listen for approaching traffic that is out of your line of vision.
- Slow down at street crossings. Check both ways before crossing.
- Use hand signals—the same as for automobile drivers—if you intend to stop or turn. Use audible signals to warn those in your path.
- Maintain full control. Avoid anything that interferes with your vision. Don't jeopardize your ability to steer by carrying anything (including people) on the handlebars.
- Keep your bicycle in good shape. Brakes, gears, saddle, wheels, and tires should always be in good condition.
- See and be seen. Use a headlight at night, and equip your bike with rear reflectors. Use side reflectors on pedals, front and rear. Wear light-colored clothing or use reflective tape at night; wear bright colors or use fluorescent tape by day.
- Be courteous to other road users. Anticipate the worst, and practice preventive cycling.
- Use a rear-view mirror.

Developing Cardiorespiratory Endurance

Cycling is an excellent way to develop and maintain cardiorespiratory endurance and a healthy body composition.

Intensity, duration, and frequency: If you've been inactive for a long time, begin your cycling program at a heart rate that is 10–20% below your target zone. Once you feel at home on your bike, try 1 mile at a comfortable speed, and then stop and check your heart rate. Increase your speed gradually until you can cycle at 12–15 miles per hour (4–5 minutes per mile), a speed fast enough to bring most new cyclists' heart rate into their target zone. Allow your pulse rate to be your guide: More highly fit individuals may need to ride faster to achieve their target heart rate. Cycling for at least 20 minutes three times a week will improve your fitness.

Calorie cost: Use Table 4 to determine the number of calories you burn during each outing. You can increase the number of calories burned by cycling faster or for a longer duration (it's usually better to increase distance rather than to add speed).

At the beginning: It may require several outings to get the muscles and joints of your legs and hips adjusted to this new activity. Begin each outing with a 10-minute warm-up that includes stretches for your hamstrings and your back and neck muscles. Until you become a skilled cyclist, select routes with the fewest hazards, and avoid heavy automobile traffic.

SAMPLE PROGRAM TABLE 4   *Calorie Costs for Bicycling*

This table gives the approximate calorie costs per pound of body weight for cycling from 5 to 60 minutes for distances of .50 mile up to 15 miles on a level terrain. To use the table, find on the horizontal line the time most closely approximating the number of minutes you cycle. Next, locate on the vertical column the approximate distance in miles you cover. The figure at the intersection represents an estimate of the calories used per minute per pound of body weight. Multiply this figure by your own body weight. Then multiply the product of these two figures by the number of minutes you cycle to get the total number of calories burned. For example, assuming you weigh 154 pounds and cycle 6 miles in 40 minutes, you would burn 260 calories: 154 × .042 (calories per pound, from table) = 6.5 × 40 (minutes) = 260 calories burned.

	Time (min)											
Distance (mi)	5	10	15	20	25	30	35	40	45	50	55	60
.50	.032											
1.00	.062	.032										
1.50		.042	.032									
2.00		.062	.039	.032								
3.00			.062	.042	.036	.032						
4.00				.062	.044	.039	.035	.032				
5.00				.097	.062	.045	.041	.037	.035	.032		
6.00					.088	.062	.047	.042	.039	.036	.034	.032
7.00						.081	.062	.049	.043	.040	.038	.036
8.00							.078	.062	.050	.044	.041	.039
9.00								.076	.062	.051	.045	.042
10.00								.097	.074	.062	.051	.045
11.00									.093	.073	.062	.052
12.00										.088	.072	.062
13.00											.084	.071
14.00												.081
15.00												.097

SOURCE: Kusinitz, I., and M. Fine. 1995. *Your Guide to Getting Fit*, 3d ed. Mountain View, Calif.: Mayfield.

As you progress: Interval training is also effective with bicycling. Simply increase your speed for periods of 4–8 minutes or for specific distances, such as 1–2 miles. Then coast for 2–3 minutes. Alternate the speed intervals and slow intervals for a total of 20–60 minutes, depending on your level of fitness. Hilly terrain is also a form of interval training.

Developing Muscular Strength and Endurance

Bicycling develops a high level of endurance and a moderate level of strength in the muscles of the lower body. To develop muscular strength and endurance of the upper body—and to make greater and more rapid gains in lower-body strength—you need to include resistance training as part of your fitness program. Use the general wellness weight training program from Chapter 4, or tailor one to fit your personal fitness goals. If one of your goals is to increase your cycling speed and performance, be sure to include exercises for the quadriceps, hamstrings, and buttocks muscles in your strength training program. No matter which exercises you include in your program, follow the general guidelines for successful and safe training:

- Train 2–3 days per week.

- Perform 1 or more sets of 8–12 repetitions of 8–10 exercises.

- Include exercises that work all the major muscle groups: neck, shoulders, chest, arms, upper and lower back, abdomen, thighs, and calves.

Depending on your schedule, you may find it more convenient to alternate between your cardiorespiratory endurance workouts and your muscular strength and endurance workouts. In other words, cycle one day and strength train the next day.

Developing Flexibility

A complete fitness program also includes exercises that develop flexibility. The best time for a flexibility workout is when your muscles are warm, as they are immediately following a session of cardiorespiratory endurance exercise or strength training. Perform the stretching routine presented in Chapter 5, or develop one that meets your own goals and preferences. Pay special attention to the hamstrings and quadriceps, which are not worked through their complete range of motion during bike riding, and to the muscles in your lower back, shoulders, and neck. As you put your stretching program together, remember these basic guidelines:

- Stretch at least 2–3 days per week, preferably when muscles are warm.

- Stretch all the major muscle groups.

- Stretch to the point of mild discomfort, and hold for 10–30 seconds.

- Repeat each stretch at least 4 times.

Swimming is one of the best activities for developing all-around fitness. Because water supports the body weight of the swimmer, swimming places less stress than weight-bearing activities on joints, ligaments, and tendons and tends to cause fewer injuries.

Equipment and Safety Guidelines

Aside from having access to a swimming pool, the only equipment required for a swimming program is a swimsuit and a pair of swimming goggles to protect the eyes from irritation in chlorinated pools.

Following these few simple rules can help keep you safe and healthy during your swimming sessions:

- Swim only in a pool with a qualified lifeguard on duty.

- Always walk carefully on wet surfaces.

- Dry your ears well after swimming. If you experience the symptoms of swimmer's ear (itching, discharge, or even a partial hearing loss), consult your physician. If you swim while recovering from swimmer's ear, protect your ears with a few drops of lanolin on a wad of lamb's wool.

- To avoid back pain, try not to arch your back excessively when you swim.

- Be courteous to others in the pool.

If you swim in a setting other than a pool with a lifeguard, remember the following important rules:

- Don't swim beyond your skill and endurance limits.

- Avoid being chilled by water colder than 70°F.

- Never drink alcohol before going swimming.

- Never swim alone.

Developing Cardiorespiratory Endurance

Any one or any combination of common swimming strokes—front crawl stroke, breaststroke, backstroke, butterfly stroke, sidestroke, or elementary backstroke—can help develop and maintain cardiorespiratory fitness. (Swimming may not be as helpful as walking, jogging, or cycling for body fat loss.)

Intensity, duration, and frequency: Because swimming is not a weight-bearing activity and is not done in an upright position, it elicits a lower heart rate per minute. Therefore, you need to adjust your target heart rate zone. To calculate your target heart rate for swimming, use this formula:

Maximum swimming heart rate (MSHR) = 205 − age
Target heart rate zone = 65–90% of MSHR

For example, a 19-year-old would calculate her target heart rate zone for swimming as follows:

MSHR = 205 − 19 = 186 bpm

Target heart rate zone for swimming:

at 65% intensity: $0.65 \times 186 = 121$ bpm

at 90% intensity: $0.90 \times 186 = 167$ bpm

Base your duration of swimming on your intensity and target calorie costs. Swim at least three times a week.

Calorie cost: Calories burned while swimming are the result of the pace: how far you swim and how fast (see Table 5). Work up to using at least 300 calories per session.

At the beginning: If you don't have much experience swimming, invest the time and money for instruction. You'll make more rapid gains in fitness if you learn correct swimming technique. If you've been sedentary and haven't done any swimming for a long time, begin your program with 2–3 weeks, three times a week, of leisurely swimming at a pace that keeps your heart rate 10–20% below your target zone. Start swimming laps of the width of the pool if you can't swim the length. To keep your heart rate below target, take rest intervals as needed. Swim one lap, then rest 15–90 seconds as needed. Start with 10 minutes of swim/rest intervals and work up to 20 minutes. How long it takes will depend on your swimming skills and muscular fitness.

As you progress: Gradually increase the duration, or the intensity, or both duration and intensity of your swimming to raise your heart rate to a comfortable level within your target zone. Gradually increase your swimming intervals and decrease your rest intervals as you progress. Once you can swim the length of the pool at a pace that keeps your heart rate on target, continue swim/rest intervals for 20 minutes. Your rest intervals should be 30–45 seconds. You may find it helpful to get out of the pool during your rest intervals and walk until you've lowered your heart rate. Next, swim two laps of the pool length per swim interval and continue swim/rest intervals for 30 minutes. For the 30-second rest interval, walk (or rest) until you've lowered your heart rate. Gradually increase the number of laps you swim consecutively and the total duration of your session until you reach your target calorie expenditure and fitness level. But take care not to swim at too fast a pace: It can raise your heart rate too high and limit your ability to sustain your swimming. Alternating strokes can rest your muscles and help prolong your swimming time. A variety of strokes will also let you work more muscle groups.

Developing Muscular Strength and Endurance

The swimming program outlined in this section will result in moderate gains in strength and large gains in endurance in the muscles used during the strokes you've chosen. To develop strength and endurance in all the muscles of the body, you need to include resistance training as part of your fitness program. Use the general wellness weight training program from Chapter 4, or tailor one to fit your personal fitness goals. To improve your swimming performance, include exercises that work key muscles. For example, if you swim primarily front crawl, include exercises to increase strength in your shoulders, arms, and upper back. (Training the muscles you use during swimming can also help prevent injuries.) Regardless of which strength training exercise you include in your program, follow the general guidelines for successful training:

- Train 2–3 days per week.

- Perform 1 or more sets of 8–12 repetitions of 8–10 exercises.

- Include exercises that work all the major muscle groups: neck, shoulders, chest, arms, upper and lower back, abdomen, thighs, and calves.

Depending on the amount of time you have for exercise, you might want to schedule your cardiorespiratory endurance workouts and your muscular strength and endurance workouts on alternate days. In other words, swim one day and strength train the next day.

Developing Flexibility

For a complete fitness program, you also need to include exercises that develop flexibility. The best time for a flexibility workout is when your muscles are warm, as they are immediately following cardiorespiratory endurance exercise or strength training. Perform the stretching routine presented in Chapter 5 or one you have created to meet your own goals and preferences. Be sure to pay special attention to the muscles you use during swimming, particularly the shoulders and back. As you put your program together, remember the basic structure of a successful flexibility program:

- Stretch at least 2–3 days per week, preferably when muscles are warm.

- Stretch all the major muscle groups.

- Stretch to the point of mild discomfort, and hold for 10–30 seconds.

- Repeat each stretch at least 4 times.

IN-LINE SKATING SAMPLE PROGRAM

In-line skating is currently the fastest growing sport in the United States. Skating is convenient and inexpensive (after the initial outlay for equipment); it can be done on city streets, on paved bike paths and trails, and in parks. If done intensively enough, skating can provide a cardiorespiratory endurance workout comparable to the workouts provided by jogging and cycling. Studies indicate that skating consumes about as many calories as jogging.

An advantage of skating over jogging is that skating is low impact, so it is less harmful to the knees and ankles. An advantage of skating over bicycling is that it works the hamstring muscle in the back of the thigh. Skating develops lower-body strength and endurance, working all the muscles of the leg and hip and strengthening the muscles and connective tissues surrounding the ankles, knees, and hips.

Equipment

To skate safely and enjoyably, you will need a pair of comfortable, sturdy, quality skates and adequate safety equipment. The skate consists of a hard polyurethane shell or outer boot; a padded foam liner; and a frame or chassis that holds the wheels, bearings, spacers, and brake. If you want to try out the sport before making a commitment, rent your skates and equipment from a skate shop. If you are buying, plan to spend about $110–$200 for skates that meet the basic needs of most recreational skaters. Shop for the best combination of price, quality, comfort, and service.

Essential safety equipment includes a helmet, elbow pads, knee pads, and wrist guards. (Wrist injuries are the most common in-line skating injury.) You may want to put reflective tape on your skates for those occasions when you don't get home before dark. Carry moleskin or adhesive bandages with you in case you start to develop a blister while skating. (For more on safety, see Appendix A.)

Technique

In-line skating uses many of the skills and techniques of ice skating, roller skating, and skiing, so if you have ever participated in any of those activities, you will probably take to in-line skating fairly readily. Many people begin in-line skating without instruction, but instruction will allow you to progress more quickly.

To begin, center your weight equally over both skates, bend your knees slightly so your nose, knees, and toes are all in the same line, and look straight ahead. Keep your weight forward over the balls of your feet; don't lean back.

To skate, use a stroke, glide, stroke, glide rhythm (rather than a series of quick, short strokes). Push with one leg while gliding with the other. Shift your body weight back and forth so it is always centered over the gliding skate.

To stop, use your brake, located on the back of the right skate in most skates. With knees bent and arms extended in front of your body, move the right foot forward, shift your weight to your left leg, and lift your right toe until the brake pad touches the ground and stops you. An alternative stop is the T-stop, in which you drag one skate behind the other at a 90-degree angle to the direction of your forward motion.

If you lose your balance and are about to fall, lower your center of gravity by bending at the waist and putting your hands on your knees. If you can't regain your balance, try to fall forward, directing the impact to your wrist guards and knee pads. Try not to fall backward.

Again, instruction can help you learn many moves and techniques that will make the sport safer and more enjoyable.

Developing Cardiorespiratory Endurance

Studies have shown that in-line skaters raise their heart rates and oxygen consumption comparably to joggers, bicyclers, and walkers. Skaters reached 60–75% of $\dot{V}O_{2max}$ by skating continuously (not pushing off and gliding for several seconds) at 10.6–12.5 mph for 20–30 minutes. It may be difficult for recreational skaters to safely skate this fast for this long, however, given the typical constraints of city and suburban streets. Experts suggest skating uphill as much as possible to reach the level of intensity that builds cardiorespiratory endurance. If you can reach and maintain higher speeds in parks or on paved paths, do so, but always skate safely. (If you belong to a gym or fitness club and want to do some indoor skating, Nautilus manufactures a piece of equipment called the Skate Machine.)

Intensity, duration, and frequency: Start your early skating sessions at a pace that keeps your heart rate about 10–20% below your target zone. Skate for 5–10 minutes, and then check your heart rate. Increase your speed gradually until you can skate at about 10 miles per hour (6 minutes per mile). Use your pulse as a guide to speed, aiming for 65% of your target heart rate zone. To achieve cardiorespiratory benefits, you will have to skate at a continuous and relatively intense pace for at least 20 minutes three times a week. The more fit you are, the more intensively you will need to skate to reach your target heart rate.

Calorie cost: Use Table 6 to determine the approximate number of calories you burn during each outing. You can increase the number of calories burned by skating faster, for a longer time, or uphill.

At the beginning: If you are a beginner, practice skating in an empty schoolyard or a parking lot. As you become confident with the basic techniques, you can move on to streets, parks, and paved bike trails. Maintain an easy pace, alternating stroking and gliding.

Begin each outing with a 5- to 10-minute warm-up of walking, jogging, or even slow skating. Once your muscles are warm, you can do some stretches to help loosen and warm up the primary muscles used during skating. These muscles include the quadriceps, hamstrings, buttocks, hips, groin, ankles, calves, and lower back. You can also save the stretches for the end of the workout.

To launch an in-line skating fitness program, aim for slow, long-distance workouts at first. Start by skating for 15 minutes, and gradually increase your sessions to 20–30 minutes of continuous skating (about 3.5–5 miles). Try to skate about 20 miles a week, or 5 miles a day (about 30 minutes) 4 days a week.

As you progress: After the first week or two, add about a mile a day, up to 40 miles per week (60 minutes a day). To increase intensity, add some hills, sprints (bursts of short, rapid striding), and interval training (periods of intensive exercise at your target heart rate alternating with timed rest periods when your heart rate drops below your target zone). Try to skate 30–60 minutes a day four or more times a week.

The harder and faster you skate, the more intensive your workout will be and the more your cardiorespiratory endurance and muscular strength will improve. The longer and more often you skate, the more your endurance will increase.

Developing Muscular Strength and Endurance

In-line skating develops the muscles in the entire upper leg, buttocks, and hip; lower back; and upper arms and shoulders when arms are swung vigorously. To make greater gains in lower-body strength and to develop the entire upper body, include resistance training in your overall fitness program. Use the general wellness weight training program from Chapter 4, or tailor one to fit your personal fitness goals. No matter which exercises you include in your program, follow the general guidelines for successful and safe training:

- Train 2–3 days per week.
- Perform 1 or more sets of 8–12 repetitions of 8–10 exercises.
- Include exercises that work all the major muscle groups: neck, shoulders, chest, arms, upper and lower back, thighs, and calves.

Depending on your schedule, you may find it more convenient to skate and weight train on alternate days.

SAMPLE PROGRAM TABLE 6
Calorie Costs for In-Line Skating

To estimate the number of calories you burn, first determine your approximate speed (use the Minutes: Seconds per Mile column if necessary), multiply the calories per minute per pound by your weight, and then multiply that figure by the number of minutes you skate. For example: assuming you weigh 145 pounds and skate at 10 mph for 30 minutes, you would burn 273 calories: 145 × .063 (calories per pound, from table) = 9.1 × 30 (minutes) = 273 calories burned. Calculations are approximate.

Speed		Calories per Minute per Pound
Miles per Hour	Minutes:Seconds per Mile	
8	7:30	.041
9	6:40	.053
10	6:00	.063
11	5:25	.072
12	5:00	.084
13	4:35	.095
14	4:20	.105
15	4:00	.115

SOURCES: Adapted from International Inline Skating Association. 1999. *Health Benefits of Inline Skating* (http://www.iisa.org/numbers/health.htm; retrieved April 7, 2000); Wallick, M. E., et al. 1995. Physiological responses to in-line skating compared to treadmill running. *Medicine and Science in Sports and Exercise* 27(2): 242–248.

Developing Flexibility

The best times for a flexibility workout are when your muscles are warm, so stretch after a short warm-up at the beginning of your skating session, or after your skating session, or after a weight training session. Use the stretching routine presented in Chapter 5, or develop one that meets your own goals and preferences. Pay particular attention to your quadriceps, hamstrings, buttocks, hips, groin, ankles, calves, and lower back. Remember these basic guidelines:

- Stretch at least 2–3 days per week, preferably when muscles are warm.
- Stretch all the major muscle groups.
- Stretch to the point of mild discomfort, and hold for 10–30 seconds.
- Repeat each stretch at least 4 times.

Name _____ Section _____ Date _____

 LAB 7-I *A Personal Fitness Program Plan and Contract*

A. I, _____, am contracting with myself to follow a physical fitness
(name)

program to work toward the following goals:

Specific or short-term goals

1. _____

2. _____

3. _____

4. _____

General or long-term goals

1. _____

2. _____

3. _____

4. _____

B. My program plan is as follows:

Activities	Components (Check ✓)					Intensity*	Duration	Frequency (Check ✓)						
	CRE	MS	ME	F	BC			M	Tu	W	Th	F	Sa	Su

*Conduct activities for achieving CRE goals at your target heart rate or RPE value.

C. My program will begin on _____. My program includes the following schedule of mini-goals. For each step
(date)

in my program, I will give myself the reward listed.

_____   _____   _____
(mini-goal 1)   (date)   (reward)

_____   _____   _____
(mini-goal 2)   (date)   (reward)

_____   _____   _____
(mini-goal 3)   (date)   (reward)

_____   _____   _____
(mini-goal 4)   (date)   (reward)

_____   _____   _____
(mini-goal 5)   (date)   (reward)

LABORATORY ACTIVITIES

D. My program will include the addition of physical activity to my daily routine (such as climbing stairs or walking to class):

1. _____

2. _____

3. _____

4. _____

5. _____

E. I will use the following tools to monitor my program and my progress toward my goals:

_____

(list any charts, graphs, or journals you plan to use)

_____

_____

I sign this contract as an indication of my personal commitment to reach my goal.

_____   _____
(your signature)   (date)

I have recruited a helper who will witness my contract and _____

_____

(list any way your helper will participate in your program)

_____

_____   _____
(witness's signature)   (date)

Nutrition

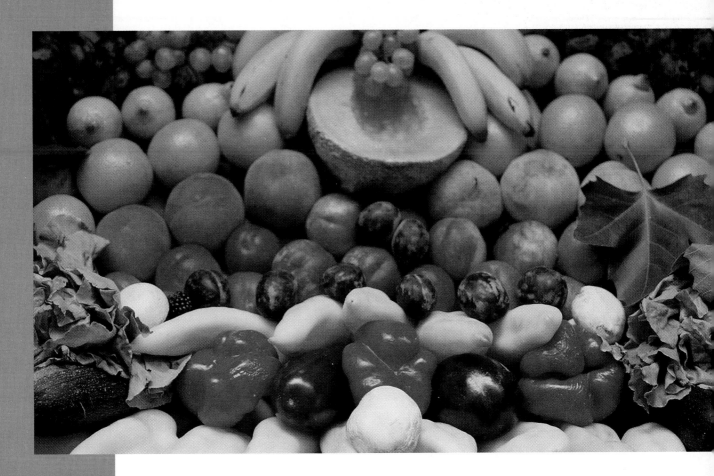

LOOKING AHEAD

After reading this chapter, you should be able to answer these questions about nutrition:

- What are the different kinds of essential nutrients, and what functions do they perform in the body?

- What guidelines have been developed to help people choose a healthy diet, avoid nutritional deficiencies, and protect themselves from diet-related chronic diseases?

- What information do consumers need to make informed choices about food?

- How can people adapt nutritional information to their own lives and circumstances?

191

Nutrition is a vital component of wellness. What you eat affects your energy level, well being, and over all health. Eating habits can also be closely linked with certain diseases, disabling conditions, and other health problems. Of particular concern is the connection between lifetime nutritional habits and the risk of the major chronic diseases, including heart disease, cancer, stroke, and diabetes. On the more positive side, however, a well-planned diet in conjunction with a fitness program can help prevent such conditions and even reverse some of them.

Creating a diet plan to support maximum fitness and protect against disease is a two-part project. First, you have to know which nutrients are necessary and in what amounts. Second, you have to translate those requirements into a diet consisting of foods you like to eat that are both available and affordable. Once you have an idea of what constitutes a healthy diet for you, you may also have to make adjustments in your current diet to bring it into line with your goals.

This chapter provides the basic principles of **nutrition.** It introduces the six classes of essential nutrients, explaining their role in the functioning of the body. It also provides different sets of guidelines that are available to help you design a healthy diet plan. Finally, it offers practical tools and advice to help you apply the guidelines to your own life, whether you are eating at home, at school, or in a restaurant. Diet is an area of your life in which you have almost total control. Using your knowledge and understanding of nutrition to create a healthy diet plan is a significant step toward wellness.

NUTRITIONAL REQUIREMENTS: COMPONENTS OF A HEALTHY DIET

When you think about your diet, you probably do so in terms of the foods you like to eat—a turkey sandwich and a glass of milk, or a steak and a baked potato. What's important for your health, though, are the nutrients contained in those foods. Your body requires proteins, fats, carbohydrates, vitamins, minerals, and water—about 45 **essential nutrients.** The word *essential* in this context means that you must get these substances from food because your body is unable to manufacture them at all, or at least not fast enough to meet your physiological needs. The six classes of nutrients, along with their functions and major sources, are listed in Table 8-1.

Nutrients are released into the body by the process of **digestion,** which breaks them down into compounds that the gastrointestinal tract can absorb and the body can use (Figure 8-1). In this form, the essential nutrients provide energy, build and maintain body tissues, and regulate body functions.

The energy in foods is expressed as **kilocalories.** One kilocalorie represents the amount of heat it takes to raise the temperature of 1 liter of water 1°C. A person needs about 2000 kilocalories a day to meet energy needs. In common usage, people usually refer to kilocalories as *calories,* which is a much smaller energy unit: 1 kilocalorie contains 1000 calories. We'll use the familiar word *calorie* in this chapter to stand for the larger energy unit.

Of the six classes of nutrients, three supply energy:

- Fats (supply the most energy) = 9 calories per gram
- Protein = 4 calories per gram
- Carbohydrates = 4 calories per gram

(Alcohol, although it is not an essential nutrient, also supplies energy, providing 7 calories per gram.) Experts advise against high fat consumption, in part because fats provide so many calories. Given the typical American diet, most Americans do not need the extra calories to meet energy needs.

Meeting our energy needs is only one of the functions of food. All the nutrients perform numerous other vital functions. In terms of quantity, water is the most significant nutrient: The body is approximately 60% water and can survive only a few days without it. Vitamins and minerals are needed in much smaller quantities, but they are still vital.

Practically all foods contain mixtures of nutrients, although foods are commonly classified according to their predominant nutrients. For example, spaghetti is considered a carbohydrate food although it contains small amounts of other nutrients. Let's take a closer look at the functions and sources of the six classes of nutrients.

Proteins—The Basis of Body Structure

Proteins form important parts of the body's main structural components: muscles and bones. Proteins also form important parts of blood, enzymes, cell membranes, and some hormones. As mentioned above, protein can also provide energy at 4 calories per gram of protein weight.

TERMS **nutrition** The science of food and how the body uses it in health and disease.

essential nutrients Substances the body must get from food because it cannot manufacture them at all or fast enough to meet its needs. These nutrients include proteins, fats, carbohydrates, vitamins, minerals, and water.

digestion The process of breaking down foods in the gastrointestinal tract into compounds the body can absorb.

kilocalorie A measure of energy content in food; 1 kilocalorie represents the amount of heat needed to raise the temperature of 1 liter of water 1°C; commonly referred to as *calorie.*

protein An essential nutrient; a compound made of amino acids that contains carbon, hydrogen, oxygen, and nitrogen.

TABLE 8-1   The Six Classes of Essential Nutrients

Nutrient	Function	Major Sources
Proteins (4 calories/gram)	Form important parts of muscles, bone, blood, enzymes, some hormones, and cell membranes; repair tissue; regulate water and acid-base balance; help in growth; supply energy	Meat, fish, poultry, eggs, milk products, legumes, nuts
Carbohydrates (4 calories/gram)	Supply energy to cells in brain, nervous system, and blood; supply energy to muscles during exercise	Grains (breads and cereals), fruits, vegetables, milk
Fats (9 calories/gram)	Supply energy; insulate, support, and cushion organs; provide medium for absorption of fat-soluble vitamins	Saturated fats primarily from animal sources, palm and coconut oils, and hydrogenated vegetable fats; unsaturated fats from grains, nuts, seeds, fish, vegetables
Vitamins	Promote (initiate or speed up) specific chemical reactions within cells	Abundant in fruits, vegetables, and grains; also found in meat and dairy products
Minerals	Help regulate body functions; aid in the growth and maintenance of body tissues; act as catalysts for the release of energy	Found in most food groups
Water	Makes up 50–70% of body weight; provides a medium for chemical reactions; transports chemicals; regulates temperature; removes waste products	Fruits, vegetables, and liquids

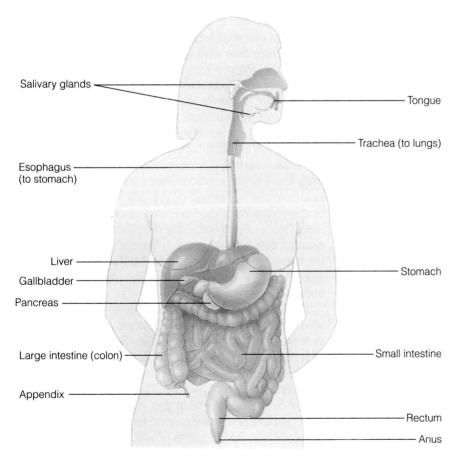

Figure 8-1 The digestive system. Food is partially broken down by being chewed and mixed with saliva in the mouth. As food moves through the digestive tract, it is mixed by muscular contractions and broken down by chemicals. After traveling to the stomach via the esophagus, food is broken down further by stomach acids. Most absorption of nutrients occurs in the small intestine, aided by secretions from the pancreas, gallbladder, and intestinal lining. The large intestine reabsorbs excess water; the remaining solid wastes are collected in the rectum and excreted through the anus.

Amino Acids The building blocks of proteins are called **amino acids**. Twenty common amino acids are found in food; nine of these are essential: histidine, isoleucine, leucine, lysine, methionine, phenylalanine, threonine, tryptophan, and valine. "Essential," again, means that they are required for normal health and growth but must be provided in the diet because the body manufactures them in insufficient quantities, if at all. The other eleven amino acids can be produced by the body as long as the necessary ingredients are supplied by foods.

Complete and Incomplete Proteins Individual protein sources are considered "complete" if they supply all the essential amino acids in adequate amounts and "incomplete" if they do not. Meat, fish, poultry, eggs, milk, cheese, and other foods from animal sources provide complete proteins. Incomplete proteins, which come from plant sources such as **legumes** and nuts, are good sources of most essential amino acids, but are usually low in one or two.

Combining two vegetable proteins, such as wheat and peanuts in a peanut butter sandwich, allows each vegetable protein to make up for the amino acids missing in the other protein. The combination yields a complete protein. Your concern with amino acids and complete protein in your diet should focus on what you consume throughout the day, rather than at each meal. It was once believed that vegetarians had to "complement" their proteins at each meal in order to receive the benefit of a complete protein. It is now known, however, that proteins consumed throughout the course of the day can complement each other to form a pool of amino acids the body can draw from to produce the necessary proteins. (Healthy vegetarian diets are discussed later in the chapter.)

Recommended Protein Intake The leading sources of protein in the American diet are (1) beef, steaks, and roasts; (2) hamburger and meatloaf; (3) white bread, rolls, and crackers; (4) milk; and (5) pork. About two-thirds of the protein in the American diet comes from animal sources; therefore, the American diet is rich in amino acids. Most Americans consume more protein than they need each day. Protein consumed beyond what the body needs is synthesized into fat for energy storage or burned for energy requirements. Consuming somewhat above our needs is not harmful, but it does contribute fat to the diet because protein-rich foods are often fat-rich as well.

Fats—Essential in Small Amounts

Fats, also known as lipids, are the most concentrated source of energy, at 9 calories per gram. The fats stored in your body represent usable energy, help insulate your body, and support and cushion your organs. Fats in the diet help your body absorb fat-soluble vitamins and add important flavor and texture to foods. Fats are the major fuel for the body during periods of rest and light activity.

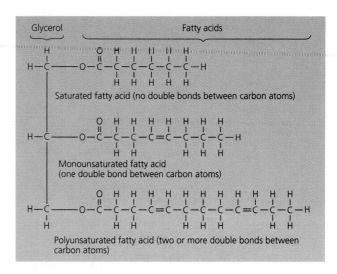

Figure 8-2 Chemical structures of saturated and unsaturated fatty acids. This example of a triglyceride consists of a molecule of glycerol with three fatty acids attached. Fatty acids can differ in the length of their carbon chains and their degree of saturation.

Two fats—linoleic acid and alpha-linolenic acid—are essential to the diet; they are key regulators of such body functions as the maintenance of blood pressure and the progress of a healthy pregnancy.

Types and Sources of Fats Most of the fats in food and in your body are in the form of triglycerides, which are composed of a glycerine molecule (an alcohol) plus three fatty acids. A fatty acid is made up of a chain of carbon atoms with oxygen attached at the end and hydrogen atoms attached along the length of the chain. Fatty acids differ in the length of their carbon atom chains and in their degree of saturation (the number of hydrogens attached to the chain). If every available bond from each carbon atom in a fatty acid chain is attached to a hydrogen atom, the fatty acid is said to be **saturated** (Figure 8-2). If not all the available bonds are taken up by hydrogens, the carbon atoms in the chain will form double bonds with each other. Such fatty acids are called unsaturated fats. If there is only one double bond, the fatty acid is called **monounsaturated.** If there are two or more double bonds, the fatty acid is called **polyunsaturated.** The essential fatty acids, linoleic and alpha-linolenic acids, are both polyunsaturated.

Food fats are often composed of both saturated and unsaturated fatty acids; the dominant type of fatty acid determines the fat's characteristics. Food fats containing large amounts of saturated fatty acids are usually solid at room temperature (these are called "fats"); they are generally found in animal products. The leading sources of saturated fat in the American diet are unprocessed animal flesh (hamburger, steak, roasts), whole milk, cheese, and hot dogs and lunch meats. Food fats containing large amounts of monounsaturated and polyunsaturated fatty acids are usually from plant sources and are liquid at room temperature (these are called "oils"). Olive, canola, safflower, and peanut oils contain mostly monounsaturated fatty acids. Corn, soybean, and cottonseed oils contain mostly polyunsaturated fatty acids. (The safflower oil available in stores has traditionally contained mostly polyunsaturated fatty acids, but in recent years, in response to market demand, manufacturers have switched to a variety of safflower oil containing mostly monounsaturated fatty acids.) There are some exceptions to the rules when it comes to saturated and unsaturated fats. A few vegetable oils, notably palm and coconut oils, are highly saturated, and the oils from many fish are rich in polyunsaturates.

Another type of fatty acid, **trans fatty acid,** is produced when hydrogen molecules are added to unsaturated vegetable oils, turning many of the double bonds in unsaturated fatty acids into single bonds like those in saturated fatty acids. This process, known as **hydrogenation,** stabilizes oils and increases their shelf life. Hydrogenation makes oils solid at room temperature and capable of withstanding the high temperatures required for deep-frying foods like french fries and doughnuts, it keeps the oil from separating out of peanut butter, and it improves the texture of foods like pie crusts and pastries. Developed in the early 1900s, hydrogenation is a commercially valuable process; however, the trans fats it produces have a negative effect on heart health, as described below.

Recommended Fat Intake You need only about 1 tablespoon (15 grams) of vegetable oil per day incorporated into your diet to supply the essential fats. The average American diet supplies considerably more than this amount; in fact, fats make up about 33% of our calorie intake. (This is the equivalent of about 75 grams, or 5 tablespoons, of fat a day.) Health experts recommend that most people reduce their fat intake to 30%, but not less than 10%, of total daily calories, with less than 10% of their intake coming from saturated fat. For reducing the risk of CVD, the American Heart Association (AHA) recommends the same limits for total and saturated fat; in addition, the AHA suggests up to 10% of total calories from polyunsaturated fat and up to 15% of total calories from monounsaturated fat. These recommendations are intended to reduce saturated fat in the diet and help keep calories under control to manage weight. For healthy Americans whose calories are under control, the AHA offers an alternative diet that is higher in monounsaturated fat (≥15%) and total fat (>30%) but continues to limit saturated fat to less than 10% of total calories. In this alternative diet, people are urged to replace saturated fat with monounsaturated fat rather than carbohydrates. This recommendation, made in 1999, reflects the growing evidence for the health-conferring benefits of monounsaturated fats.

The fat content of many common foods is given in Figure 8-3. The box "Setting Goals for Fat, Protein, and Carbohydrate Intake" explains how to set a daily goal for fat consumption.

Fats and Health Different types of fats have very different effects on health. Many studies have examined the effects of dietary fat intake on blood **cholesterol** levels and the risk of heart disease. Saturated and trans fatty acids raise blood levels of **low-density lipoprotein (LDL),** or "bad" cholesterol, thereby increasing a person's risk of heart disease. Unsaturated fatty acids, on the other hand, lower LDL. Monounsaturated fatty acids, such as those found in olive and canola oils, may also help maintain levels of **high-density lipoprotein (HDL),** or "good" cholesterol, providing even greater benefits for heart health.

A growing body of evidence is showing that trans fats may be as bad for heart health as saturated fats—and possibly even worse. Like saturated fats, trans fats raise levels of artery-clogging LDL; in addition, they lower levels of HDL. The net effect of trans fats on the ratio of bad-to-good cholesterol may be twice that caused by saturated fats. Health experts are particularly troubled by trans fats because their effects are not widely known by the public; in fact, many foods with trans fats appear to be healthy choices because they contain vegetable oil. Most of the trans fats in the American diet come from margarine, fried fast food, and packaged and prepared foods, especially

TERMS

amino acids The building blocks of proteins.

legumes Vegetables such as peas and beans that are high in fiber and are also important sources of protein.

saturated fat A fat with no carbon-carbon double bonds; solid at room temperature.

monounsaturated fat A fat with one carbon-carbon double bond; liquid at room temperature.

polyunsaturated fat A fat containing two or more carbon-carbon double bonds; liquid at room temperature.

trans fatty acid A type of unsaturated fatty acid produced during the process of hydrogenation; trans fats have an atypical shape that affects their chemical activity.

hydrogenation A process by which hydrogens are added to unsaturated fats, increasing the degree of saturation and turning liquid oils into solid fats. Hydrogenation produces a mixture of saturated fatty acids and standard and trans forms of unsaturated fatty acids.

cholesterol A waxy substance found in the blood and cells and implicated in heart disease.

low-density lipoprotein (LDL) Blood fat that transports cholesterol to organs and tissues; excess amounts result in the accumulation of fatty deposits on artery walls.

high-density lipoprotein (HDL) Blood fat that helps transport cholesterol out of the arteries, thereby protecting against heart disease.

	0–10%	10–30%	30–50%	50–75%	75–100%
Breads, cereals, rice, and pasta	Many dry cereals and breads, rice, pasta, tortillas, pretzels	Plain popcorn, hot cereals, some breads	Granola, buttered popcorn, crackers, biscuits, muffins	Croissants	
Vegetables and fruits	Most fresh, frozen, canned, and dried fruits and vegetables		French fries, onion rings	Potato chips, coconut	Avocado, olives
Milk, yogurt, and cheese	Fat-free milk, yogurt, and cottage cheese	Low-fat cottage cheese and yogurt, low-fat (1%) and reduced-fat (2%) milk, buttermilk	Whole milk, regular ice cream	Most cheeses, rich ice cream	Half-and-half, cream cheese, sour cream, heavy cream
Meat, poultry, fish, dry beans, eggs, nuts	Skinless turkey breast, haddock, cod, most dry beans, egg whites	Skinless white meat chicken, halibut, shrimp, clams, tuna in water, red snapper, trout, low-fat tofu	Beef top round, broiled steak, ham, skinless dark meat poultry, salmon, mackerel, swordfish	Roast beef, ground chuck; pork, lamb and veal chops; poultry with skin; tuna in oil; regular tofu; eggs	Salami, bacon, hot dogs, spareribs, most nuts and seeds, peanut butter, egg yolks
Combination foods	Clear soup (bouillon)	Most broth-based soups, vegetarian chili	Hamburger, lasagna, chili with meat, potato salad, vegetable and cheese pizza, macaroni and cheese, enchilada	Cheeseburger; meat pizza; large meat, poultry, or cheese sandwich; taco salad	
Fats, oils, and sweets	Hard candy, chewing gum			Chocolate bar	Butter, margarine, vegetable oil, mayonnaise, salad dressing

Figure 8-3 Percentage of total calories from fat for selected foods.

snack foods and sweets. Dairy and beef fat contain small amounts of trans fatty acids, but many people already limit their consumption of beef and dairy products to avoid saturated fats, so those sources are not as troubling to health experts.

The FDA has proposed that information on trans fat be provided on the Nutrition Facts panel of food labels and on the Supplements Facts panel of dietary supplement labels. The amount of trans fat would be added to the amount of saturated fat per serving, and an asterisk after the heading "Saturated Fat" would refer to a footnote stating that the product "Includes__g trans fat." The proposal would also add limits on trans fat to allowable health claims, such as "low saturated fat" and "lean." Until these rules go into effect, consumers can check food labels for such ingredients as "partially hydrogenated oil" and "vegetable shortening," both of which indicate that the product contains trans fat.

To protect your heart, limit your consumption of both saturated and trans fats. (Americans consume more saturated fat than trans fat—11% versus 2–4% of total calories.) The best way to reduce saturated fat is to lower your

intake of meat and full-fat dairy products (whole milk, cream, butter, cheese, ice cream). The best way to reduce trans fats is to lower your intake of deep-fried foods and baked goods made with hydrogenated vegetable oils, to use liquid oils rather than margarine, and to use squeeze or tub margarine rather than stick margarine. The softer or more liquid the margarine, the less trans fat it is likely to contain. Some margarines are labeled low-trans or trans-free, and some contain added plant sterols, compounds that may even lower cholesterol levels in people who have high cholesterol.

Although saturated and trans fats pose health hazards, some fats are turning out to be beneficial. Monounsaturated fatty acids, as found in avocados, most nuts, and olive, canola, peanut, and safflower oils, improve blood cholesterol levels and may help protect against some cancers. **Omega-3 fatty acids**, a form of polyunsaturated fat found primarily in fish, may be even more healthful. Omega-3s are produced when the endmost double bond of a polyunsaturated fat occurs three carbons from the end of the fatty acid chain. (The polyunsaturated fatty acid shown in Figure 8-2 is an omega-3 form.) Omega-3s reduce the tendency of blood to clot and help heart muscles beat in a steady rhythm, thus aiding in the prevention of heart attacks. They also reduce the body's inflammatory response. To increase omega-3 fatty acids in the diet, experts recommend two or more servings of fish a week, especially salmon, tuna, trout, mackerel, herring, sardines,

TERMS omega-3 fatty acids Polyunsaturated fatty acids commonly found in fish oils that are beneficial to cardiovascular health; the endmost double bond occurs three carbons from the end of the fatty acid chain.

TACTICS AND TIPS   *Setting Goals for Fat, Protein, and Carbohydrate Intake*

Setting Daily Goals

To meet the recommendations for nutrient intakes, start by setting some overall daily goals.

1. Determine approximately how many calories you consume each day. Depending on your activity level, daily needs range from about 2200 to 3500 calories for men and from about 1600 to 2500 for women.

2. Set percentage goals or limits for your intake of fat, protein, and carbohydrate. Those recommended for the general public are 30% or less of total daily calories from fat, 10–15% of total daily calories from protein, and 55% of total daily calories from carbohydrate. If your diet already meets these goals, you may want to set more challenging marks, such as raising your daily carbohydrate consumption to 60% of total calories.

3. Change your limits or goals from percentages to grams for easy tracking. A person who eats about 2200 calories per day could calculate her or his goals as follows:

Fat: 2200 calories per day × 30% = 660 calories of fat per day

660 calories ÷ 9 calories per gram = **73 g of fat per day**

Protein: 2200 calories per day × 15% = 330 calories of protein per day

330 calories ÷ 4 calories per gram = **83 g of protein per day**

Carbohydrate: 2200 calories per day × 55% = 1210 calories of carbohydrate per day

1210 calories ÷ 4 calories per gram = **303 g of carbohydrate per day**

(Remember, there are 9 calories per gram of fat and 4 calories per gram of protein and carbohydrate.)

Evaluating an Individual Food Item

You can do the same type of calculations to evaluate a particular food item, to determine whether it is high or low in protein, fat, or carbohydrate. For example, suppose you want to determine how high in fat peanut butter is. First, you need to know the total number of calories and grams of fat it contains. Multiply the grams of fat by 9 (because there are 9 calories in a gram of fat), and then divide that number by the total calories. For a tablespoon of peanut butter (8 grams of fat and 95 calories), you would calculate as follows: 8 × 9 = 72; 72 ÷ 95 = 0.76, or 76% of calories from fat. This means peanut butter is relatively high in fat. If your overall daily fat consumption goal is 70 grams of fat, a tablespoon of peanut butter would represent 11% of your daily target.

Of course, you can still eat high-fat foods. But it makes good sense to limit the size of your portions and to balance your intake with low-fat foods. For example, a tablespoon of peanut butter eaten on whole-wheat bread and served with a banana, carrot sticks, and a glass of nonfat milk makes a nutritious lunch—high in protein and carbohydrate, low in fat. Three tablespoons of peanut butter on high-fat crackers with potato chips, cookies, and whole milk is a less healthy combination. So although it's important to evaluate individual food items, it is more important to look at them in the context of your overall diet.

Monitoring Your Progress

Depending on your current diet and health needs, you may choose to focus on a particular goal, such as that for fat or protein. For prepared foods, food labels list the number of grams of fat, protein, and carbohydrate. The breakdown for many common foods and for popular fast-food items can be found in Appendixes B and C. Nutrition information is also posted in many grocery stores, published in inexpensive nutrition guides, and available online. By checking these resources, you can keep a running total of the grams of fat, protein, and carbohydrate you eat and determine how close you are to meeting your goals.

and anchovies. Lesser amounts of omega-3s are found in plant sources, including dark-green leafy vegetables; walnuts; flaxseeds; and canola, walnut, and flaxseed oils.

Another form of polyunsaturated fat, omega-6 fatty acid, is produced when the endmost double bond of a polyunsaturate occurs at the sixth carbon atom. Most of the polyunsaturated fats currently consumed by Americans are omega-6s, primarily from corn oil and soybean oil. Foods rich in omega-6s are important because they contain the essential nutrient linoleic acid, but nutritionists recommend that people reduce the proportion of omega-6s they consume in favor of omega-3s. To make this adjustment, use canola or flaxseed oil rather than corn or soybean oil, and watch out for soybean oil in mayonnaise, margarine, and salad dressings.

Dietary fat can affect other health factors besides cholesterol levels. Diets high in fatty red meats are associated with an increased risk of certain forms of cancer, especially colon cancer. A high-fat diet can also make weight management more difficult. Because fat is a concentrated source of calories, a high-fat diet is often a high-calorie diet that can lead to weight gain. In addition, there is some evidence that calories from fat are more easily converted to body fat than calories from protein or carbohydrate.

	Type of Fatty Acid	Found in[a]	Recommended Percentage of Total Calories	Possible Effects on Health
Keep Intake Low	SATURATED	Animal fats (especially fatty meats and poultry fat and skin) Butter, cheese, and other high-fat dairy products Palm and coconut oils	<10%	Raises total cholesterol and "bad" (LDL) cholesterol levels Increases risk of heart disease May increase risk of colon and prostate cancers
	TRANS	French fries and other deep-fried fast foods Stick margarines, shortening Packaged cookies and crackers Processed snacks and sweets	Not yet determined	Raises total cholesterol and "bad" (LDL) cholesterol levels Lowers "good" (HDL) cholesterol levels May increase risk of heart disease and breast cancer
Choose Moderate Amounts	MONOUNSATURATED	Olive, canola, and safflower oils Avocados, olives Peanut butter (without added fat) Many nuts, including almonds, cashews, pecans, pistachios	≤15%	Lowers total cholesterol and "bad" (LDL) cholesterol levels May reduce blood pressure and lower triglyceride levels (a risk factor for CVD) May reduce risk of heart disease, stroke, and some cancers
	POLYUNSATURATED (two groups)[b]			
	Omega-3 fatty acids	Fatty fish, including salmon, white albacore tuna, mackerel, anchovies, and sardines Lesser amounts in walnut, flaxseed, canola, and soybean oils; tofu; walnuts; flaxseeds; and dark-green, leafy vegetables	≤10% total for all poly-unsaturated fats	Reduces blood clotting and inflammation, and inhibits abnormal heart rhythms Lowers triglyceride levels (a risk factor for CVD) May lower blood pressure in some people May reduce risk of fatal heart attack and some cancers
	Omega-6 fatty acids	Corn, soybean, and cottonseed oils (often used in margarine, mayonnaise, and salad dressing)		Lowers total cholesterol and "bad" (LDL) cholesterol levels May lower "good" (HDL) cholesterol levels May reduce risk of heart disease May slightly increase risk of cancer if omega-6 intake is high and omega-3 intake is low

Recommended Percentage of Total Calories   **≤30%[c]**

[a] Food fats contain a combination of types of fatty acids in various proportions; for example, canola oil is composed mainly of monounsaturated fatty acids (62%) but also contains polyunsaturated (32%) and saturated (6%) fatty acids. Food fats are categorized here according to their predominant fatty acid.

[b] The essential fatty acids are polyunsaturated: linoleic acid is an omega-6 fatty acid and alpha-linolenic acid is an omega-3 fatty acid.

[c] Totals higher than 30% may be appropriate for some people, as long as the extra calories come from monounsaturated fat, intake of saturated fat is less than 10%, and body weight is maintained at a healthy level.

Figure 8-4   Types of fatty acids and their effects on health.   SOURCES: Allison, D. B., et al. 1999. Estimated intakes of *trans* fatty and other fatty acids in the U.S. population. *Journal of the American Dietetic Association* 99.166–174. American Heart Association. 1996. *Dietary Guidelines for Healthy American Adults.* Medical/Scientific Statement. Dallas, Tex.: American Heart Association.

Although more research is needed on the precise effects of different types and amounts of fat on overall health, a great deal of evidence points to the fact that most people benefit from lowering their overall fat intake to recommended levels and substituting unsaturated fats, particularly monounsaturated fats, for saturated and trans fats. The types of fatty acids, their effects on health, and recommended amounts are summarized in Figure 8-4.

Carbohydrates—An Ideal Source of Energy

Carbohydrates are needed in the diet primarily to supply energy to body cells. Some cells, such as those in the brain and other parts of the nervous system and in the blood, use only carbohydrates for fuel. During high-intensity exercise, muscles also get most of their energy from carbohydrates.

Simple and Complex Carbohydrates   Carbohydrates are classified into two groups: simple and complex. Simple carbohydrates contain only one or two sugar units in each molecule; they include sucrose (table sugar), fructose (fruit sugar, honey), maltose (malt sugar), and lactose (milk sugar). They provide much of the sweetness in foods and are found naturally in fruits and milk and are added to soft drinks, fruit drinks, candy, and sweet desserts. There is no evidence that any type of simple sugar is more nutritious than any other.

Starches and most types of dietary fiber are complex carbohydrates; they consist of chains of many sugar molecules. Starches are found in a variety of plants, especially grains (wheat, rye, rice, oats, barley, millet), legumes, and tubers (potatoes and yams). Most other vegetables contain a mix of starches and simple carbohydrates. Dietary fiber is found in fruits, vegetables, and grains.

During digestion in the mouth and small intestine, the body breaks down starches and double sugars into single sugar molecules, such as **glucose,** for absorption into the bloodstream. Once the glucose is absorbed, cells take it up and use it for energy. The liver and muscles also take up glucose and store it in the form of a starch called **glycogen.** The muscles use glycogen as fuel during endurance events or long workouts. Carbohydrates consumed in excess of the body's energy needs are changed into fat and stored. Whenever calorie intake exceeds calorie expenditure, fat storage can lead to weight gain. This is true whether the excess calories come from carbohydrates, proteins, fat, or alcohol.

Nutritionists distinguish between refined, or processed, carbohydrates and unrefined, or whole, carbohydrates. During processing, whole grains are stripped of their nutrient-rich inner germ and outer bran parts, leaving just the starchy middle layer. The refining process turns brown rice into white rice, whole-wheat flour into white flour, and so on. Unrefined carbohydrates are preferable to refined ones for several reasons. Unrefined carbohydrates retain the fiber, vitamins, and minerals that are stripped out of processed carbohydrates. They take longer to chew and digest, and they enter the bloodstream more slowly. This slower digestive pace makes people feel full sooner and for a longer period, lessening the likelihood that they will overeat and gain weight. It also helps keep blood sugar and insulin levels low, which may decrease the risk of diabetes.

Whole grains also have a positive effect on overall health and reduce the risk of heart disease and cancer. The USDA allows food manufacturers to claim that foods that are 51% or more whole grain help fight heart disease and certain cancers. The benefit seems to come not just from dietary fiber but from an abundance of antioxidant vitamins and phytochemicals acting together to provide protection from disease. For all these reasons, whole grains are recommended over refined ones.

Recommended Carbohydrate Intake   Health experts recommend that Americans consume about 55% of their total daily calories from carbohydrates, especially complex carbohydrates. The American Heart Association recommends that this intake include at least three servings a day of whole-grain foods.

Experts also recommend that Americans alter the proportion of simple and complex carbohydrates in the diet, lowering simple carbohydrate intake from 25% to about 15% of total daily calories. The bulk of simple carbohydrates should come from fruits, which are excellent sources of vitamins and minerals, and milk, which is high in protein and calcium. Sweets, candy, soft drinks, and sweetened fruit drinks are high in simple sugars but low in other nutrients; in other words, they add empty calories to the diet.

On average, Americans consume more than 250 grams of carbohydrates a day, well above the minimum requirement of 50–100 grams. Nevertheless, experts recommend that people increase their consumption of carbohydrates to meet the suggested 55% of total daily calories. As mentioned in the discussion of fats, however, the American Heart Association has suggested an alternative diet for people who have calorie consumption under control. Evidence indicates that substituting monounsaturated fats rather than carbohydrates for saturated fats in the diet may have a positive effect on risk for heart disease. In this diet, people may consume more than 30% of their daily calories from fat—and thus less than 55% from carbohydrates—provided 15% or more of the fat calories are from monounsaturated fat.

Athletes in training can especially benefit from high-carbohydrate diets (60–70% of total daily calories), which enhance the amount of carbohydrates stored in their muscles (as glycogen) and therefore provide more carbohydrate fuel for use during endurance events or long workouts. In addition, carbohydrates consumed during prolonged athletic events can help fuel muscles and extend the availability of the glycogen stored in muscles. (For more on the special nutritional needs of athletes, see pp. 214–215.)

Dietary Fiber—A Closer Look

Dietary fiber consists of carbohydrate plant substances that are difficult or impossible for humans to digest. Instead, fiber passes through the intestinal tract and provides bulk for feces in the large intestine, which in turn facilitates elimination. In the large intestine, some types of fiber are broken down by bacteria into acids and gases, which explains why consuming too much fiber can lead to intestinal gas.

Types of Dietary Fiber   Nutritionists classify dietary fiber as soluble or insoluble. **Soluble fiber** slows the body's absorption of glucose and binds cholesterol-containing compounds in the intestine, lowering blood cholesterol levels and reducing the risk of cardiovascular disease. **Insoluble**

---

carbohydrate   An essential nutrient; sugars, starches, and dietary fiber are all carbohydrates.

glucose   A simple sugar; the body's basic fuel.

glycogen   A starch stored in the liver and muscles.

dietary fiber   Carbohydrates and other substances in plants that are difficult or impossible for humans to digest.

soluble fiber   Fiber that dissolves in water or is broken down by bacteria in the large intestine.

insoluble fiber   Fiber that does not dissolve in water and is not broken down by bacteria in the large intestine.

TERMS

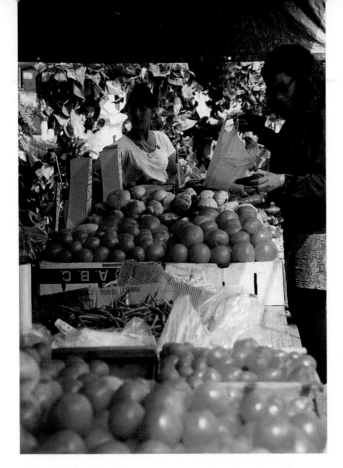

Our bodies require adequate amounts of all essential nutrients—water, proteins, carbohydrates, fats, vitamins, and minerals—to grow and function properly. Choosing foods to satisfy these nutritional requirements is an important part of a healthy lifestyle.

fiber binds water, making the feces bulkier and softer so they pass more quickly and easily through the intestines.

Both kinds of fiber contribute to disease prevention. A diet high in soluble fiber can help people manage diabetes and high blood cholesterol levels. A diet high in insoluble fiber can help prevent a variety of health problems, including constipation, hemorrhoids, and **diverticulitis.** Some studies have linked diets high in fiber-rich fruits, vegetables, and grains with a lower risk of some kinds of cancer; however, it is unclear whether fiber or other food components are responsible for this reduction in risk.

Sources of Dietary Fiber   All plant foods contain some dietary fiber, but fruits, legumes, oats (especially oat

bran), barley, and psyllium (found in some laxatives) are particularly rich in it. Wheat (especially wheat bran), cereals, grains, and vegetables are all good sources of insoluble fiber. However, the processing of packaged foods can remove fiber, so it's important to depend on fresh fruits and vegetables and foods made from whole grains as sources of dietary fiber.

Recommended Intake of Dietary Fiber   Most experts believe the average American would benefit from an increase in daily fiber intake. Currently, most Americans consume about 16 grams of fiber a day, whereas the recommended daily amount is 20–35 grams of fiber—not from supplements, which should be taken only under medical supervision.

To increase the amount of fiber in your diet, try the following:

- Look for breads, crackers, and cereals that list whole grain first in the ingredient list: Whole-wheat flour, whole-grain oats, and whole-grain rice are whole grains; wheat flour is not.
- Eat whole, unpeeled fruits rather than drinking fruit juice. Top cereals, yogurt, and desserts with berries, apple slices, or other fruit.
- Include beans in soups and salads. Combine raw vegetables with pasta, rice, or beans in salads.
- Substitute bean dip for cheese-based or sour cream–based dips or spreads. Use raw vegetables rather than chips for dipping.

Vitamins—Organic Micronutrients

Vitamins are organic (carbon-containing) substances required in very small amounts to promote specific chemical reactions within living cells (Table 8-2). Humans need 13 vitamins. Four are fat-soluble (A, D, E, and K), and nine are water-soluble (C and the eight B-complex vitamins: thiamin, riboflavin, niacin, vitamin B-6, folate, vitamin B-12, biotin, and pantothenic acid). Solubility affects how a vitamin is absorbed, transported, and stored in the body. The water-soluble vitamins are absorbed directly into the bloodstream, where they travel freely; excess water-soluble vitamins are detected by the kidneys and excreted in urine. Fat-soluble vitamins require a more complex digestive process; they are usually carried in the blood by special proteins and are stored in the body in fat tissues rather than excreted.

Functions of Vitamins   Vitamins help chemical reactions take place. They provide no energy to the body directly but help unleash the energy stored in carbohydrates, proteins, and fats. Vitamins are critical in the production of red blood cells and the maintenance of the nervous, skeletal, and immune systems. Some vitamins also form substances that act as **antioxidants**, which help preserve

	TABLE 8-2	*Facts About Vitamins*		

Vitamin	Important Dietary Sources	Major Functions	Signs of Prolonged Deficiency	Toxic Effects of Megadoses
Fat-Soluble				
Vitamin A	Liver, milk, butter, cheese, and fortified margarine; carrots, spinach, and other orange and deep-green vegetables and fruits	Maintenance of vision; skin; linings of the nose, mouth, digestive and urinary tracts; immune function	Night blindness; dry, scaling skin; increased susceptibility to infection; loss of appetite; anemia; kidney stones	Headache, vomiting and diarrhea, vertigo, double vision, bone abnormalities, liver damage, miscarriage and birth defects
Vitamin D	Fortified milk and margarine, fish liver oils, butter, egg yolks (sunlight on skin also produces vitamin D)	Development and maintenance of bones and teeth, promotion of calcium absorption	Rickets (bone deformities) in children; bone softening, loss, and fractures in adults	Kidney damage, calcium deposits in soft tissues, depression, death
Vitamin E	Vegetable oils, whole grains, nuts and seeds, green leafy vegetables, asparagus, peaches	Protection and maintenance of cellular membranes	Red blood cell breakage and anemia, weakness, neurological problems, muscle cramps	Relatively nontoxic, but may cause excess bleeding or formation of blood clots
Vitamin K	Green leafy vegetables; smaller amounts widespread in other foods	Production of factors essential for blood clotting	Hemorrhaging	Anemia, jaundice
Water-Soluble				
Vitamin C	Peppers, broccoli, spinach, brussels sprouts, citrus fruits, strawberries, tomatoes, potatoes, cabbage, other fruits and vegetables	Maintenance and repair of connective tissue, bones, teeth, and cartilage; promotion of healing; aid in iron absorption	Scurvy, anemia, reduced resistance to infection, loosened teeth, joint pain, poor wound healing, hair loss, poor iron absorption	Urinary stones in some people, acid stomach from ingesting supplements in pill form, nausea, diarrhea, headache, fatigue
Thiamin	Whole-grain and enriched breads and cereals, organ meats, lean pork, nuts, legumes	Conversion of carbohydrates into usable forms of energy, maintenance of appetite and nervous system function	Beriberi (symptoms include muscle wasting, mental confusion, anorexia, enlarged heart, abnormal heart rhythm, nerve changes)	None reported
Riboflavin	Dairy products, enriched breads and cereals, lean meats, poultry, fish, green vegetables	Energy metabolism; maintenance of skin, mucous membranes, and nervous system structures	Cracks at corners of mouth, sore throat, skin rash, hypersensitivity to light, purple tongue	None reported
Niacin	Eggs, poultry, fish, milk, whole grains, nuts, enriched breads and cereals, meats, legumes	Conversion of carbohydrates, fats, and protein into usable forms of energy	Pellagra (symptoms include diarrhea, dermatitis, inflammation of mucous membranes, dementia)	Flushing of the skin, nausea, vomiting, diarrhea, liver dysfunction, glucose intolerance
Vitamin B-6	Eggs, poultry, fish, whole grains, nuts, soybeans, liver, kidney, pork	Protein and neurotransmitter metabolism; red blood cell synthesis	Anemia, convulsions, cracks at corners of mouth, dermatitis, nausea, confusion	Neurological abnormalities and damage
Folate	Green leafy vegetables, yeast, oranges, whole grains, legumes, liver	Amino acid metabolism, synthesis of RNA and DNA, new cell synthesis	Anemia, weakness, fatigue, irritability, shortness of breath, swollen tongue	Masking of vitamin B-12 deficiency
Vitamin B-12	Eggs, milk, meats, other animal foods	Synthesis of red and white blood cells; other metabolic reactions	Anemia, fatigue, nervous system damage, sore tongue	None reported
Biotin	Cereals, yeast, egg yolks, soy flour, liver; widespread in foods	Metabolism of fats, carbohydrates, and proteins	Rash, nausea, vomiting, weight loss, depression, fatigue, hair loss	None reported
Pantothenic acid	Animal foods, whole grains, legumes; widespread in foods	Metabolism of fats, carbohydrates, and proteins	Fatigue, numbness and tingling of hands and feet, gastrointestinal disturbances	None reported

SOURCES: Food and Nutrition Board. 2000. *Dietary Reference Intakes for Vitamin C, Vitamen E, Selenium, and Carotenoids.* Washington, D.C.: National Academy Press. Food and Nutrition Board. 1998. *Dietary Reference Intakes for Thiamin, Riboflavin, Niacin, Vitamin B$_6$, Folate, Vitamin B$_{12}$, Pantothenic Acid, and Choline.* Washington, D.C.: National Academy Press. National Research Council. 1989. *Recommended Dietary Allowances,* 10th ed. Washington, D.C.: National Academy Press. Copyright © 1989 by the National Academy of Sciences. Adapted with permission from the National Academy Press, Washington, D.C. Shils, M. E., et al., eds. 1998. *Modern Nutrition in Health and Disease,* 9th ed. Baltimore Md.: Williams & Wilkins.

healthy cells in the body. Key vitamin antioxidants include vitamin E, vitamin C, and the vitamin A derivative beta-carotene. (The actions of antioxidants are described later in the chapter.)

Sources of Vitamins The human body does not manufacture most of the vitamins it requires and must obtain them from foods. Vitamins are abundant in fruits, vegetables, and grains. In addition, many processed foods, such as flour and breakfast cereals, are enriched with certain vitamins during the manufacturing process. A few vitamins are made in certain parts of the body: The skin makes vitamin D when it is exposed to sunlight, and intestinal bacteria make biotin and vitamin K.

Vitamin Deficiencies and Excesses If your diet lacks sufficient amounts of a particular vitamin, characteristic symptoms of deficiency develop (see Table 8-2). For example, vitamin A deficiency can cause blindness, and vitamin B-6 deficiency can cause seizures. Vitamin deficiency diseases are most often seen in developing countries; they are relatively rare in the United States because vitamins are readily available from our food supply. However, intakes below recommended levels can have adverse effects on health even if they are not low enough to cause a deficiency disease. For example, low intake of folate increases a woman's chance of giving birth to a baby with a neural tube defect (a congenital malformation of the central nervous system).

Extra vitamins in the diet can be harmful, especially when taken as supplements. High doses of vitamin A are toxic and increase the risk of birth defects, for example. Vitamin B-6 can cause irreversible nerve damage when taken in large doses. Megadoses of fat-soluble vitamins are particularly dangerous because the excess will be stored in the body rather than excreted, increasing the risk of toxicity. Even when supplements are not taken in excess, relying on them for an adequate intake of vitamins can be a problem: There are many substances in foods other than vitamins and minerals, and some of these compounds may have important health effects. Later in the chapter we discuss specific recommendations for vitamin intake and when a supplement is advisable. For now, keep in mind that it's best to obtain most of your vitamins from foods rather than supplements.

TERMS **minerals** Inorganic compounds needed in small amounts for regulation, growth, and maintenance of body tissues and functions.

anemia A deficiency in the oxygen-carrying material in the red blood cells.

osteoporosis A condition in which the bones become thin and brittle and break easily.

free radical An electron-seeking compound that can react with fats, proteins, and DNA, damaging cell membranes and mutating genes in its search for electrons; produced through chemical reactions in the body and by exposure to environmental factors such as sunlight and tobacco smoke.

When preparing foods, remember that vitamins in vegetables can be easily lost. To retain their value, eat or process vegetables immediately after buying them. If you can't do this, then store them in a cool place, covered to retain moisture—either in the refrigerator (for a few days) or in the freezer (for a longer term).

Minerals—Inorganic Micronutrients

Minerals are inorganic (non–carbon-containing) compounds you need in small amounts to help regulate body functions, aid in the growth and maintenance of body tissues, and help release energy (Table 8-3). There are about 17 essential minerals. The major minerals, those that the body needs in amounts exceeding 100 milligrams, include calcium, phosphorus, magnesium, sodium, potassium, and chloride. The essential trace minerals, those that you need in minute amounts, include copper, fluoride, iodide, iron, selenium, and zinc.

Characteristic symptoms develop if an essential mineral is consumed in a quantity too small or too large for good health. The minerals most commonly lacking in the American diet are iron, calcium, zinc, and magnesium. Focus on good food choices for these nutrients (see Table 8-3). Lean meats are rich in iron and zinc, whereas low-fat or nonfat dairy products are excellent choices for calcium. Plant foods are good sources of magnesium. Iron-deficiency **anemia** is a problem in some age groups, and researchers fear poor calcium intakes are sowing the seeds for future **osteoporosis**, especially in women. See the box "Osteoporosis" to learn more.

Water—A Vital Component

Water is the major component in both foods and the human body: You are composed of about 60% water. Your need for other nutrients, in terms of weight, is much less than your need for water. You can live up to 50 days without food but only a few days without water.

Water is distributed all over the body, among lean and other tissues and in urine and other body fluids. Water is used in the digestion and absorption of food and is the medium in which most of the chemical reactions take place within the body. Some water-based fluids like blood transport substances around the body, while other fluids serve as lubricants or cushions. Water also helps regulate body temperature.

Water is contained in almost all foods, particularly in liquids, fruits, and vegetables. The foods and fluids you consume provide 80–90% of your daily water intake; the remainder is generated through metabolism. You lose water each day in urine, feces, and sweat and through evaporation in your lungs. To maintain a balance between water consumed and water lost, you need to take in about 1 milliliter of water for each calorie you burn—about 2 liters, or 8 cups, of fluid per day—more if you live in a hot climate or engage in vigorous exercise.

Thirst is one of the body's first signs of dehydration

TABLE 8-3 **Facts About Selected Minerals**

Mineral	Important Dietary Sources	Major Functions	Signs of Prolonged Deficiency	Toxic Effects of Megadoses
Calcium	Milk and milk products, tofu, fortified orange juice and bread, green leafy vegetables, bones in fish	Maintenance of bones and teeth, control of nerve impulses and muscle contraction	Stunted growth in children, bone mineral loss in adults; urinary stones	Constipation, calcium deposits in soft tissues, inhibition of mineral absorption
Fluoride	Fluoride-containing drinking water, tea, marine fish eaten with bones	Maintenance of tooth and bone structure	Higher frequency of tooth decay	Increased bone density, mottling of teeth, impaired kidney function
Iron	Meat, legumes, eggs, enriched flour, dark-green vegetables, dried fruit, liver	Component of hemoglobin, myoglobin, and enzymes	Iron-deficiency anemia, weakness, impaired immune function, gastrointestinal distress	Liver and kidney damage, joint pains, sterility, disruption of cardiac function, death
Iodine	Iodized salt, seafood	Essential part of thyroid hormones, regulation of body metabolism	Goiter (enlarged thyroid), cretinism (birth defect)	Depression of thyroid activity, hyperthyroidism in susceptible people
Magnesium	Widespread in foods and water (except soft water); especially found in grains, legumes, nuts, seeds, green vegetables	Transmission of nerve impulses, energy transfer, activation of many enzymes	Neurological disturbances, cardiovascular problems, kidney disorders, nausea, growth failure in children	Nausea, vomiting, diarrhea, central nervous system depression, coma; death in people with impaired kidney function
Phosphorus	Present in nearly all foods, especially milk, cereal, legumes, meat, poultry, fish	Bone growth and maintenance, energy transfer in cells	Impaired growth, weakness, kidney disorders, cardiorespiratory and nervous system dysfunction	Drop in blood calcium levels, calcium deposits in soft tissues
Potassium	Meats, milk, fruits, vegetables, grains, legumes	Nerve function and body water balance	Muscular weakness, nausea, drowsiness, paralysis, confusion, disruption of cardiac rhythm	Cardiac arrest
Selenium	Seafood, meat, eggs, whole grains	Protection of cells from oxidative damage, immune response	Muscle pain and weakness, heart disorders	Hair and nail loss, nausea and vomiting, weakness, irritability
Sodium	Salt, soy sauce, salted foods, tomato juice	Body water balance, acid-base balance, nerve function	Muscle weakness, loss of appetite, nausea, vomiting; deficiency is rare	Edema, hypertension in sensitive people
Zinc	Whole grains, meat, eggs, liver, seafood (especially oysters)	Synthesis of proteins, RNA, and DNA; wound healing; immune response; ability to taste	Growth failure, loss of appetite, impaired taste acuity, skin rash, impaired immune function, poor wound healing	Vomiting, impaired immune function, decline in blood HDL levels, impaired copper absorption

SOURCES: Food and Nutrition Board. 2000. *Dietary Reference Intakes for Vitamin C, Vitamen E, Selenium, and Carotenoids.* Washington, D.C.: National Academy Press. Food and Nutrition Board. 1997. *Dietary Reference Intakes for Calcium, Phosphorus, Magnesium, Vitamin D, and Fluoride.* Washington, D.C.: National Academy Press. National Research Council. 1989. *Recommended Dietary Allowances,* 10th ed. Washington, D.C.: National Academy Press. Copyright © 1989 by the National Academy of Sciences. Reprinted with permission from National Academy Press, Washington, D.C. Shils, M. E., et al., eds. 1998. *Modern Nutrition in Health and Disease,* 9th ed. Baltimore, Md.: Williams & Wilkins.

that we can actually recognize. However, by the time we are actually thirsty, our cells have been needing fluid for quite some time. A good motto to remember, especially when exercising, is: Drink *before* you're thirsty. If the thirst mechanism is faulty, as it may be during illness or vigorous exercise, hormonal mechanisms can help conserve water by reducing the output of urine. Severe dehydration causes weakness and can lead to death.

Other Substances in Food

There are many substances in food that are not essential nutrients but that may influence health.

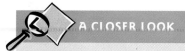

Osteoporosis is a condition in which the bones become dangerously thin and fragile over time. It currently afflicts some 25 million Americans, 80% of them women, and results in about 1.5 million bone fractures each year. The incidence of osteoporosis may double in the next 25 years as the population ages.

The bones in your body are continually being broken down and rebuilt in order to adapt to mechanical strain. About 20% of your body's bone mass is replaced each year. In the first few decades of life, bones become thicker and stronger as they are rebuilt. Most of your bone mass (95%) is built by age 18. After bone mass peaks between the ages of 25 and 35, the rate of bone loss exceeds the rate of replacement, and bones become less dense. In osteoporosis, this loss of density becomes so severe that bones become very fragile.

Fractures are the most serious consequence of osteoporosis; up to 25% of all people who suffer a hip fracture die within a year. Other problems associated with osteoporosis are loss of height and a stooped posture caused by vertebral fractures, severe back and hip pain, and breathing problems caused by changes in the shape of the skeleton.

Who Is at Risk?

Women are at greater risk than men for osteoporosis because they have 10–25% less bone in their skeleton. As they lose bone mass with age, women's bones become dangerously thin sooner than men's bones. Bone loss accelerates in women during the first 5–10 years after the onset of menopause because of a drop in estrogen production. (Estrogen improves calcium absorption and reduces the amount of calcium the body excretes.)

Other risk factors include a family history of osteoporosis, early menopause (before age 45), abnormal menstruation, a history of anorexia, and a thin, small frame. Thyroid medication, corticosteroid drugs for asthma or arthritis, and certain other medications can also have a negative impact on bone mass. African American women tend to have a lower risk of osteoporosis than women from other ethnic groups.

What Can You Do?

To prevent osteoporosis, the best strategy is to build as much bone as possible during your young years and then do everything you can to maintain it as you age. Up to 50% of bone loss is determined by controllable lifestyle factors.

Ensure Adequate Intake of Calcium and Vitamin D   Consuming an adequate amount of calcium is important throughout life to build and maintain bone mass. Americans average 600–800 mg of calcium per day, only about half of what is recommended. Milk, yogurt, and calcium-fortified orange juice, bread, and cereals are all good sources. Nutritionists suggest that you obtain calcium from foods first and then take supplements only if needed to make up the difference.

Vitamin D is necessary for bones to absorb calcium; a daily intake of 400–800 IU is recommended by the National Osteoporosis Foundation. Vitamin D can be obtained from foods (milk and fortified cereals, for example) and is manufactured by the skin when it is exposed to sunlight. Adequate intake of vitamin K has also been linked to a lower risk of bone fractures. Other nutrients important for maintenance of bone strength include vitamin C, potassium, magnesium, and isoflavones (estrogen-like plant substances in soy foods). Micronutrients common in fruit and vegetables, including zinc, boron, and manganese, may also help prevent osteoporosis.

Exercise   Weight-bearing aerobic activities help build and maintain bone mass throughout life, but they must be performed regularly to have lasting effects. Strength training is also helpful: It improves bone density, muscle mass, strength, and balance, protecting against both bone loss and falls, a major cause of fractures. Even low-intensity strength training has been shown to improve density—even in women in their 70s.

Don't Smoke, and Drink Alcohol Only in Moderation   Smoking reduces the body's estrogen levels and is linked to earlier menopause and more rapid postmenopausal bone loss. Alcohol reduces the body's ability to absorb calcium and may interfere with estrogen's bone-protecting effects.

Be Moderate in Your Consumption of Protein, Sodium, Caffeine, and Vitamin A   A high intake of protein and sodium has been shown to increase calcium loss in the urine and may lead to loss of calcium from the skeleton. Caffeine may also cause small losses of urinary calcium, and experts often recommend that heavy caffeine consumers take special care to include calcium-rich foods in their diet. Excessive consumption of vitamin A in the form of retinol—the form most common in multivitamins—can threaten bone health. Take no more than 100% of the Daily Value for vitamin A, with most of that coming from beta-carotene rather than retinol.

Manage Depression and Stress   Some women with depression experience significant bone loss that may increase their risk of fractures. Researchers haven't identified the mechanism, but it may be linked to increases in the stress hormone cortisol.

After Menopause, Consider Testing and Treatment   The National Osteoporosis Foundation recommends bone mineral density testing for all women over age 65 as well as younger postmenopausal women who have a fracture or who have one or more osteoporosis risk factors. Results of bone mineral density testing can be used to gauge an individual's risk of fracture and help determine an appropriate course of action.

Hormone replacement therapy (HRT) combats bone loss as well as menopausal symptoms and heart disease. However, estrogen acts on many tissues in the body, and HRT is not without side effects and risks, including a slight increase in the risk of breast cancer. Compounds called selective estrogen receptor modulators, or SERMs, have been found to act like estrogen on some body tissues but not others. Researchers hope to develop SERMs that have all of estrogen's beneficial effects without the associated risks. Although currently not as effective as HRT in preventing bone loss, SERMs such as raloxifene (Evista) may be a good choice for some women. Other drug treatments include alendronate (Fosamax) and calcitonin (Miacalcin), which slow the resorption of bone by the body, and fluoride, which helps build bone in women who already have osteoporosis.

Antioxidants When the body uses oxygen or breaks down certain fats as a normal part of metabolism, it gives rise to substances called **free radicals.** Environmental factors such as cigarette smoke, exhaust fumes, radiation, excessive sunlight, certain drugs, and stress can increase free radical production. A free radical is a chemically unstable molecule that is missing an electron; it will react with any molecule it encounters from which it can take an electron. In their search for electrons, free radicals react with fats, proteins, and DNA, damaging cell membranes and mutating genes. Because of this, free radicals have been implicated in aging, cancer, cardiovascular disease, and other degenerative diseases.

Antioxidants found in foods can help protect the body by blocking the formation and action of free radicals and repairing the damage they cause. For this reason, smokers are advised to consume an extra 35 milligrams a day of vitamin C. Some antioxidants, such as vitamin C, vitamin E, and selenium, are also essential nutrients; others, such as carotenoids, found in yellow, orange, and dark-green leafy vegetables, are not. Many fruits and vegetables are rich in antioxidants.

Phytochemicals Antioxidants are a particular type of **phytochemical,** a substance found in plant foods that may help prevent chronic disease. Researchers have just begun to identify and study all the different compounds found in foods, and many preliminary findings are promising. For example, certain proteins found in soy foods may help lower cholesterol levels. Sulforaphane, a compound isolated from broccoli and other **cruciferous vegetables,** may render some carcinogenic compounds harmless. Allyl sulfides, a group of chemicals found in garlic and onions, appear to boost the activity of cancer-fighting immune cells. Further research on phytochemicals may extend the role of nutrition to the prevention and treatment of many chronic diseases.

If you want to increase your intake of phytochemicals, it is best to obtain them by eating a variety of fruits and vegetables rather than relying on supplements. Like many vitamins and minerals, isolated phytochemicals may be harmful if taken in high doses. In addition, it is likely that their health benefits are the result of chemical substances working in combination. The role of phytochemicals in disease prevention is discussed in Chapters 11 and 12.

NUTRITIONAL GUIDELINES: PLANNING YOUR DIET

The second part of putting together a healthy food plan—after you've learned about necessary nutrients—is choosing foods that satisfy nutritional requirements and meet your personal criteria. Various tools have been created by scientific and government groups to help people design healthy diets. Two well-known standards are the **Recommended Dietary Allowances (RDAs)** and the **Dietary Reference Intakes (DRIs),** both of which provide recommendations for nutrient intake designed to prevent nutritional deficiencies and reduce the risk of chronic disease. Another tool, the **Food Guide Pyramid,** translates these nutrient recommendations into a balanced food-group plan that includes all essential nutrients. To provide further guidance, **Dietary Guidelines for Americans** have been established to address the prevention of diet-related chronic diseases. Together, these tools make up a complete set of resources for dietary planning.

Recommended Dietary Allowances (RDAs) and Dietary Reference Intakes (DRIs)

The Food and Nutrition Board of the National Academy of Sciences establishes the RDAs, DRIs, and related guidelines. The RDAs were developed as standards to prevent nutritional deficiency diseases such as anemia. First published in 1941, the RDAs have been updated periodically to keep pace with new research findings; the most recent version was published in 1989.

Scientific knowledge about nutrition has increased dramatically since the inception of the RDAs, and current research focuses not just on the prevention of nutrient deficiencies but also on the role of nutrients in preventing chronic diseases such as osteoporosis, cancer, and cardiovascular disease. This expanded focus is the basis for the development of a new system of recommendations, the Dietary Reference Intakes. The DRIs, which will eventually replace the RDAs, include standards for both recommended intakes and maximum safe intakes.

TERMS

phytochemical A naturally occurring substance found in plant foods that may help prevent and treat chronic diseases such as heart disease and cancer; *phyto* means plant.

cruciferous vegetables Vegetables of the cabbage family, including cabbage, broccoli, brussels sprouts, kale, and cauliflower.

Recommended Dietary Allowances (RDAs) Amounts of certain nutrients considered adequate to prevent deficiencies in most healthy people; will eventually be replaced by the Dietary Reference Intakes (DRIs).

Dietary Reference Intakes (DRIs) An umbrella term for four types of nutrient standards: Adequate Intake (AI), Estimated Average Requirement (EAR), and Recommended Dietary Allowance (RDA) set levels of intake considered adequate to prevent nutrient deficiencies and reduce the risk of chronic disease; Tolerable Upper Intake Level (UL) sets the maximum daily intake that is unlikely to cause health problems.

Food Guide Pyramid A food-group plan that provides practical advice to ensure a balanced intake of the essential nutrients.

Dietary Guidelines for Americans General principles of good nutrition intended to help prevent certain diet-related diseases.

- Recommended nutrient intakes can be expressed as three different types of standards—Adequate Intake (AI), Estimated Average Requirement (EAR), and Recommended Dietary Allowance (RDA)—depending on the intended use of the standard and the amount of scientific information available. Regardless of the type of standard used, the DRI represents the best available estimate of intake for optimal health.

- The Tolerable Upper Intake Level (UL), sets the maximum daily intake by a healthy person that is unlikely to cause health problems. Because of lack of data, ULs have not been set for all nutrients. This does not mean that people can tolerate chronic intakes of these vitamins above recommended levels, and there is no established benefit from consuming nutrients at levels above the AI or RDA.

The DRIs are being issued in stages, and they have not yet been established for all vitamins and minerals. Those vitamins and minerals for which DRIs have been set are listed at the end of the chapter, in Nutritional Resources. There you can also find a list of nutrient upper intake levels for adults and an abridged version of the 1989 RDAs, including nutrients for which DRIs have not yet been set.

Should You Take Supplements? The aim of the RDAs and DRIs is to guide you in meeting your nutritional needs primarily with food rather than with vitamin and mineral supplements. This goal is important because recommendations have not yet been set for some essential nutrients, and so these nutrients are not included in most supplements. Supplements also lack potentially beneficial phytochemicals that are found only in whole foods. Experts generally agree that most Americans can obtain most of the vitamins and minerals they need to prevent deficiencies by consuming a varied, nutritionally balanced diet. Ongoing research is examining whether supplements of particular vitamins and minerals should be recommended for their potential disease-fighting properties, as for antioxidants like vitamin E.

The question of whether to take supplements is a serious one. Some vitamins and minerals are dangerous when ingested in excess, as shown in Nutritional Resources. Large doses of particular nutrients can also cause health problems by affecting the absorption of other vitamins and minerals. For all these reasons, you should think carefully about whether to take supplements; consider consulting a physician or registered dietitian.

In 1998, the Food and Nutrition Board recommended supplements of particular nutrients for the following groups:

- Women who are capable of becoming pregnant should take 400 micrograms a day of folic acid from fortified foods and/or supplements in addition to getting folate from a varied diet. Research indicates that this level of folate intake will reduce the risk of neural tube defects, which occur early in pregnancy. Since 1998, enriched breads, flours, cornmeals, rice, noodles, and other grain products have been fortified with small amounts of folic acid. Folate is found naturally in green leafy vegetables, legumes, citrus fruits and juices, and most berries.

- People over age 50 should consume foods fortified with vitamin B-12, B-12 supplements, or a combination of the two to meet the majority of the DRI of 2.4 milligrams of B-12 daily. Up to 30% of people over 50 may have problems absorbing vitamin B-12; the consumption of supplements and fortified foods can overcome this problem and help prevent a deficiency.

Supplements may also be recommended in other cases. Women with heavy menstrual flow may need extra iron to compensate for the monthly loss. Some vegetarians may need extra calcium, iron, zinc, and vitamin B-12. Newborns need a single dose of vitamin K, administered under the direction of a physician. People who consume few calories, who have certain diseases, or who take certain drugs may also need specific nutrients; it is important to consult a physician because some vitamins and minerals can block the actions of some medications.

In deciding whether to take a supplement, consider whether you already regularly consume a fortified breakfast cereal. If you do decide to take a supplement, choose a balanced formulation that contains 50–100% of the adult Daily Value for vitamins and minerals. Avoid supplements containing large doses of particular nutrients.

Daily Values Because the RDAs are far too cumbersome to use as a basis for food labels, the U.S. Food and Drug Administration (FDA) developed another set of dietary standards, the Daily Values. On food labels, **Daily Values** are expressed as a percentage of a 2000-calorie diet, an average daily caloric intake for Americans. Using this single set of recommendations on food labels helps make nutrition information more accessible to the consumer. Food labels are described in more detail later in the chapter.

The Food Guide Pyramid

Many of us learned about food groups in grade school. We learned that by choosing foods from each group, we could have a healthy diet. The fundamental principles of this food guide are moderation, variety, and balance—a theme echoed throughout this chapter. A diet is balanced if it contains appropriate amounts of each nutrient, and

TERMS **Daily Values** A simplified version of the RDAs used on food labels; also included are values for nutrients with no established RDA.

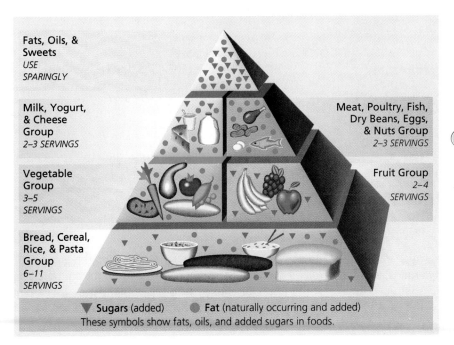

Figure 8-5 The Food Guide Pyramid: A guide to daily food choices. The Pyramid is an outline of what to eat each day—not a rigid prescription, but a general guide that lets you choose a healthful diet that's right for you. It calls for eating a variety of foods to get the nutrients you need and at the same time the right amount of calories to maintain a healthy weight. The Pyramid also focuses on fat because many Americans eat too much fat, especially saturated fat. SOURCE: USDA. Center for Nutrition Policy and Information. 1996. *Food Guide Pyramid.* USDA Home and Garden Bulletin no. 252.

choosing foods from each of the food groups helps ensure that balance.

The latest version of the food-group plan is the U.S. Department of Agriculture's Food Guide Pyramid (Figure 8-5). It is based on a recommended number of servings from six food groups. A range of servings is given for each group. The smaller number is for people who consume about 1600 calories a day, such as many sedentary women; the larger number is for those who consume about 2800 calories a day, such as active men. Serving sizes and examples of foods are described below for each group.

It is important to choose a variety of foods within each group because different foods have different combinations of nutrients: For example, within the vegetable group, potatoes are high in vitamin C, whereas spinach is a rich source of vitamin A. Foods also vary in their amount of calories and nutrients, and people who do not need many calories should focus on nutrient-dense foods within each group (foods that are high in nutrients relative to the amount of calories they contain). Many foods you eat contain nutrients from more than one food group.

Bread, Cereals, Rice, and Pasta (6–11 Servings)

Foods from this group are usually low in fat and rich in complex carbohydrates, dietary fiber, and many vitamins and minerals, including thiamin, riboflavin, iron, niacin, folate, and zinc. Although 6–11 servings may seem like a large amount of food, many people eat several servings at a time. A single serving is the equivalent of the following:

- 1 slice of bread or half a hamburger bun, English muffin, or bagel
- 1 small roll, biscuit, or muffin
- 1 ounce of ready-to-eat cereal
- ½ cup cooked cereal, rice, or pasta
- 5–6 small or 2–3 large crackers

If you are one of the many people who have trouble identifying an ounce of cereal or half a cup of rice, see the strategies in the box "Judging Serving Sizes." Choose foods that are typically made with little fat or sugars (bread, rice, pasta) over those that are high in fat and sugars (croissants, chips, cookies, doughnuts). For maximum nutrition, choose at least three servings from whole grains, such as whole-wheat bread, high-fiber cereal, whole-wheat pasta, and brown rice. For shopping suggestions, see the box "Adding Whole-Grain Foods to Your Diet."

Vegetables (3–5 Servings)

Vegetables are rich in carbohydrates, dietary fiber, vitamin A, vitamin C, folate, iron, magnesium, and other nutrients. They are also naturally low in fat. A serving of vegetables is equivalent to the following:

- 1 cup raw leafy vegetables
- ½ cup raw or cooked vegetables
- ½ cup tomato sauce
- ¾ cup vegetable juice
- ½ cup cooked dry beans

Good choices from this group include dark-green leafy vegetables such as spinach, chard, and collards; deep-orange and red vegetables such as carrots, winter squash, red bell peppers, and tomatoes; broccoli, cauliflower, and other cruciferous vegetables; peas; green beans; potatoes; and corn. Dry beans (legumes) such as pinto, navy, kidney, and black beans can be counted as servings of vegetables *or* as alternatives to meat.

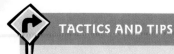
Studies have shown that most people underestimate the size of their food portions, in many cases by as much as 50%. If you need to retrain your eye, try using measuring cups and spoons and an inexpensive kitchen scale when you eat at home. With a little practice, you'll learn the difference between 3 and 8 ounces of chicken or meat and what a half-cup of rice really looks like. For quick estimates, use these equivalents:

- 1 teaspoon of margarine = the tip of your thumb.

- 1 ounce of cheese = your thumb or four dice stacked.

- 3 ounces of chicken or meat = a deck of cards or an audio-cassette tape.

- ½ cup of rice or cooked vegetables = an ice cream scoop or one-third of a soda can.

- 2 tablespoons of peanut butter = a Ping-Pong ball.

- 1 cup of pasta = a woman's fist or a tennis ball.

- 1 medium potato = a computer mouse.

Fruits (2–4 Servings)   Like vegetables, fruits are rich in carbohydrates, dietary fiber, and many vitamins, especially vitamin C. They are low in fat and sodium. The serving sizes used in the Pyramid are as follows:

- 1 medium (apple, banana, peach, orange, pear) or 2 small (apricot, plum) whole fruit(s)

- 1 melon wedge

- ½ cup berries, cherries, or grapes

- ½ grapefruit

- ½ cup chopped, cooked, canned, or frozen fruit

- ¾ cup fruit juice (100% juice)

- ¼ cup dried fruit

Good choices from this group are citrus fruits and juices, melons, pears, apples, bananas, and berries. Choose whole fruits often—they are higher in fiber and often lower in calories than fruit juices. Fruit *juices* typically contain more nutrients than fruit *drinks*. For canned fruits, choose those packed in their own juice rather than in syrup.

Milk, Yogurt, and Cheese (2–3 Servings)   Foods from this group are high in protein, carbohydrate, calcium, riboflavin, potassium, and zinc. To limit the fat in your diet, choose servings of low-fat or nonfat items from this group:

- 1 cup milk or yogurt

- 1½ ounces cheese

- 2 ounces processed cheese

Cottage cheese is lower in calcium than most other cheeses, and 1 cup of cottage cheese counts as only half a serving for this food group. Ice cream is also lower in calcium than many other dairy products (1 cup is equivalent to ⅔ serving); in addition, it is high in sugar and fat.

Meat, Poultry, Fish, Dry Beans, Eggs, and Nuts (2–3 Servings   This food group provides protein, niacin, iron, vitamin B-6, zinc, and thiamin; the animal foods in the group also provide vitamin B-12. The Pyramid recom-

mends 2–3 servings each day of foods from this group. The total amount of these servings should be the equivalent of 5–7 ounces of cooked lean meat, poultry, or fish a day. Many people misjudge what makes up a single serving for this food group:

- 2–3 ounces cooked lean meat, poultry, or fish (an average hamburger or a medium chicken breast half is about 3 ounces; 4 slices of bologna, 6 slices of hard salami, or ½ cup of drained canned tuna counts as about 2 ounces)

- The following portions of nonmeat foods are equivalent to 1 ounce of lean meat: ½ cup cooked dry beans (if not counted as a vegetable), 1 egg, 2 tablespoons peanut butter, ⅓ cup nuts, ¼ cup seeds, and ½ cup tofu

To limit your intake of fat and saturated fat, choose lean cuts of meat and skinless poultry, eat nuts and seeds in moderation, and watch your serving sizes carefully. Choose at least one serving of plant proteins every day.

Fats, Oils, and Sweets   The tip of the Pyramid includes fats, oils, and sweets—foods such as salad dressings, oils, butter, margarine, gravy, mayonnaise, soft drinks, sugar, candy, jellies and jams, syrups, and sweet desserts. Foods from the tip of the Pyramid provide calories but few nutrients; they should not replace foods from the other groups. The total amount of fats, oils, and sweets you consume should be determined by your overall energy needs.

The colored triangles and circles in the Pyramid appear in all the other food groups to remind you that food choices in those groups can also be high in fats and added sugars. ("Added sugars" are sugars added in processing, not those found naturally in fruits and milk.) Foods that come from animals (the meat and milk groups) are naturally higher in fats than foods that come from plants, which is why it's important to choose lean meats and low-fat dairy products. Foods that come from plants are lower in fat, but they are often prepared in ways that make them higher-fat choices, such as french fries, baked potatoes

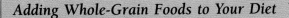
Whole-grain foods—wheat, corn, oats, rice, barley—are good weapons against heart disease and certain cancers, as well as a factor in living longer. Whole grains are low in fat and cholesterol, too, and so can be a good choice for managing weight. Federal dietary guidelines recommend 6–11 servings of grain products every day, with at least 3 of these servings from whole grains. How do you add whole-grain foods to your diet? Here are some tips.

Read Labels

If more than 51% of the food's ingredients are whole grain, the package may have the words "whole grain," "whole wheat," or "may reduce the risk of heart disease and certain cancers." The list of ingredients should have a whole grain as the first ingredient.

Read Beyond a Food's Description

Don't be misled by a packaged food's description. Products described using words like the following tend to contain mostly refined grains: cracked wheat; made with whole grain; made with whole wheat; multigrain; oat bran; oatmeal, pumpernickel, or rye bread; 7-bran, 12-bran, and so on; 7-grain, 8-grain, 9-grain, 12-grain; 5-seed; stoned wheat; unbleached wheat flour; wheat; wheatberry. When in doubt, always check the list of ingredients, looking for the word "whole" as the first word.

Include Whole-Grain Foods on Your Grocery List

Today many supermarkets carry whole-grain foods. Here's a whole-grain grocery list to give you a few ideas. To increase your health quotient, look for low-fat versions of cereals and snacks. And for those harder-to-find items, try your local health food store.

- *Wheat bread:* Look for sandwich bread, pitas, and tortillas with "whole wheat" listed as the first ingredient.
- *Rye bread:* Check the label for "whole rye."
- *Corn tortillas:* Check the label for "whole corn."
- *Breakfast cereals (whole-grain varieties only):* Bran (including some raisin brans), muesli, oatmeal (all kinds: old-fashioned, quick-cooking, instant), shredded wheat, and many name-brand varieties.
- *Rice:* Brown only.
- *Snacks:* Crispbread crackers (such as Ry-Krisp), popcorn, popcorn cakes, rice cakes, some tortilla chips (check first ingredient for "whole corn"), Triscuits, Wheat Thins.
- *Harder-to-find whole-grain items:* Whole-wheat bagels, English muffins, breakfast bars, cookies, couscous, crackers, hamburger buns, pizza crust, pretzels, oat cakes (a sweet snack), pancake mix, pasta.

with sour cream and cheese, fettuccine Alfredo, and baked goods like cookies and pies. Added sugars are common in the milk group (ice cream, sweetened yogurt), the fruit group (canned fruit in syrup), and the grain group (baked goods). Reduced-fat versions of prepared foods are often *very* high in added sugars and consequently just as high in calories as their full-fat versions.

The average American diet currently includes more fat and added sugars than recommended. The Pyramid suggests that Americans limit the fat in their diets to 30% of total calories. You will consume about half this amount if you eat the recommended number of servings from each food group, select the lowest-fat choices, and add no fat during cooking or at the table. Additional fat, up to 30% of total calories, is considered discretionary in that you can decide whether to get it from higher-fat food choices or additions to your foods. As mentioned earlier, the American Heart Association has stated that consuming more than 30% of calories from fat may confer heart health benefits for people who manage their weight through calorie control and who have low saturated fat intake—if the extra calories come from monounsaturated fats.

Added sugars are less of a concern to health than fat, but consumption of large amounts of sugars adds empty calories to the diet and can make weight management more difficult. Americans are consuming more sugar than

ever; consumption of soft drinks has increased more than 100% since the 1970s. Overconsumption of fat and added sugars leaves fewer calories available for healthier food choices from the five major food groups. For example, the average daily diet among American women includes about 9 teaspoons (36 grams) of added sugars and 5 grams of fat above recommended limits (Table 8-4). The 200 calories in these extra sugars and fats could be better used to increase the number of servings from the food groups for which women typically fall short of Pyramid recommendations.

General strategies for controlling intake of fat and added sugars include choosing lower-fat foods within each food group, eating fewer foods that are high in sugar and low in other nutrients, and limiting the amount of fats and sugars added to foods during cooking or at the table.

The Food Guide Pyramid is a general guide to what you should eat every day. By eating a balanced variety of foods from each of the six food groups and including some plant proteins, you can ensure that your daily diet is adequate in all nutrients. A diet using low-fat food choices contains only about 1600 calories but meets all known nutritional needs, except possibly for iron in some women who have heavy menstrual periods. For these women, foods fortified in iron, such as breakfast cereals, can make up the deficit.

	Recommended Diets at Three Calorie Levels[a]			Average American Diet	
				Women (1600 calories)	Men (2400 calories)
	1600	2200	2800		
Grain group (servings)	6	9	11	5.5	7.9
Vegetable group (servings)	3	4	5	3.1	4.1
Fruit group (servings)	2	3	4	1.5	1.5
Dairy group (servings)[b]	2–3	2–3	2–3	1.1	1.5
Meat group (ounces)[c]	5	6	7	3.9	6.4
Total fat (grams)[d]	53	73	93	58.1	90.1
Total added sugars (teaspoons)[d,e]	6	12	18	15.4	22.3

[a]The bottom of the recommended range of servings (1600 calories) is about right for many sedentary women and older adults. The middle range (2200 calories) is about right for most children, teenage girls, active women, and many sedentary men. The top of the range (2800 calories) is about right for teenage boys, many active men, and some very active women.
[b]Women who are pregnant or lactating, teenagers, and young adults to age 24 need 3 servings.
[c]The Pyramid recommends 2–3 servings a day, the equivalent of 5–7 ounces of cooked lean meat, poultry, or fish (see p. 208).
[d]Values for total fat and added sugars include fat and added sugars that are in food choices from the five major food groups as well as fat and added sugars from foods in the Fats, Oils, and Sweets group. The total for added sugars does not include sugars that occur naturally in foods such as fruit and milk. The recommended fat totals are based on a limit of 30% of total calories as fat.
[e]A teaspoon of sugar is equivalent to 4 grams (16 calories).

SOURCES: Agricultural Research Service. 1999. *Pyramid Servings Data: Results from USDA's Continuing Survey of Food Intakes by Individuals.* Beltsville, Md.: Food Surveys Research Group (http://www.barc.usda.gov/bhnrc/foodsurvey/pdf/3yr_py.pdf; retrieved May 5, 2000). Shaw, A., et al. 1997. *Using the Food Guide Pyramid: A Resource for Nutrition Educators.* USDA Center for Nutrition Policy and Promotion (http://www.nal.usda.gov/fnic/Fpyr/guide.pdf; retrieved April 18, 2000).

Dietary Guidelines for Americans

To provide further guidance for choosing a healthy diet, the U.S. Department of Agriculture and the U.S. Department of Health and Human Services have issued Dietary Guidelines for Americans, most recently in 2000. Following these guidelines promotes health and reduces risk for chronic diseases. Ten Dietary Guidelines are provided, organized under three messages, the "ABCs for Health":

Aim for fitness.

Build a healthy base.

Choose sensibly.

What follows is a brief summary of the guidelines.

Aim for Fitness   The two guidelines in this category emphasize a lifestyle that combines sensible eating with regular physical activity.

- *Aim for a healthy weight.* Evaluate your body weight, especially in light of any risk factors you may have for disease. (See Chapter 6 for instructions on evaluating your body weight.) If you are at a healthy weight, aim to avoid weight gain. Do so by eating vegetables, fruits, and whole grains with little added fat or sugar and selecting sensible portion sizes. If you are overweight, first aim to prevent further weight gain, and then lose weight to improve your health. Aim to lose weight gradually—about 10% of your weight over about 6 months. Loss of ½ to 2 pounds a week is usually safe. Your health is more likely to improve over the long term if you achieve and maintain a healthy weight rather than lose and regain several times. But even if you have regained weight in the past, it's worthwhile to try again.

- *Be physically active every day.* Become active if you are inactive, and maintain or increase physical activity if you are already active. Aim to accumulate at least 30 minutes of physical activity most days, preferably every day. (Children and adolescents need at least 60 minutes of physical activity every day.) Moderate physical activity is any activity that requires about as much energy as walking 2 miles in 30 minutes. You can do the activity all at once or spread it out over two or three periods during the day. Choose activities that you enjoy and can do regularly. Aerobic activities and activities for strength and flexibility are especially beneficial.

Physical activity and nutrition work together for better health. For example, physical activity increases the amount of calories you use, which in turn makes it easier to get the nutrients you need. For those who have intentionally lost weight, being active makes it easier to maintain the weight loss. However, 30 minutes a day may not be enough to lose weight or maintain weight loss; increase activity to 45 minutes a day for weight maintenance.

Build a Healthy Base

The four guidelines in this category provide a foundation for healthy eating.

- *Let the Pyramid guide your food choices.* To ensure that you get all the nutrients and other substances you need, choose the recommended number of daily servings from each of the five major food groups shown in the Food Guide Pyramid. Healthy eating patterns start with plant foods, represented in the three food groups at the base of the Pyramid: grains, fruits, and vegetables. Plan your meals around a variety of foods from these groups.

  People's food choices are affected by culture, family background, religion, moral beliefs, the cost and availability of food, life experience, food intolerances, and allergies. The Pyramid provides a good guide to healthy eating no matter how the foods are prepared or combined. However, if you avoid all foods from any of the five groups, be sure to get enough nutrients from other groups. For example, if you do not eat dairy products because of intolerance to lactose, choose other foods that are good sources of calcium, and make sure you get enough vitamin D. If you avoid animal products, be sure you get enough iron, vitamin B-12, calcium, and zinc.

- *Eat a variety of grains daily, especially whole grains.* Make grains the foundation of your diet (whole-grain and refined breads, cereals, pasta, and rice). Eat six or more servings daily, but if your calorie needs are low, eat only six servings of a sensible size. Include several servings of whole grains daily, choosing a variety of grains, such as whole wheat, brown rice, oats, and whole corn. Prepare or choose grain products with little added saturated fat and moderate or low amounts of added sugar.

- *Eat a variety of fruits and vegetables daily.* Different fruits and vegetables are rich in different nutrients, so it's important to choose a variety. Eat at least two servings of fruit and three servings of vegetables daily. Choose fresh, frozen, dried, or canned forms and a variety of colors and kinds. Favor dark-green leafy vegetables, bright orange fruits and vegetables, and cooked dried peas and beans.

- *Keep food safe to eat.* Safe foods are those that pose little risk of foodborne illness, whether from harmful bacteria, viruses, parasites, or chemical contaminants. Follow these steps to keep your food safe: (1) Wash hands and surfaces often. (2) Separate raw, cooked, and ready-to-eat foods while shopping, preparing, and storing. (3) Cook food to a safe temperature. Use a thermometer when cooking animal products. (4) Refrigerate perishable foods promptly —within 2 hours of purchasing or preparing, within 1 hour if the air temperature is above 90°F. Use refrigerated leftovers within 3–4 days. (5) Follow safety instructions on the label. (6) Serve meat, poultry, eggs, and fish just before eating, and chill leftovers as soon as you are finished. Keep hot foods above 140°F and cold foods below 40°F. (7) If in doubt, throw it out. If food has been left out for too long or refrigerated for too long, it may not be safe to eat even if it looks and smells fine.

Choose Sensibly

The four guidelines in this category help you make sensible choices that promote health and reduce the risk of certain chronic diseases.

- *Choose a diet low in saturated fat and cholesterol and moderate in total fat.* (*Moderate* means no more than 30% of calories.) Limit use of animal fats, hard margarines (unless labeled trans-fatty-acid free), and partially hydrogenated shortenings; use vegetable oils instead. Choose fat-free or low-fat dairy products, cooked dried beans and peas, fish, and lean meats and poultry. Use food labels to help you choose foods lower in fat, saturated fat, and cholesterol. Refer to the box "Reducing the Fat in Your Diet" for some specific suggestions.

- *Choose beverages and foods to moderate your intake of sugars.* Sugar doesn't cause hyperactivity, but it does promote tooth decay. Keep your teeth and gums healthy by rinsing your mouth after you eat sugar or starches, including dried fruit, and brush and floss regularly. Limit your consumption of foods with added sugars. Drink water rather than sweetened drinks, and don't let sodas and other sweets crowd out more nutritious foods, such as low-fat milk or other sources of calcium.

- *Choose and prepare foods with less salt.* You can reduce your chances of developing high blood pressure by consuming less salt. Aim for a moderate salt intake, about 1 teaspoon a day (2400 mg of sodium). Use herbs and spices rather than salt to enhance flavors, and limit your use of high-sodium foods like soy sauce, ketchup, mustard, pickles, and olives. Read food labels to identify foods lower in sodium, especially prepared foods.

- *If you drink alcoholic beverages, do so in moderation.* Excess alcohol consumption alters judgment and can lead to dependency and other serious health

- Be moderate in your consumption of foods high in fat, especially those high in saturated and trans fat, including fast food, commercially prepared baked goods and desserts, meat, poultry, nuts and seeds, and regular dairy products (see Figure 8-3).

- When you do eat high-fat foods, limit your portion sizes, and balance your intake with foods low in fat.

- Choose lean cuts of meat, and trim any visible fat from meat before and after cooking. Remove skin from poultry before or after cooking.

- Replace whole milk with skim or low-fat milk in puddings, soups, and baked products. Substitute plain low-fat yogurt, blender-whipped cottage cheese, or buttermilk in recipes that call for sour cream.

- To reduce saturated and trans fat, use vegetable oil instead of butter or margarine. Use tub or squeeze margarine instead of stick margarine. Look for margarines that are free of trans fat.

- To achieve the recommended proportions of unsaturated fat in your diet, favor monounsaturated fats over polyunsaturated fats and, in choosing polyunsaturated fats, favor omega-3 forms over omega-6 forms.

- Season vegetables with herbs and spices rather than with sauces, butter, or margarine.

- Try lemon juice on salad, or use a yogurt-based salad dressing instead of mayonnaise or sour cream dressings.

- Steam, boil, or bake vegetables, or stir-fry them in a small amount of vegetable oil.

- Roast, bake, or broil meat, poultry, or fish so that fat drains away as the food cooks.

- Use a nonstick pan for cooking so that added fat will be unnecessary; use a vegetable spray for frying.

- Chill broths from meat or poultry until the fat becomes solid. Spoon off the fat before using the broth.

- Eat a low-fat vegetarian main dish at least once a week.

problems. Drinking in moderation is defined as no more than one drink a day for women and no more than two drinks a day for men. People who should not drink at all include individuals who cannot restrict their drinking to moderate levels, women who are or may become pregnant, individuals who plan to drive or operate machinery, and individuals taking certain medications that can interact with alcohol. Never drink if it puts you or others at risk.

The Vegetarian Alternative

Some people choose a diet with one essential difference from the diets we've already described: Foods of animal origin (meat, poultry, fish, eggs, milk) are eliminated or restricted. Today, about 12 million Americans follow a vegetarian diet. Most do so because they think foods of plant origin are a more natural way to nourish the body. Some do so for religious, health, ethical, or philosophical reasons. If you choose to be a vegetarian, you can be confident of meeting your nutritional needs by following a few basic rules. (Vegetarian diets for children and pregnant women warrant individual professional guidance.)

Types of Vegetarian Diets There are a variety of vegetarian styles; the wider the variety of the diet eaten, the easier it is to meet nutritional needs. **Vegans** eat only plant foods. **Lacto-vegetarians** eat plant foods and dairy products. **Lacto-ovo-vegetarians** eat plant foods, dairy products, and eggs. Finally, **partial vegetarians, semivegetarians,** or **pesco-vegetarians** eat plant foods, dairy products, eggs, and usually a small selection of poultry, fish, and other seafood. Including some animal protein in a diet makes planning much easier, but it is not necessary for health.

A Food-Group Plan for Vegetarians A food-group plan has been developed for lacto-vegetarians; it includes 6–11 servings from grains and 2–4 servings from legumes, nuts, and seeds. Add to this 3–5 servings from the vegetable group, 2–4 servings from the fruit group, and 2 or more servings from the milk, yogurt, and cheese group to complete the plan. By following this plan, lacto-vegetarians should have no problem obtaining an adequate diet. Consuming fruits with most meals is especially helpful, because any vitamin C present will improve iron absorption (the iron in plants is more difficult to absorb than the iron in animal sources).

In contrast to those who eat dairy products, vegans must do much more special diet planning to obtain all essential nutrients. A vegan must take special care to con-

TERMS **vegan** A vegetarian who eats no animal products at all.

lacto-vegetarian A vegetarian who includes milk and cheese products in the diet.

lacto-ovo-vegetarian A vegetarian who eats no meat, poultry, or fish, but does eat eggs and milk products.

partial vegetarian, semivegetarian, or **pesco-vegetarian** A vegetarian who includes eggs, dairy products, and small amounts of poultry and seafood in the diet.

sume adequate amounts of protein, riboflavin, vitamin D, vitamin B-12, calcium, iron, and zinc; good strategies for obtaining these nutrients include the following:

- Eat proteins from a wide variety of sources, and include a few protein sources at each meal. A good rule of thumb is 11 servings of grains and 4 servings of legumes, nuts, and seeds daily. Soy milk, tofu (soybean curd), and tempeh (a cultured soy product) make important nutrient contributions to this diet plan.

- Obtain riboflavin from green leafy vegetables, whole grains, yeast, and legumes.

- Obtain vitamin D by spending 5–15 minutes a day out in the sun, from vitamin D–fortified products like rice milk or soy milk, or from a supplement.

- Obtain vitamin B-12 (found only in animal foods) from a supplement or from foods fortified with vitamin B-12, such as special yeast products, soy milk, and breakfast cereals.

- Obtain calcium from fortified tofu; dark-green leafy vegetables; nuts; tortillas made from lime-processed corn; and fortified orange juice, bread, and soy milk.

- Obtain iron from whole grains, fortified bread and breakfast cereals, dried fruits, spinach, brewer's yeast, nuts, and legumes.

- Obtain zinc from whole grains, nuts, and legumes.

It takes a little planning and common sense to put together a good vegetarian diet. If you are a vegetarian or are considering becoming one, devote some extra time and thought to your diet. It's especially important that you eat as wide a variety of foods as possible to ensure that all of your nutritional needs are satisfied. Consulting with a registered dietitian will make your planning even easier.

Dietary Challenges for Special Population Groups

The Food Guide Pyramid and Dietary Guidelines for Americans provide a basis that everyone can use to create a healthy diet. However, some population groups face special dietary challenges.

Women   Women tend to be smaller and to weigh less than men, meaning they have lower energy needs and therefore consume fewer calories. Because of this, women have more difficulty getting adequate amounts of all the essential nutrients and need to focus on nutrient-dense foods. Two nutrients of special concern are calcium and iron, minerals for which many women fail to meet the RDAs. Low calcium intake may be linked to the development of osteoporosis in later life. The *Healthy People 2010* report sets a goal of increasing from 40% to 75% the proportion of women age 20–49 who meet the dietary rec-

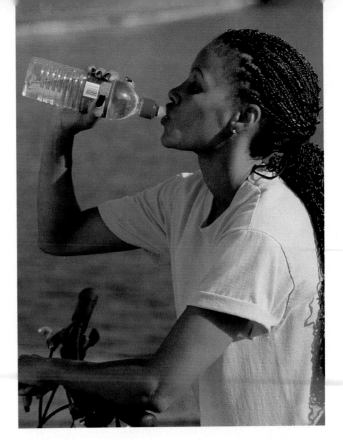

No matter what your dietary choices or challenges, you need to include water in your daily diet. Drink about 8 cups of fluid a day—more if you live in a hot climate or if you exercise vigorously.

ommendation for calcium. Nonfat and low-fat dairy products and fortified cereal, bread, and orange juice are good choices. Iron is also a concern: Menstruating women have higher iron requirements than other groups, and a lack of iron in the diet can lead to iron-deficiency anemia. Lean red meat, green leafy vegetables, and fortified breakfast cereals are good sources of iron. As discussed earlier, all women capable of becoming pregnant should consume adequate folate from fortified foods and/or supplements.

Men   Men are seldom thought of as having nutritional deficiencies because they generally have high-calorie diets. However, many men have a diet that does not follow the Food Guide Pyramid but that includes more red meat and fewer fruits, vegetables, dairy products, and grains than recommended. This dietary pattern is linked to heart disease and some types of cancer. A high intake of calories can lead to weight gain in the long term if a man's activity level decreases as he ages. Men should use the Food Guide Pyramid as a basis for their overall diet and focus on increasing their consumption of fruits, vegetables, and grains to obtain vitamins, minerals, dietary fiber, and phytochemicals.

College Students   Foods that are convenient for college students are not always the healthiest choices. It is easy

General Guidelines

- Eat slowly, and enjoy your food.

- Eat a colorful, varied diet. The more colorful your diet is, the more varied and rich in fruits and vegetables it will be. Many Americans eat few fruits and vegetables, despite the fact that these foods are typically inexpensive, delicious, rich in nutrients, and low in fat and calories.

- Eat breakfast. You'll have more energy in the morning and be less likely to grab an unhealthy snack later on.

- Choose healthy snacks—fruits, vegetables, grains, and cereals—as often as you can.

- Combine physical activity with healthy eating. You'll look and feel better and have a much lower risk of many chronic diseases. Even a little exercise is better than none.

Eating in the Dining Hall

- Choose a meal plan that includes breakfast, and don't skip it.

- If menus are posted or distributed, decide what you want to eat before getting in line, and stick to your choices. Consider what you plan to do and eat for the rest of the day before making your choices.

- Ask for large servings of vegetables and small servings of meat and other high-fat main dishes. Build your meals around grains and vegetables.

- Choose leaner poultry, fish, or bean dishes rather than high-fat meats and fried entrees.

- Ask that gravies and sauces be served on the side; limit your intake.

- Choose broth-based or vegetable soups rather than cream soups.

- Drink nonfat milk, water, mineral water, or fruit juice rather than heavily sweetened fruit drinks or whole milk.

- Choose fruit for dessert rather than pastries, cookies, or cakes.

- Do some research about the foods and preparation methods used in your dining hall or cafeteria. Discuss any food and nutrition suggestions you have with your food service manager.

Eating in Fast-Food Restaurants

- Most fast-food chains can provide a brochure with a nutritional breakdown of the foods on the menu. Ask for it. (See also the information in Appendix C.)

- Order small single burgers with no cheese instead of double burgers with many toppings. If possible, ask for them broiled instead of fried.

- Ask for items to be prepared without mayonnaise, tartar sauce, sour cream, or other high-fat sauces. Ketchup, mustard, and fat-free mayonnaise or sour cream are better choices and are available at many fast-food restaurants.

- Choose whole-grain buns or bread for burgers, hot dogs, and sandwiches.

- Choose chicken items made from chicken breast, not processed chicken.

- Order vegetable pizzas.

- At the salad bar, choose a low-fat dressing. Put the dressing on the side and dip your fork into it—don't pour it over your salad. Avoid heavily dressed potato and pasta salads. Don't put croutons and bacon on vegetable salads.

- If you order french fries or onion rings, get the smallest size and/or share them with a friend.

Eating on the Run

Are you chronically short of time? The following healthy and filling items can be packed for a quick snack or meal: fresh or dried fruit, fruit juices, raw fresh vegetables, plain bagels, bread sticks, fig bars, low-fat cheese sticks or cubes, low-fat crackers or granola bars, nonfat or low-fat yogurt, pretzels, rice or corn cakes, plain popcorn, soup (if you have access to a microwave), or water.

---

for students who eat in buffet-style dining halls to overeat, and the foods offered are not necessarily high in essential nutrients and low in fat. The same is true of meals at fast-food restaurants, another convenient source of quick and inexpensive meals for busy students. Although no food is entirely "bad," consuming a wide variety of foods is critical for a healthy diet. See the box "Eating Strategies for College Students" for tips on making healthy eating convenient and affordable.

Older Adults   As people age, they tend to become less active, so they require fewer calories to maintain their

weight. At the same time, the absorption of nutrients tends to be lower in older adults because of age-related changes in the digestive tract. Thus, they must consume nutrient-dense foods to meet their nutritional requirements. As discussed earlier, foods fortified with vitamin B-12 and/or B-12 supplements are recommended for people over age 50. Because constipation is a common problem, consuming foods high in dietary fiber is another important goal.

Athletes   Key dietary concerns for athletes are meeting their increased energy requirements and drinking enough fluids during practice and throughout the day to remain fully hydrated. Individuals engaged in vigorous training programs expend more energy (calories) than sedentary and moderately active individuals and may have energy needs ranging from 2000 to more than 6000 calories a day. For athletes, the American Dietetic Association recommends a diet with 60–65% of calories coming from carbohydrate, 10–15% from protein, and no more than 30% from fat.

Endurance athletes involved in competitive events lasting longer than 90 minutes may benefit from increasing carbohydrate intake to 65–70% of total calories; this increase should come in the form of complex, rather than simple, carbohydrates. High carbohydrate intake builds and maintains muscle glycogen stores, resulting in greater endurance and delayed fatigue during competitive events. Some endurance athletes engage in "carbohydrate loading"—a practice that involves increasing carbohydrate intake in the days before a competition.

Athletes for whom maintaining low body weight and body fat is important—such as skaters, gymnasts, and wrestlers—should consume adequate calories and nutrients and avoid falling into unhealthy patterns of eating. The combination of low levels of body fat, high physical activity, disordered eating habits, and, in women, amenorrhea, is associated with stress fractures and other injuries and with osteoporosis. Eating disorders are discussed in Chapter 9.

Strenuous exercise can lead to rapid loss of fluids. Endurance athletes should consume at least 16 ounces (2 cups) of fluid about 2 hours before a workout, followed by another 16 ounces about 20 minutes before exercise. In hot and humid conditions, an additional 4–6 ounces should be consumed every 15 minutes during a workout. Athletes should consume enough fluids during activity so that their body weight remains relatively constant before and after an exercise session. For workouts lasting less than 60–90 minutes, cool water is an appropriate fluid replacement; for longer workouts or for exercise in especially hot and humid conditions, a commercial sports beverage that contains carbohydrates may be beneficial.

There is no evidence that consuming supplements containing vitamins, minerals, protein, or specific amino acids will build muscle or improve sports performance. Strength and muscle are built with exercise, not extra protein, and carbohydrates provide the fuel needed for muscle-building exercise. Strenuous physical activity does increase the need for protein and some vitamins and minerals; however, the increased energy intake of athletes more than compensates for this increased need. (Indeed, the protein intake in the average American diet is already about 50% above the RDA, representing 16% of total calories.) For athletes, the American Dietetic Association recommends a daily protein intake of 1.0–1.5 grams per kilogram of body weight, up from the RDA of 0.8 gram per kilogram. A 160-pound athlete consuming 3500 calories a day needs to obtain only 12% of total calories from protein to achieve the upper end of the protein range for athletes. A balanced high-carbohydrate, moderate-protein, low-fat diet can provide all the nutrients athletes need.

People with Special Health Concerns Many Americans have special health concerns that affect their dietary needs. For example, women who are pregnant or breastfeeding require extra calories, vitamins, and minerals. People with diabetes benefit from a well-balanced diet that is low in simple sugars, high in complex carbohydrates, and relatively rich in monounsaturated fats. And people with high blood pressure need to limit their sodium consumption and control their weight. If you have a health problem or concern that may require a special diet, discuss your situation with a physician or registered dietitian.

NUTRITIONAL PLANNING: MAKING INFORMED CHOICES ABOUT FOOD

Now that you know the nutrients you need and the amounts required for maximum wellness, you are almost ready to create a diet that works for you. Depending on your needs and dietary habits, you may have some specific areas of concern you want to address first, such as interpreting food labels, understanding food additives, or avoiding foodborne illnesses. We turn to these and other topics next.

Food Labels—A Closer Look

Consumers can get help in applying the principles of the Food Guide Pyramid and the Dietary Guidelines for Americans from food labels. Since 1994, all processed foods regulated by either the FDA or the USDA have included standardized nutrition information on their labels. Every food label shows serving sizes and the amount of fat, saturated fat, cholesterol, protein, dietary fiber, and sodium in each serving. To make intelligent choices about food, learn to read and understand food labels (see the box "Using Food Labels." Research has shown that people who read food labels eat less fat.

Because most meat, poultry, fish, fruits, and vegetables are not processed, they were not covered by the 1994 law. You can obtain information on the nutrient content of these items from basic nutrition books, registered dietitians, nutrient analysis computer software, the World Wide Web, and the companies that produce or distribute these foods. Also, supermarkets often have large posters

Food labels are designed to help consumers make food choices based on the nutrients that are most important to good health. A food label states how much fat, saturated fat, cholesterol, protein, dietary fiber, and sodium the food contains. In addition to listing nutrient content by weight, the label puts the information in the context of a daily diet of 2000 calories that includes no more than 65 grams of fat (approximately 30% of total calories). For example, if a serving of a particular product has 13 grams of fat, the label will show that the serving represents 20% of the daily fat allowance. If your daily diet contains fewer or more than 2000 calories, adjust these calculations accordingly. Refer to p. 197 for instructions on setting nutrient intake goals.

Food labels contain uniform serving sizes. This means that if you look at different brands of salad dressing, for example, you can compare calories based on the serving amount. Regulations also require that foods meet strict definitions if their packaging includes the terms "light," "low-fat," or "high-fiber" (see below). Health claims such as "good source of dietary fiber" or "low in saturated fat" on packages are signals that those products can wisely be included in your diet. Overall, the food label is an important tool to help you choose a diet that conforms to the Food Guide Pyramid and the Dietary Guidelines.

Selected Nutrient Claims and What They Mean

Healthy A food that is low in fat, is low in saturated fat, has no more than 360–480 mg of sodium and 60 mg of cholesterol, *and* provides 10% or more of the Daily Value for vitamin A, vitamin C, protein, calcium, iron, or dietary fiber.

Light or lite One-third fewer calories or 50% less fat than a similar product.

Reduced or fewer At least 25% less of a nutrient than a similar product; can be applied to fat ("reduced fat"), saturated fat, cholesterol, sodium, and calories.

Extra or added At least 10% more of the Daily Value of a particular nutrient per serving than a similar product.

Good source 10–19% of the Daily Value for a particular nutrient.

High, rich in, or excellent source of 20% or more of the Daily Value for a particular nutrient.

Low calorie 40 calories or fewer per serving.

High fiber 5 g or more of fiber per serving.

Good source of fiber 2.5–4.9 g of fiber per serving.

Fat-free Less than 0.5 g of fat per serving.

Low-fat 3 g of fat or less per serving.

Saturated fat–free Less than 0.5 g of saturated fat and 0.5 g of trans fatty acids per serving.

Low saturated fat 1 g or less of saturated fat per serving and no more than 15% of total calories.

Cholesterol-free Less than 2 mg of cholesterol and 2 g or less of saturated fat per serving.

Low cholesterol 20 mg or less of cholesterol and 2 g or less of saturated fat per serving.

Low sodium 140 mg or less of sodium per serving.

Very low sodium 35 mg or less of sodium per serving.

Lean Cooked seafood, meat, or poultry with less than 10 g of fat, 4.5 g or less of saturated fat, and 95 mg of cholesterol per serving.

Extra lean Cooked seafood, meat, or poultry with less than 5 g of fat, 2 g of saturated fat, and 95 mg of cholesterol per serving.

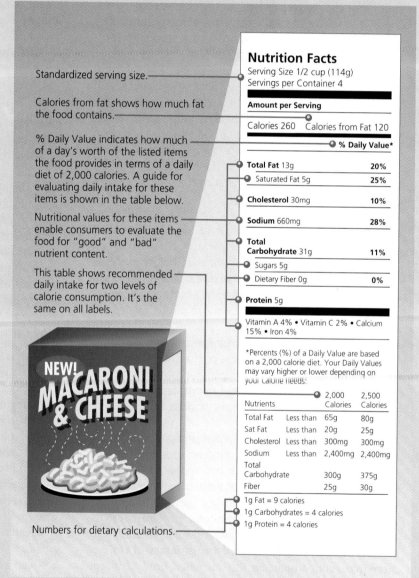

Standardized serving size.

Calories from fat shows how much fat the food contains.

% Daily Value indicates how much of a day's worth of the listed items the food provides in terms of a daily diet of 2,000 calories. A guide for evaluating daily intake for these items is shown in the table below.

Nutritional values for these items enable consumers to evaluate the food for "good" and "bad" nutrient content.

This table shows recommended daily intake for two levels of calorie consumption. It's the same on all labels.

Numbers for dietary calculations.

Nutrition Facts
Serving Size 1/2 cup (114g)
Servings per Container 4

Amount per Serving

Calories 260   Calories from Fat 120

	% Daily Value*
Total Fat 13g	**20%**
Saturated Fat 5g	25%
Cholesterol 30mg	**10%**
Sodium 660mg	**28%**
Total Carbohydrate 31g	**11%**
Sugars 5g	
Dietary Fiber 0g	0%
Protein 5g	

Vitamin A 4% • Vitamin C 2% • Calcium 15% • Iron 4%

*Percents (%) of a Daily Value are based on a 2,000 calorie diet. Your Daily Values may vary higher or lower depending on your calorie needs:

Nutrients		2,000 Calories	2,500 Calories
Total Fat	Less than	65g	80g
Sat Fat	Less than	20g	25g
Cholesterol	Less than	300mg	300mg
Sodium	Less than	2,400mg	2,400mg
Total Carbohydrate		300g	375g
Fiber		25g	30g

1g Fat = 9 calories
1g Carbohydrates = 4 calories
1g Protein = 4 calories

NEW! MACARONI & CHEESE

or pamphlets listing the nutrient contents of these foods. Lab 8-3 gives you the opportunity to compare foods using the information provided on their labels.

Dietary Supplement Labels—New Requirements

Dietary supplements include vitamins, minerals, amino acids, and herbs and other plant-derived substances. Although dietary supplements are often thought to be safe and "natural," they do contain powerful, bioactive chemicals that have the potential for harm. About one-quarter of all pharmaceutical drugs are derived from botanical sources, and even essential vitamins and minerals can have toxic effects if consumed in excess.

In the United States, supplements are not considered drugs and are not regulated the way drugs are. Before they are approved by the FDA and put on the market, drugs undergo clinical studies to determine safety, effectiveness, side effects and risks; possible interactions with other substances; and appropriate dosages. The FDA does not authorize or test dietary supplements, nor does it any longer track adverse reactions, and supplements are not required to demonstrate either safety or effectiveness before they are marketed. Although dosage guidelines exist for some of the compounds in dietary supplements, dosages for many are not well established.

Many ingredients in dietary supplements are classified by the FDA as "generally recognized as safe," but some have been found to be dangerous on their own or to interact with prescription or over-the-counter drugs in dangerous ways. Garlic supplements, for example, can cause bleeding if taken with anticoagulant ("blood-thinning") medications. Even products that are generally considered safe can have side effects—St. John's wort, for example, increases the skin's sensitivity to sunlight.

There are also key differences between drugs and supplements in their manufacture. FDA-approved medications are standardized for potency, and quality control and proof of purity are required. Dietary supplement manufacture is not so closely regulated, and there is no guarantee that a product even contains a given ingredient, let alone in the appropriate amount. The potency of herbal supplements can vary widely due to differences in growing and harvesting conditions, preparation methods, and storage. Contamination and misidentification of plant compounds are also potential problems.

In an effort to provide consumers with more reliable and consistent information about supplements, the FDA has developed new labeling regulations. Since March 1999, labels similar to those found on foods have been required for dietary supplements; for more information, see the box "Using Dietary Supplement Labels."

Remember that dietary supplements are no substitute for a healthy diet. Supplements do not provide all the known—or yet-to-be-discovered—benefits of whole foods. Supplements should also not be used as a replacement for medical treatment for serious illnesses.

Food Additives—Benefits and Risks

Today, some 2800 substances are intentionally added to foods for one or more of the following reasons: (1) to maintain or improve nutritional quality, (2) to maintain freshness, (3) to help in processing or preparation, or (4) to alter taste or appearance. Additives make up less than 1% of our food. The most widely used are sugar, salt, and corn syrup; these three, plus citric acid, baking soda, vegetable colors, mustard, and pepper, account for 98% by weight of all food additives used in the United States.

Some additives may be of concern for certain people, either because they are consumed in large quantities or because they cause some type of allergic reaction. Additives having potential health concerns include the following:

- *Nitrates and nitrites:* Used to protect meats from contamination from the microorganism that causes botulism. Consumption of these substances is associated with the synthesis of cancer-causing agents in the stomach, but the cancer risk appears to be low, except for people with low stomach acid output (such as some older people). The use of nitrates or nitrites is allowed in small quantities.

- *BHA and BHT:* Used to help maintain the freshness of foods. Some studies indicate a potential link between BHT and an increased risk of certain cancers. The FDA is reviewing the use of BHT and BHA, but any risk to the diet from these agents is low. Many manufacturers have stopped using BHT and BHA.

- *Sulfites:* Used to keep vegetables from turning brown. They can cause severe allergic reactions in some people. The FDA strictly limits the use of sulfites and requires any foods containing sulfites to be clearly labeled.

- *Monosodium glutamate (MSG):* Typically used as a flavor enhancer. MSG may cause some people to experience episodes of high blood pressure and sweating. If you are sensitive to MSG, check food labels when shopping, and ask that it not be added to dishes you order in restaurants.

Food additives pose no significant health hazard to most people because the levels used are well below any that could produce toxic effects. Eat a variety of foods in moderation. If you have any sensitivity to an additive, check food labels when you shop, and ask questions when you eat out.

Foodborne Illness—An Increasing Threat

Many people worry about additives or pesticide residues in their food. However, the greatest threat to the safety of the food supply comes from microorganisms that cause foodborne illnesses. Raw or undercooked animal products, such as chicken, hamburger, and oysters, pose the greatest risk for contamination. In 1999 the CDC estimated that 76 million Americans become sick each

Since 1999, specific types of information have been required on the labels of dietary supplements. In addition to basic information about the product, labels include a "Supplement Facts" panel, modeled after the "Nutrition Facts" panel used on food labels (see the figure). Under the Dietary Supplement Health and Education Act (DSHEA) and food labeling laws, supplement labels can make three types of health-related claims:

- *Nutrient-content claims,* such as "high in calcium," "excellent source of vitamin C," or "high potency." The claims "high in" and "excellent source of" mean the same as they do on food labels. A "high potency" single-ingredient supplement must contain 100% of its Daily Value; a "high potency" multi-ingredient product must contain 100% or more of the Daily Value of at least two-thirds of the nutrients present for which Daily Values have been established.

- *Disease claims,* if they have been authorized by the FDA or another authoritative scientific body. The association between adequate calcium intake and lower risk of osteoporosis is an example of an approved disease claim.

- *Structure-function claims,* such as "antioxidants maintain cellular integrity" or " this product enhances energy levels." Because these claims are not reviewed by the FDA, they must carry a disclaimer (see the sample label).

Tips for Choosing and Using Dietary Supplements

- Check with your physician before taking a supplement. Many are not meant for children, older adults, women who are pregnant or breastfeeding, people with chronic illnesses, or people taking prescription or OTC medications.

- Choose brands made by nationally known food and drug manufacturers or "house brands" from large retail chains. Due to their size and visibility, such sources are likely to have higher manufacturing standards.

- Look for the *USP* or *NF* designation, indicating that the product meets some minimum safety and purity standard developed by the United States Pharmacopeia. (The United States Pharmacopeia develops standards for purity and potency for pharmaceutical drugs and has also set standards for vitamins, minerals, and some herbal products.)

- Follow the cautions, instructions for use, and dosage given on the label.

- If you experience side effects, discontinue use of the product and contact your physician. Report any serious reactions to the FDA's MedWatch monitoring program (800-FDA-1088; http://www.fda.gov/medwatch).

For More Information About Dietary Supplements

Blumenthal, M., ed. 1998. *The Complete German Commission E Monographs: Therapeutic Guide to Herbal Medicines.* Tallahassee, Fla.: Integrative Medicines. *(Herbal products have been studied more thoroughly in Germany; Commission E is the German equivalent of the FDA.)*

Herbal Rx: The promises and the pitfalls. 1999. *Consumer Reports,* March.

O'Hara, M., et al. 1998. A review of 12 commonly used medicinal herbs. *Archives of Family Medicine* 7:523–536.

Physician's Desk Reference. 1998. *PDR for Herbal Medicines.* Montvale, N.J.: Medical Economics.

Robbers, J. E., and V. E. Tyler. 1998. *Tyler's Herbs of Choice: The Therapeutic Use of Phytomedicinals,* 2d ed. Binghamton, N.Y.: Haworth Press.

U.S. Pharmacopeia. 1996. *The USP Guide to Vitamins and Minerals.* New York: Avon.

FDA Information About Dietary Supplements (http://vm.cfsan.fda.gov/~dms/supplmnt.html).

National Institutes of Health Office of Dietary Supplements (http://odp.od.riih.gov/ods)

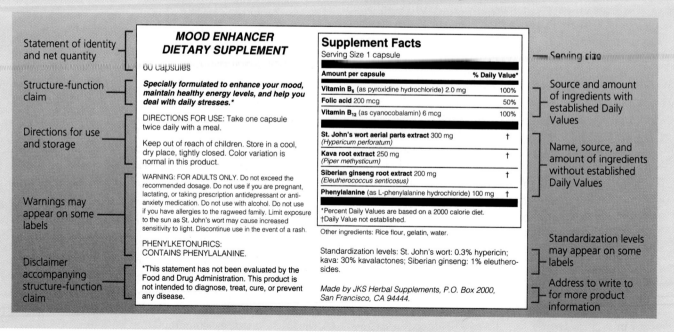

Statement of identity and net quantity

Structure-function claim

Directions for use and storage

Warnings may appear on some labels

Disclaimer accompanying structure-function claim

MOOD ENHANCER DIETARY SUPPLEMENT

60 capsules

Specially formulated to enhance your mood, maintain healthy energy levels, and help you deal with daily stresses.*

DIRECTIONS FOR USE: Take one capsule twice daily with a meal.

Keep out of reach of children. Store in a cool, dry place, tightly closed. Color variation is normal in this product.

WARNING: FOR ADULTS ONLY. Do not exceed the recommended dosage. Do not use if you are pregnant, lactating, or taking prescription antidepressant or anti-anxiety medication. Do not use with alcohol. Do not use if you have allergies to the ragweed family. Limit exposure to the sun as St. John's wort may cause increased sensitivity to light. Discontinue use in the event of a rash.

PHENYLKETONURICS: CONTAINS PHENYLALANINE.

*This statement has not been evaluated by the Food and Drug Administration. This product is not intended to diagnose, treat, cure, or prevent any disease.

Supplement Facts
Serving Size 1 capsule

Amount per capsule	% Daily Value*
Vitamin B₆ (as pyroxidine hydrochloride) 2.0 mg	100%
Folic acid 200 mcg	50%
Vitamin B₁₂ (as cyanocobalamin) 6 mcg	100%
St. John's wort aerial parts extract 300 mg (*Hypericum perforatum*)	†
Kava root extract 250 mg (*Piper methysticum*)	†
Siberian ginseng root extract 200 mg (*Eleutherococcus senticosus*)	†
Phenylalanine (as L-phenylalanine hydrochloride) 100 mg	†

*Percent Daily Values are based on a 2000 calorie diet.
†Daily Value not established.

Other ingredients: Rice flour, gelatin, water.

Standardization levels: St. John's wort: 0.3% hypericin; kava: 30% kavalactones; Siberian ginseng: 1% eleutherosides.

Made by JKS Herbal Supplements, P.O. Box 2000, San Francisco, CA 94444.

Serving size

Source and amount of ingredients with established Daily Values

Name, source, and amount of ingredients without established Daily Values

Standardization levels may appear on some labels

Address to write to for more product information

year as a result of foodborne illness, 325,000 are hospitalized, and 5000 die. These estimates are higher for illnesses but lower for deaths than previous estimates. In most cases, foodborne illness produces acute gastroenteritis, characterized by diarrhea, vomiting, fever, and weakness. People often mistake foodborne illness for a bout of the flu. Although the effects of foodborne illness are usually not serious, some groups, such as children and older people, are at risk for severe complications, including rheumatic diseases, kidney failure, seizures, blood poisoning, and death.

Causes of Foodborne Illnesses

Most cases of foodborne illness are caused by **pathogens,** disease-causing microorganisms that contaminate food, usually from improper handling. The threats are numerous and varied; among them are the sometimes deadly *Escherichia coli* (*E. coli*) O157:H7 in meat and apple juice; *Salmonella* in eggs, on vegetables, and on poultry; *Vibrio* in shellfish; *Cyclospora* and hepatitis A virus on fruit; *Cryptosporidium* in drinking water; *Campylobacter jejuni* in meat and poultry; and *Listeria monocytogenes* in lunch meats, sausages, and hot dogs.

Statistics reveal high levels of contamination in many foods. Currently, it is estimated that at least 10% of all ground beef and 25% of all chicken sold in the United States are contaminated with pathogenic bacteria. Problems have increased both because of changes in food production methods—most food is now produced on huge, crowded farms and ranches and transported long distances—and because of changes in people's eating habits—more people are eating out. Additionally, the number of virulent and drug-resistant pathogens is rising, partly because of the widespread use of antibiotics to stimulate growth in animals. An antibiotic-resistant strain of *Salmonella* was recently identified, raising concerns about a potential increase in serious illness from this pathogen.

Recently, the U.S. government has been taking steps to reduce levels of contamination, including more precise national surveillance and closer inspection at several levels. As a result, the number of food recalls has increased; the 1998 recall of 35 million pounds of hot dogs and lunch meat from one plant due to possible *Listeria* contamination was one of the largest recalls to date. Improved surveillance also led to the decline of foodborne illness caused by two of the leading pathogens between 1996 and 1998—cases of *Salmonella* infection declined by 14% and of *Campylobacter* by 8%. Additionally, in 1999 the government addressed some of its food-safety advice specifically to certain high-risk groups, including pregnant women, young children, elderly people, and individuals with weakened immune systems, such as people with AIDS and chemotherapy patients. Some pathogens, such as *Listeria,* seem to cause serious illness only in such high-risk individuals.

Preventing and Treating Foodborne Illness

Increased monitoring of foods will not, however, eliminate all contamination. The key to protecting yourself from foodborne illness is to handle, cook, and store foods in ways that prevent bacteria from spreading and multiplying. When handling foods, keep these tips in mind:

- Don't buy food in containers that leak, bulge, or are severely dented. Refrigerated foods should be cold, and frozen foods should be solid.

- Refrigerate perishable items as soon as possible after purchase. Use or freeze fresh meats within 3–5 days and fresh poultry, fish, and ground meat within 1–2 days.

- Thaw frozen food in the refrigerator or in the microwave oven, not on the kitchen counter.

- Thoroughly wash your hands with soapy water for 20 seconds before and after handling food, especially raw meat, fish, poultry, or eggs.

- Make sure counters, cutting boards, dishes, and other equipment are thoroughly cleaned before and after use. If possible, use separate cutting boards for meat and for foods that will be eaten raw, such as fruits and vegetables. Wash dishcloths and kitchen towels frequently.

- Thoroughly rinse and scrub fruits and vegetables with a brush, if possible, or peel off the skin.

- Cook foods thoroughly, especially beef, poultry, fish, pork, and eggs. Cooking kills most microorganisms, as long as an appropriately high temperature is reached. The USDA now recommends that consumers, especially high-risk individuals, use a food thermometer to verify that hamburgers are cooked to 160°F. When eating out, order red meat cooked "well-done."

- Cook stuffing separate from poultry; or wash poultry thoroughly, stuff immediately before cooking, and transfer the stuffing to a clean bowl immediately after cooking.

- Store foods below 40°F. Do not leave cooked or refrigerated foods, such as meats or salads, at room temperature for more than 2 hours. Use cooked leftovers within 3–4 days.

- Don't eat raw animal products, including raw eggs in Caesar salad, hollandaise sauce, or eggnog. Use only pasteurized milk and juice, and look for pasteurized eggs, which are now available in some states.

- Cook eggs until they're firm, and fully cook foods containing eggs. Store eggs in the coldest part of the refrigerator, not on the door, and use them within 3–5 weeks.

pathogen A microorganism that causes disease. **TERMS**

- Because of possible contamination with *E. coli* O157:H7 and *Salmonella*, avoid raw sprouts, or eat them only after submerging them in boiling water for 10 seconds.
- If you are in a high-risk group, the government recommends extra precautions to protect yourself from *Listeria*: Heat any ready-to-eat meat, including lunch meats, sausages, and hot dogs, in a pot, oven, or pan (but not a microwave) until it's steaming hot. *Listeria* continues to grow in refrigerated foods, so throw away any ready-to-eat meats if their expiration date has passed.
- According to the USDA, "When in doubt, throw it out."

If you think you have a foodborne illness, drink plenty of clear fluids to prevent dehydration, and rest to speed recovery. See a physician for a fever higher than 102°F, blood in the stool, or dehydration, especially if symptoms persist for more than 2–3 days. In cases of suspected botulism—characterized by symptoms such as double vision, paralysis, dizziness, and vomiting—consult a physician immediately.

Irradiated Foods—A Technique of Biotechnology

Irradiation is a tool of biotechnology being used to protect consumers from foodborne illness. Subjecting products to radiation significantly reduces the risk of foodborne disease caused by various pathogens, among them *E. coli* O157:H7 and several *Salmonella* species. In the United States, where irradiation is categorized as an additive, approval of irradiated foods is regulated by Congress. Since 1963, the government has allowed the irradiation of certain foods that are available commercially. This growing list includes wheat and flour (1963), pork (1985), some vegetables and spices (1986), raw poultry (1992), and, most recently, red meats (2000).

Even though irradiation has been generally endorsed by agencies such as the World Health Organization and the American Medical Association, skepticism exists. Those who oppose irradiation say that essential nutrients in food may be destroyed, that eating food that's been irradiated may cause cancer or other debilitating conditions, and that irradiation may be hazardous to the employees and residents of the area surrounding a food irradiation site. However, studies haven't conclusively identified any harmful effects of food irradiation. In fact, studies indicate that when consumers are educated about the benefits of irradiated foods, most want

to buy it. Without consumer education, many remain skeptical.

All primary irradiated foods (meat, vegetables, and so on) are labeled with the flower-like radura symbol and a brief informational label. Spices and any food that is merely an ingredient do not have to be labeled.

Organic Foods—Stricter Standards for a Booming Industry

The term *organic foods* refers generally to foods produced naturally, without the use of toxic chemicals. In 1990, Congress directed the USDA to establish a national standard for the production, processing, and certification of organic foods. Under the USDA's auspices, an organic standards board was set up. Since then, it has been developing the guidelines that will regulate all crops—from produce, grains, meat, dairy, and eggs to processed foods.

In recent years, advances in biotechnology and new agricultural practices have organic farmers and some consumers rallying for stricter standards—not only for produce but for red meat and poultry as well. Today, "organic foods" can be genetically manipulated, irradiated, and fertilized with sewage sludge; livestock can be given hormones and antibiotics with no labeling required. Some people have ethical concerns, too. A number of consumers want chicken and livestock raised in open-air environments, not closed, cramped quarters. In 1999, the USDA responded to many of these concerns with tighter ruling on what makes a food **certified organic:** To qualify as organic, foods must be raised without pesticides or herbicides and processed without preservatives. Livestock and poultry cannot be given growth hormones or treated with antibiotics, and 100% of their feed must be organic. In addition, foods cannot be certified organic if they have been irradiated or genetically modified.

The production of organic foods is a booming industry. There are now more than 10,000 U.S. farms raising organic crops and livestock. Since 1990, U.S. sales of organic foods have grown by 20% a year, reaching $3.3 billion in 1996 and $6.5 billion in 2000. Sales of organic dairy products are increasing by more than 100% annually.

A PERSONAL PLAN: APPLYING NUTRITIONAL PRINCIPLES

You've learned the basics of good nutrition, know how to interpret food and supplement labels, and have some guidelines for protecting yourself from environmental contaminants and foodborne illness. With this foundation, you can now put together a diet that works for you. Based on your particular nutrition and health status, there probably is an ideal diet for you, but there is no single

TERMS **irradiation** The treatment of foods with gamma rays, X rays, or high-voltage electrons to kill potentially harmful pathogens and increase shelf life.

certified organic A designation applied to foods grown and produced according to strict guidelines limiting the use of pesticides and nonorganic ingredients.

There is no one ethnic diet that clearly surpasses all others in providing people with healthful foods. Every diet has its advantages and disadvantages, and within each cuisine, some foods are better choices. It is in the area of personal choice that individuals can make a difference in their own health. The dietary guidelines described in this chapter can be applied to any ethnic cuisine. For additional guidance, refer to the healthy choices listed below.

	Cooking Methods/ Terms	Meats (Proteins)	Healthy Sauces or Accompaniments	Grains
Chinese	Steamed	Chicken without skin	(Choose no MSG)	Steamed rice
	Jum (poached)	Fresh fish fillets, shrimp, scallops	Hoisin sauce	
	Lightly stir-fried	Lean beef	Oyster Sauce	
	Chu		Hot and spicy tomato sauce	
	Kow (roasted)		Sweet-and-sour sauce	
	Shu (barbecued)		Hot mustard sauce	
			Reduced-sodium soy sauce	
French	Steamed	Fresh fish, shrimp, scallops (without sauces)	Dinner salad with vinegar or lemon juice	(Without cream or added butter or other fat)
	Poached	Steamed mussels		Rice
		Chicken breast, without skin		Noodles
				Crusty bread
Italian	Grilled (often fish or vegetables)	Lean meats	Red sauces: spicy marinara sauce (arrabiata), marinara sauce, or cacciatore	Rice
	Lightly sauteed	Fresh seafood		Pasta (noodles, spaghetti)
			Light red sauce, light red or white wine sauce, light mushroom sauce	
			Red clam sauce	
			Primavera (with vegetables, no cream sauce)	
			Florentine (with spinach)	
			Piccata (with lemon)	
Middle Eastern	Grilled on a skewer	Spiced ground meat	Special garlic sauce	Couscous
	Marinated and barbecued	Mashed chickpeas	Blended with Middle Eastern spices	Rice or bulgur (cracked wheat)
	Baked	Fava beans	With tomatoes, onions, green peppers, and cucumbers	
	Charbroiled or charcoal broiled		With chopped parsley and onion	
			Stuffed with rice	

(continued)

	Cooking Methods/ Terms	Meats (proteins)	Healthy Sauces or Accompaniments	Grains
Japanese	Yakimono (broiled)	Chicken	Grilled vegetables	Rice
	Grilled	Fish or shrimp teriyaki, broiled in sauce	House salad with fresh ginger and cellophane noodles	Menrui or soba noodles
	Nabemono (boiled)		Tofu or bean curd	
Indian	Broiled	Chicken or shrimp kabob	Marinated in yogurt or spices	Basmati rice
	Tandoori (cooked in a clay oven)	Lentils, garbanzo beans, beans	Cooked with green vegetables, onions, tomatoes, peppers, and mushrooms	Baked leavened bread
	Tikka (pan-roasted)		Masala	
			Paneer	
			Cooked with curry, marinated in spices	
			Saag (with spinach)	
			Garnished with dried fruits	
Mexican	Grilled	Shredded spicy chicken	Chili vegetarian tomato sauce	Rice
	Marinated	Ceviche (raw fish marinated in lime juice and mixed with spices)	Enchilada sauce	Soft corn or wheat flour tortillas
	Simmered	Black beans	Salsa (hot red tomato sauce)	
			Salsa verde (green chili sauce)	
			Picante sauce	
			Shredded lettuce, diced tomatoes	
Thai	Barbecued	Seafood dishes	Fish sauce	Rice
	Sauteed	Chicken	Hot sauce	Noodles
	Broiled		Basil sauce, basil or sweet basil leaves	
	Boiled		Lime sauce or lime juice	
	Steamed, braised, marinated		Chili sauce or crushed dried chili flakes	
	Charbroiled		Thai spices	
			Bed of mixed vegetables	
			Scallions and onions	
			Napa cabbage, bamboo shoots, black mushrooms, ginger, garlic	

SOURCES: Adapted from National Heart, Lung, and Blood Institute. 1998. Tips for Healthy Multicultural Dining Out. In *Clinical Guidelines on the Identification, Evaluation, and Treatment of Overweight and Obesity in Adults,* Appendix A.3.b. Bethesda, Md.: National Institutes of Health.

type of diet that provides optimal health for everyone. Many cultural dietary patterns can meet people's nutritional requirements (see the box "Ethnic Foods: Healthy Choices"). Every individual needs to customize a food plan based on age, gender, weight, activity level, medical risk factors—and, of course, personal tastes.

Assessing and Changing Your Diet

The first step in planning a healthy diet is to examine what you currently eat. Labs 8-1 and 8-2 are designed to help you analyze your current diet and compare it with optimal dietary goals. (This analysis can be completed using either Appendix B or a nutritional analysis software program.)

Next, experiment with additions and substitutions to your current diet to bring it closer to your goals. If you are consuming too much fat, for example, try substituting fruit for a calorie-rich dessert. If you aren't getting enough iron, try adding some raisins to your cereal or garbanzo beans to your salad. If you need to plan your diet from the ground up, use the Food Guide Pyramid and the Dietary Guidelines.

To put your plan into action, use the behavioral self-management techniques and tips described in Chapter 1. If you identify several changes you want to make, focus on one at a time. You might start, for example, by substituting nonfat or low-fat milk for whole milk. When you become used to that, you can try substituting whole-wheat bread for white bread. The information on eating behavior in Lab 8-1 will help you identify and change unhealthy patterns of eating.

Staying Committed to a Healthy Diet

Beyond knowledge and information, you also need support in difficult situations. Keeping to your plan is easiest when you choose and prepare your own food at home. For meals prepared at home, advance planning is the key: mapping out meals and shopping appropriately, cooking in advance when possible, and preparing enough food for leftovers later in the week. A tight budget does not necessarily make it more difficult to eat healthy meals. It makes good health sense and good budget sense to use only small amounts of meat and to have a few meatless meals each week.

In restaurants, keeping to food plan goals becomes somewhat more difficult. Portion sizes in restaurants tend to be larger than serving sizes of the Food Guide Pyramid, but by remaining focused on your goals, you can eat only part of your meal and take the rest home for a meal later in the week. Don't hesitate to ask questions when you're eating in a restaurant. Most restaurant personnel are glad to explain how menu selections are prepared and to make small adjustments, such as serving salad dressings and sauces on the side so they can be avoided or used sparingly. To limit your fat intake, order meat or fish broiled or grilled rather than fried or sauteed, choose rice or a plain baked potato over french fries, and select a clear soup rather than a creamy one. Desserts that are irresistible can, at least, be shared.

Strategies like these can be helpful, but small changes cannot change a fundamentally high-fat, high-calorie meal into a moderate, healthful one. Often, the best advice is to bypass a steak with potatoes au gratin for a flavorful but low-fat entree. Many of the selections offered in ethnic restaurants are healthy choices (refer to the box on ethnic foods on pp. 221–222 for suggestions).

Fast-food restaurants offer the biggest challenge to a healthy diet. Surveys show that about 70% of 18- to 24-year-olds and 64% of 25- to 34-year-olds visit a fast-food restaurant at least once a week. Fast-food meals are often high in calories, total fat, saturated fat, trans fat, sodium, and sugar; they may be low in fiber and in some vitamins and minerals (see Appendix C). If you do eat at a fast-food restaurant, make sure the rest of your meals that day are low-fat meals.

Knowledge of food and nutrition is essential to the success of your program. The information provided in this chapter should give you the tools you need to design and implement a diet that promotes long-term health and well-being. If you need additional information or have questions about nutrition, be sure the source you consult is reliable.

COMMON QUESTIONS ANSWERED

Which should I eat—butter or margarine? Both butter and margarine are concentrated sources of fat, containing about 11 grams of fat and 100 calories per tablespoon. Butter is higher in saturated fat, which raises levels of artery-clogging LDL ("bad" cholesterol). Each tablespoon of butter has about 8 grams of saturated fat; margarine has about 2. Butter also contains cholesterol, which margarine does not.

Margarine, on the other hand, contains trans fat, which not only raises LDL but lowers HDL ("good" cholesterol). A tablespoon of stick margarine contains about 2 grams of trans fat. Butter contains a small amount of trans fat as well. Although butter has a combined total of saturated and trans fats that is twice that of stick margarine, the trans fat in stick margarine may be worse for you. Clearly, you should avoid both butter and stick margarine. To solve this dilemma, remember that softer is better. The softer or more liquid a margarine or spread is, the less hydrogenated it is and the less trans fat it contains.

(continued)

Tub and squeeze margarines contain less trans fat than stick margarines; some margarines are modified to be low-trans or trans-free and are labeled as such. Vegetable oils are even better choice for cooking and for table use (such as olive oil for dipping bread) because most are low in saturated fat and completely free of trans fats.

The Food Guide Pyramid seems to recommend such a large number of servings. How can I possibly follow its recommendations without gaining weight? First of all, consider how many servings from each food group are appropriate for you. The suggested number of servings is given as a range, 6–11 servings of grain products, 3–5 of vegetables, and so on. The smaller number of servings is for people who consume about 1600 calories a day, such as many sedentary women. The larger number is for those who consume about 2800 calories a day, such as active men. If the smaller number of servings is appropriate for you, concentrate on choosing nutrient-dense foods—those that are rich in nutrients but relatively low in calories, such as most grains, fruits, and vegetables.

Second, compare the serving sizes of the foods you eat with those used in the Food Guide Pyramid (see pp. 206–209). Some of the Pyramid's serving sizes are smaller than what you might typically eat. For example, many people eat a cup or more of pasta or rice in a meal, which would correspond to 2 or more servings from the grain products group. You'll probably find that your current diet already includes the minimum number of servings from most of the food groups. If not, you may find that you are eating too many servings from one group and not enough from another. Make small changes in your eating habits and food choices to bring your diet into line with the recommendations in the Pyramid, paying particular attention to your consumption of fat and added sugars. The Food Guide Pyramid is designed to help you balance your food choices to ensure good health. Strategies for successful weight management are described in detail in the next chapter.

What are functional foods, and will eating them make me healthier? Functional foods are foods with added ingredients that are thought to offer a health benefit above and beyond their inherent nutritional value. The added ingredients can be nutrients, such as calcium in orange juice; herbs, such as St. John's wort in split pea soup; or other substances, such as plant sterols in margarine. Functional foods, also called "nutraceuticals," are flooding the market, with retail sales now topping $10 billion a year. Health claims include preventing depression, enhancing relaxation, boosting memory, and promoting a healthy heart. One product, Brain Gum, promises to help people remember names, faces, phone numbers, and where they've put their eyeglasses.

Don't assume that eating these highly marketed foods will make you healthier. Consider especially the nutritional value of the product you're buying. Orange juice with added calcium is hard to fault. Other products may not be all they advertise. It's best to look closely at the Nutrition Facts label of a product before buying it. You may find out that the fortified food is largely junk food and can't take the place of fresh fruits and vegetables, which usually have no label, little advertising, and no unknown long-term effects.

An exception to this rule may be two new FDA-approved margarines that have been modified so they actually lower blood cholesterol levels. The two products, Johnson & Johnson's Benecol and Lipton's Take Control, contain substances from plants that are structurally similar to cholesterol and thus interfere with the absorption of cholesterol in the intestines. Some research has shown that they lower LDL cholesterol without also lowering HDL cholesterol. Even here, though, some cautions are in order. The products are intended to *replace* the fats in the diet, not supplement them. Additionally, they may lower cholesterol only in people whose diets are high in fat and cholesterol; they probably don't have much effect on people who already consume a low-fat diet. Finally, they cost several times as much as regular margarine.

What exactly are genetically modified foods? Are they safe? How can I recognize them on the shelf, and how can I know when I'm eating them? Genetically modified (GM) foods are foods derived from a plant by altering its DNA. Scientists use this technique in hopes of benefiting humans—by producing seeds that are more resistant to pests, last longer, or grow larger. Some genetically modified food may contain bacterial, viral, or other genes not native to the food.

In the United States, many consumers see GM products as safe and beneficial, leading to less pesticide use and increased production. The process of producing GM foods, known as agricultural biotechnology, is reviewed and approved by several federal agencies before the food is commercially released. The U.S. Department of Agriculture's Animal and Plant Health Inspection Service (APHIS) has regulated all field-testing of genetically modified plants since 1987, and about 50 genetically altered plant varieties are now commercially available.

Yet even with safety testing of GM foods, there is no way to accurately predict whether a new food will cause allergies or have some other unintended consequences. In response to some consumer concerns about safety, the USDA has directed that certified organic foods cannot include genetically modified foods.

Currently, almost half of all U.S. plantings are genetically altered; therefore eating GM foods is unavoidable in this country and has been since about 1996. It is virtually impossible to recognize GM foods. FDA officials require labeling only if a food's nutritional content is altered significantly, a potential allergic reaction is identified, or a new food additive is involved that is different from those already in foods. Of the 50 or so GM foods commercially available, the major crops are cotton (about half is genetically modified), soybeans (about half), and corn (about one-third). Products made from them include juice, soda, nuts, tuna, frozen pizza, spaghetti sauce, crackers, cookies, salad dressing, and soup. Even in health food stores, products such as tofu and canola oil often contain GM ingredients.

Remember that foods in the country have one of the highest food safety records in the world. If you are concerned about possible unintended consequences of eating GM foods, buy only foods marked *certified organic*.

SUMMARY

- Food choices made in youth can significantly affect a person's health in later years. Making good choices is an important part of everyday life.

- The six classes of nutrients are carbohydrates, proteins, fats, vitamins, minerals, and water.

- The 45 nutrients essential to humans are released into the body through digestion. Nutrients in foods provide energy, measured in kilocalories (commonly called calories); build and maintain body tissues; and regulate body functions.

- Protein, an important component of body tissue, is composed of amino acids; nine are essential to a diet. Foods from animal sources provide complete proteins; plants provide incomplete proteins.

- Fat, the major body fuel at times of rest and light activity, also insulates the body and cushions the organs; 1 tablespoon of vegetable oil per day supplies the essential fats. For most people, dietary fat should be limited to 30% or less of total calories, and unsaturated fats should be favored over saturated and trans fats.

- Carbohydrates provide energy to the brain, nervous system, and blood and to muscles during high-intensity exercise. Naturally occurring simple carbohydrates and unrefined complex carbohydrates should be favored over added sugars and refined carbohydrates. Dietary fiber includes plant substances that are difficult or impossible for the human body to digest. It helps reduce cholesterol levels and promotes the passage of wastes through the intestines.

- The 13 essential vitamins are organic substances that promote specific chemical and cell processes and act as antioxidants. The 17 known essential minerals are inorganic substances that regulate body functions, aid in growth and tissue maintenance, and help in the release of energy from food. Deficiencies in vitamins and minerals can cause severe symptoms over time, but excess doses are also dangerous.

- Water, distributed in body tissues and fluids, aids in digestion and food absorption, allows chemical reactions to take place, serves as a lubricant or cushion, and helps regulate body temperature.

- Foods contain other substances, such as phytochemicals, that may not be essential nutrients but that may protect against chronic diseases.

- The Recommended Dietary Allowances, Dietary Reference Intakes, Food Guide Pyramid, and Dietary Guidelines for Americans provide standards and recommendations for getting all essential nutrients from a varied, balanced diet and for eating in ways that protect against chronic disease.

- Basic recommendations for a healthy diet include eating a variety of foods; balancing food intake with energy expenditure; increasing complex carbohydrates; reducing all fat, especially saturated fat; and limiting sugar, salt, alcohol, and smoked and nitrate-cured foods.

- A vegetarian diet requires special planning but can meet all human nutritional needs.

- Different population groups, such as college students and athletes, face special dietary challenges and should plan their diets to meet their particular needs.

- Consumers can get help applying nutritional principles by reading the standardized labels that appear on all packaged foods and on dietary supplements.

- Food additives maintain or improve nutritional quality and freshness and help in food processing, although they may alter taste and appearance. Foodborne illnesses are a greater threat to health than additives. Food irradiation is an effective but controversial approach to preventing foodborne illness.

- Some consumer concerns about food safety have led the U.S. government to tighten national standards for foods that may be labeled *certified organic*.

- Although nutritional basics are well established, no single diet provides wellness for everyone. Individuals should focus on their particular needs and adapt general dietary principles to meet them.

FOR MORE INFORMATION

For reliable nutrition advice, talk to a faculty member in the nutrition department on your campus, a registered dietitian (R.D.), or your physician. Many large communities have a telephone service called Dial a Dietitian. By calling this number, you can receive free nutrition information from an R.D.

Experts on quackery suggest that you steer clear of anyone who puts forth any of the following false statements:

- Most diseases are caused primarily by faulty nutrition.

- Large doses of vitamins are effective against many diseases.

- Hair analysis can be used to determine a person's nutritional state.

- A computer-scored nutritional deficiency test is a basis for prescribing vitamins.

Any practitioner—licensed or not—who sells vitamins in his or her office should be thoroughly scrutinized.

Books

American Dietetic Association. 1999. *The Essential Guide to Nutrition and the Foods We Eat: Everything You Need to Know About the Foods You Eat*. New York: HarperCollins. *An excellent review of current nutrition information and issues.*

Consumer Guide Editors. 1998. *Complete Book of Vitamins and Minerals*, rev. ed. New York: Signet. *A comprehensive review of vitamins and minerals.*

Havala, S. 1999. *The Complete Idiot's Guide to Being a Vegetarian.* Indianapolis, Ind.: Macmillan. *Provides information on the benefits of vegetarian diets and how to plan healthy meals.*

Nelson, M. 2000. *Strong Women, Strong Bones: Everything You Need to Know to Prevent, Treat, and Beat Osteoporosis.* New York: Putnam. *A comprehensive, up-to-date guide to preventing and treating osteoporosis through exercise and nutrition.*

Wardlaw, G. M. 1999. *Perspectives in Nutrition*, 4th ed. Boston: McGraw-Hill. *An easy-to-understand review of major concepts in nutrition.*

Woodruff, S. 2000. *The Best-Kept Secrets of Healthy Cooking.* Garden City Park, N.Y.: Avery. *A collection of more than 600 low-fat and fatfree recipes by a best-selling cookbook author.*

Newsletters

Environmental Nutrition
P.O. Box 420235, Palm Coast, FL 32142; 800-829-5384
Nutrition Action Health Letter
1875 Connecticut Ave., N.W., Suite 300, Washington DC 20009; 202-332-9110 (http://www.cspinet.org)
Tufts University Health and Nutrition Letter
P.O. Box 420235, Palm Coast, FL 32142; 800-274-7581

Organizations, Hotlines, and Web Sites

American Dietetic Association. Provides a wide variety of educational materials on nutrition.
800-366-1655 (for general nutrition information and referrals to registered dietitians)
900-CALL-AN-RD (for customized answers to nutrition questions)
http://www.eatright.org
Ask the Dietitian. Questions and answers on many topics relating to nutrition.
http://www.dietitian.com
CyberDiet. Provides a variety of resources, including a profile that calculates calorie and nutrient needs and a database that provides nutrition information in food label format.
http://www.CyberDiet.com
FDA Center for Food Safety and Applied Nutrition. Offers information about topics such as food labeling, food additives, and foodborne illness.
http://vm.cfsan.fda.gov
Food Safety Hotlines. Provide information on the safe purchase, handling, cooking, and storage of food.
888-723-3366 (FDA)
800-535-4555 (USDA)
Gateway to Government Food Safety Information. Provides access to government resources relating to food safety, including consumer advice and information on specific pathogens.
http://www.foodsafety.gov
Health Canada: Food and Nutrition. Provides information about Canada's Food Guide to Healthy Eating as well as advice for people with special dietary needs.
http://www.hc-sc.gc.ca/english/food.htm
Meals Online. A searchable database of more than 10,000 recipes.
http://www.my-meals.com

National Academies' Food and Nutrition Board. Provides information about the Dietary Reference Intakes and related guidelines.
http://www4.nationalacademies.org/IOM/IOMHome.nsf/Pages/Food+and+Nutrition+Board
National Osteoporosis Foundation. Provides up-to-date information on the causes, prevention, detection, and treatment of osteoporosis.
202-223-2226
http://www.nof.org
Tufts University Nutrition Navigator. Provides descriptions and ratings for many nutrition-related Web pages.
http://navigator.tufts.edu
USDA Center for Nutrition Policy and Promotion. Click on "Interactive Healthy Eating Index" for an online assessment of your diet for one day and a comparison of your diet with the Food Guide Pyramid. Also provides RDAs and advice.
http://www.usda.gov/cnpp
USDA Food and Nutrition Information Center. Provides a variety of materials relating to the Dietary Guidelines, food labels, Food Guide Pyramid, and many other topics; Web site includes extensive links.
301-504-5719
http://www.nal.usda.gov/fnic
Vegetarian Resource Group. Information and links for vegetarians and people interested in learning more about vegetarian diets.
http://www.vrg.org

You can obtain nutrient breakdowns of individual food items from the following sites:

Nutrition Analysis Tool, University of Illinois, Urbana/Champaign
http://www.nat.uiuc.edu
USDA Food and Nutrition Information Center
http://www.nal.usda.gov/fnic/foodcomp
See also the resources listed in Chapters 9, 11, and 12.

SELECTED BIBLIOGRAPHY

Agricultural Research Service. 2000. *Report of the Dietary Guidelines Advisory Committee on Dietary Guidelines for Americans, 2000* (http://www.ars.usda.gov/dgac; retrieved May 5, 2000).

Alberts, D. S., et al. 2000. Lack of effect of a high-fiber cereal supplement on the recurrence of colorectal adenomas. *New England Journal of Medicine* 342(16): 1156–1162.

Allison, D. B., et al. 1999. Estimated intakes of trans fatty and other fatty acids in the U.S. population. *Journal of the American Dietetic Association* 99(2): 166–174.

American Heart Association. 1996. Dietary guidelines for healthy American adults. *Circulation* 94:1795–1800.

Balluz, L. S., et al. 2000. Vitamin and mineral supplement use in the United States: Results from the third National Health and Nutrition Examination Survey. *Archives of Family Medicine* 9(3): 258–262.

Barnard, N. D., et al. 2000. Effectiveness of a low-fat vegetarian diet in altering serum lipids in healthy premenopausal women. *American Journal of Cardiology* 85(8): 969–972.

Bruhn, C. M. 1999. Consumer perceptions and concerns about food contaminants. *Advanced Experiments in Medical Biology* 459:1–7.

Centers for Disease Control and Prevention. 1998. Osteoporosis among estrogen-deficient women—United States, 1988–1994. *Morbidity and Mortality Weekly Report* 47(45): 969–973.

Chatenoud, L., et al. 1998. Whole-grain food intake and cancer risk. *International Journal of Cancer* 77(1): 24–28.

Commission on Dietary Supplement Labels. 1997. *Report of the Commission on Dietary Supplement Labels, November 1997.* Washington, D.C.: U.S. Government Printing Office (Stock No. 017-001-00531-2).

Department of Health and Human Services. 2000. *Dietary Guidelines for Americans, 2000.* USDA Home and Garden Bulletin no. 232.

Food and Nutrition Board. 1998. *Proposed Definition and Plan for Review of Dietary Antioxidants and Related Compounds.* Washington, D.C.: National Academy Press.

Food Safety and Inspection Service. 1999. Listeria monocytogenes and *Listeriosis* (http://www.fsis.usda.gov/OA/pubs/listeria.htm; retrieved May 5, 2000).

A fresh look at chicken safety. 1998. *Consumer Reports,* October.

Giguere, Y., and F. Rousseau. 2000. The genetics of osteoporosis: 'Complexities and difficulties.' *Clinical Genetics* 57(3): 161–169.

Going with the grain. 1999. *Cancer Outlook* 5(1). Peckham Publishing publication no. 014-513.

Guthrie, J. S., and J. S. Morton. 2000. Food sources of added sweeteners in the diets of Americans. *Journal of the American Dietetic Association* 100:43–48, 51.

Hallikainen, M. A., and M. I. Uusitupa. 1999. Effects of 2 low-fat stanol ester–containing margarines on serum cholesterol concentrations as part of a low-fat diet in hypercholesterolemic subjects. *American Journal of Clinical Nutrition* 69(3): 403–410.

Henkel, J. 1998. *Irradiation: A Safe Measure for Safer Food.* Reprint no. 98-2320. Washington, D.C.: U.S. Food and Drug Administration.

Holman, R. T. 1998. The slow discovery of the importance of omega-3 essential fatty acids in human health. *Journal of Nutrition* 128(2 Suppl.): 427S–433S.

Jacobs, D. R., et al. 1999. Is whole-grain intake associated with reduced total and cause-specific death rates in older women? The Iowa Women's Health Study. *American Journal of Public Health* 89:322–329.

Jacobson, M. F., B. Silverglade, and I. R. Heller. 2000. Functional foods: Health boon or quackery? *Western Journal of Medicine* 172(1): 8–9

Kleiner, S. M. 1999. Water: An essential but overlooked nutrient. *Journal of the American Dietetic Association* 99(2): 200–206.

Knekt, P., et al. 1999. Risk of colorectal and other gastro-intestinal cancers after exposure to nitrate, nitrite and N-nitroso compounds: A follow-up study. *International Journal of Cancer* 80(6): 852–856.

Kris-Etherton, P. M. 1999. AHA Science Advisory: Monounsaturated fatty acids and risk of cardiovascular disease. *Circulation* 100(11): 1253–1258.

Many protective nutrients needed to keep bones healthy and fracture-free. 1999. *Environmental Nutrition* 22(12): 1, 6.

National Osteoporosis Foundation. 1998. *Physician's Guide to Prevention and Treatment of Osteoporosis.* Washington, D.C.: National Osteoporosis Foundation.

Nelson, G. J. 1998. Dietary fat, trans fatty acids, and risk of coronary heart disease. *Nutrition Reviews* 56(8): 250–252.

Neuhouser, M. L., A. R. Kristal, and R. E. Patterson. 1999. Use of food nutrition labels is associated with lower fat intake. *Journal of the American Dietetic Association* 99(1): 45–50, 53.

The new foods: Functional or dysfunctional? 1999. *Consumer Reports on Health* 11(6): 1–5.

Olsen, S. J., et al. 2000. Surveillance for foodborne-disease outbreaks—United States, 1993–1997. *Morbidity and Mortality Weekly Report, CDC Surveillance Summary* 49(1): 1–62.

Poison plants? Genetically modified plants, grown over much of the U.S., remain controversial. 1999. *Scientific American Explore!* 5 July.

Schatzkin, A., et al. 2000. Lack of effect of a low-fat, high-fiber diet on the recurrence of colorectal adenomas. *New England Journal of Medicine* 342(16): 1149–1155.

Shaw, A., et al. 1997. *Using the Food Guide Pyramid: A Resource for Nutrition Educators.* USDA Center for Nutrition Policy and Promotion (http://www.nal.usda.gov/fnic/Fpyr/guide.pdf; retrieved April 18, 2000.

Shils, M. E., et al., eds. 1998. *Modern Nutrition in Health and Disease,* 9th ed. Baltimore, Md.: Williams & Wilkins.

Thompson, L. 2000. Are bioengineered foods safe? *FDA Consumer,* January–February.

Van Beneden, C. A., et al. 1999. Multinational outbreak of *Salmonella enterica* serotype Newport infections due to contaminated alfalfa sprouts. *Journal of the American Medical Association* 281(2): 158–162.

Van Loan, M. D. 1998. What makes good bones? Factors affecting bone health. *ACSM Health and Fitness Journal* 2(4): 27–34.

Volpe, S. L. 1998. Butter vs margarine. What should we eat? *Healthline* 17(4):6–7.

Wardlaw, G. M. 1999. *Perspectives in Nutrition,* 4th ed. Boston: McGraw-Hill.

Whole-Grain Goodness—Three Are Key! 1994. Chicago: National Center for Nutrition and Dietetics.

Wood, O. B., and C. M. Bruhn. 2000. Position of the American Dietetic Association: Food irradiation. *Journal of the American Dietetic Association* 100(2): 246–253.

TABLE I	*Dietary Reference Intakes (DRIs): Recommended Levels for Individual Intake*

Life Stage	Group	Calcium (mg/day)	Phosphorus (mg/day)	Magnesium (mg/day)	Vitamin D (μg/day)[a,b]	Fluoride (mg/day)	Thiamin (mg/day)	Riboflavin (mg/day)
Infants	0–5 months	210	100	30	5	0.01	0.2	0.3
	6–11 months	270	275	75	5	0.5	0.3	0.4
Children	1–3 years	500	**460**	**80**	5	0.7	**0.5**	**0.5**
	4–8 years	800	**500**	**130**	5	1	**0.6**	**0.6**
Males	9–13 years	1300	**1250**	**240**	5	2	**0.9**	**0.9**
	14–18 years	1300	**1250**	**410**	5	3	**1.2**	**1.3**
	19–30 years	1000	**700**	**400**	5	4	**1.2**	**1.3**
	31–50 years	1000	**700**	**420**	5	4	**1.2**	**1.3**
	51–70 years	1200	**700**	**420**	10	4	**1.2**	**1.3**
	>70 years	1200	**700**	**420**	15	4	**1.2**	**1.3**
Females	9–13 years	1300	**1250**	**240**	5	2	**0.9**	**0.9**
	14–18 years	1300	**1250**	**360**	5	3	**1.0**	**1.0**
	19–30 years	1000	**700**	**310**	5	3	**1.1**	**1.1**
	31–50 years	1000	**700**	**320**	5	3	**1.1**	**1.1**
	51–70 years	1200	**700**	**320**	10	3	**1.1**	**1.1**
	>70 years	1200	**700**	**320**	15	3	**1.1**	**1.1**
Pregnancy	≤18 years	1300	**1250**	**400**	5	3	**1.4**	**1.4**
	19–30 years	1000	**700**	**350**	5	3	**1.4**	**1.4**
	31–50 years	1000	**700**	**360**	5	3	**1.4**	**1.4**
Lactation	≤18 years	1300	**1250**	**360**	5	3	**1.5**	**1.6**
	19–30 years	1000	**700**	**310**	5	3	**1.5**	**1.6**
	31–50 years	1000	**700**	**320**	5	3	**1.5**	**1.6**

NOTE: This table includes Dietary Reference Intakes for those nutrients for which DRIs had been set through June 2000. The table includes values for the type of DRI standard—Adequate Intake (AI) or Recommended Dietary Allowance (RDA)—that has been established for that particular nutrient and life stage. RDAs are shown in **bold type**.

[a]As cholecalciferol. 1 μg cholecalciferol = 40 IU vitamin D.

[b]In the absence of adequate exposure to sunlight.

[c]As niacin equivalents. 1 mg of niacin = 60 mg of tryptophan.

[d]As dietary folate equivalents (DFE). 1 DFE = 1 μg food folate = 0.6 μg of folic acid (from fortified food or supplement) consumed with food = 0.5 μg of synthetic (supplemental) folic acid taken on an empty stomach.

[e]Although AIs have been set for choline, there are few data to assess whether a dietary supply of choline is needed at all stages of the life cycle, and it may be that the choline requirement can be met by endogenous synthesis at some of these stages.

[f]As α-Tocopherol.

[g]Since 10–30% of older people may malabsorb food-bound B-12, it is advisable for those older than 50 years to meet their RDA mainly by consuming foods fortified with B-12 or a B-12-containing supplement.

[h]Smokers are advised to consume an extra 35 mg/day of vitamin C.

[i]In view of evidence linking folate intake with neural tube defects in the fetus, it is recommended that all women capable of becoming pregnant consume 400 μg of synthetic folic acid from fortified food and/or supplements in addition to intake of food folate from a varied diet.

[j]It is assumed that women will continue consuming 400 μg of folic acid until their pregnancy is confirmed and they enter prenatal care, which ordinarily occurs after the end of the periconceptional period—the critical time for formation of the neural tube.

SOURCES: Food and Nutrition Board. Institute of Medicine. National Academy of Sciences. 1997. *Dietary Reference Intakes for Calcium, Phosphorus, Magnesium, Vitamin D, and Fluoride*. Washington, D.C.: National Academy Press. Food and Nutrition Board. Institute of Medicine. National Academy of Sciences. 1998. *Dietary Reference Intakes for Thiamin, Riboflavin, Niacin, Vitamin B$_6$, Folate, Vitamin B$_{12}$, Pantothenic Acid, Biotin, and Choline*. Washington, D.C.: National Academy Press. Food and Nutrition Board. Institute of Medicine. National Academy of Sciences. 2000. *Dietary Reference Intakes for Vitamin C, Vitamin E, Selenium, and Carotenoids*. Washington, D.C.: National Academy Press. Copyright © 1998 by the National Academy of Sciences. Reprinted with permission from National Academy Press, Washington, D.C.

| TABLE 1 | | | *Dietary Reference Intakes (DRIs) (continued)* | | | | | | | |

Niacin (mg/day)[c]	Vitamin B-6 (mg/day)	Folate (μg/day)[d]	Vitamin B-12 (μg/day)	Pantothenic Acid (mg/day)	Biotin (μg/day)	Choline (mg/day)[e]	Vitamin C (mg/d)	Vitamin E (mg/d)[f]	Selenium (μg/d)
2	0.1	65	0.4	1.7	5	125	40	4	15
3	0.3	80	0.5	1.8	6	150	50	6	20
6	0.5	150	0.9	2	8	200	15	6	20
8	0.6	200	1.2	3	12	250	25	7	30
12	1.0	300	1.8	4	20	375	45	11	40
16	1.3	400	2.4	5	25	550	75[h]	15	55
16	1.3	400	2.4	5	30	550	90[h]	15	55
16	1.3	400	2.4	5	30	550	90[h]	15	55
16	1.7	400	2.4[g]	5	30	550	90[h]	15	55
16	1.7	400	2.4[g]	5	30	550	90[h]	15	55
12	1.0	300	1.8	4	20	375	45	11	40
14	1.2	400[i]	2.4	5	25	400	65[h]	15	55
14	1.3	400[i]	2.4	5	30	425	75[h]	15	55
14	1.3	400[i]	2.4	5	30	425	75[h]	15	55
14	1.5	400[i]	2.4[g]	5	30	425	75[h]	15	55
14	1.5	400	2.4[g]	5	30	425	75[h]	15	55
18	1.9	600[j]	2.6	6	30	450	80	15	60
18	1.9	600[j]	2.6	6	30	450	85	15	60
18	1.9	600[j]	2.6	6	30	450	85	15	60
17	2.0	500	2.8	7	35	550	115	19	70
17	2.0	500	2.8	7	35	550	120	19	70
17	2.0	500	2.8	7	35	550	120	19	70

| TABLE 2 | *Tolerable Nutrient Upper Intake Levels for Adults* |

Nutrient	Upper Intake Level
Calcium	2500 mg/day
Phosphorus	4000 mg/day
Magnesium (nonfood sources)	350 mg/day
Vitamin D	50 μg/day
Fluoride	10 mg/day
Niacin	35 mg/day
Vitamin B-6	100 mg/day
Folate	1000 μg/day
Choline	3500 mg/day
Vitamin C	2000 mg/day
Vitamin E	1000 mg/day
Selenium	400 μg/day

This table includes the adult Tolerable Upper Intake Level (UL) standard of the Dietary Reference Intakes (DRIs). For some nutrients, there is insufficient data on which to develop a UL. This does not mean that there is no potential for adverse effects from high intake, and when data about adverse effects are limited, extra caution may be warranted. In healthy individuals, there is no established benefit from nutrient intakes above the RDA or AI.

SOURCES: Food and Nutrition Board. Institute of Medicine. National Academy of Sciences. 1997. *Dietary Reference Intakes for Calcium, Phosphorus, Magnesium, Vitamin D, and Fluoride.* Washington, D.C.: National Academy Press. Food and Nutrition Board. Institute of Medicine. National Academy of Sciences. 1998. *Dietary Reference Intakes for Thiamin, Riboflavin, Niacin, Vitamin B$_6$, Folate, Vitamin B$_{12}$, Pantothenic Acid, Biotin, and Choline.* Washington, D.C.: National Academy Press. Food and Nutrition Board. Institute of Medicine. National Academy of Sciences. 2000. *Dietary Reference Intakes for Vitamin C, Vitamin E, Selenium, and Carotenoids.* Washington, D.C.: National Academy Press. Copyright © 1998 by the National Academy of Sciences. Reprinted with permission from National Academy Press, Washington, D.C.

TABLE 3	Recommended Dietary Allowances, Revised 1989[a,b,c] (Abridged)						
			Vitamins		**Minerals**		
Category	**Age (years) or Condition**	**Protein (g/kg)**[d]	*Vitamin A (μg RE)*[e]	*Vitamin K (μg)*	*Iron (mg)*	*Zinc (mg)*	*Iodine (μg)*
Infants	0.0–0.5	2.2	375	5	6	5	40
	0.5–1.0	1.6	375	10	10	5	50
Children	1–3	1.2	400	15	10	10	70
	4–6	1.1	500	20	10	10	90
	7–10	1.0	700	30	10	10	120
Males	11–14	1.0	1000	45	12	15	150
	15–18	0.9	1000	65	12	15	150
	19–24	0.8	1000	70	10	15	150
	25–50	0.8	1000	80	10	15	150
	51+	0.8	1000	80	10	15	150
Females	11–14	1.0	800	45	15	12	150
	15–18	0.8	800	55	15	12	150
	19–24	0.8	800	60	15	12	150
	25–50	0.8	800	65	15	12	150
	51+	0.8	800	65	10	12	150
Pregnant		+10g	800	65	30	15	175
Lactating	1st 6 Months	+15g	1300	65	15	19	200
	2nd 6 Months	+12g	1200	65	15	16	200

[a]This table includes RDAs for those nutrients for which DRIs had not yet been established as of April 2000. The allowances, expressed as average daily intakes over time, are intended to provide for individual variations among most normal people as they live in the United States under usual environmental stresses. Diet should be based on a variety of common foods in order to provide other nutrients for which human requirements have been less well defined.

[b]Estimated Safe and Adequate Daily Dietary Intakes (ESADDIs) for adults: 1.5–3.0 mg copper; 2.0–5.0 mg manganese; 50–200 μg chromium; 75–250 mg molybdenum. (For information on other age groups, see National Research Council. 1989. *Recommended Dietary Allowances,* 10th ed. Washington, D.C.: National Academy Press.)

[c]Estimated Minimum Requirements of healthy adults: 500 mg sodium; 750 mg chloride; 2000 mg potassium. (For information on other age groups, see *Recommended Dietary Allowances,* 10th ed.)

[d]The RDA for protein is expressed as grams of protein per kilogram of body weight. To calculate the RDA, multiply body weight in kilograms (1 kilogram = 2.2 pounds) by the appropriate number from the protein column. For example, a 19-year-old male who weighs 165 pounds would calculate his protein RDA as follows: 165 lb ÷ 2.2 kg/lb = 75 kg × 0.8 g/kg (from table) = 60 g protein per day. For pregnant or lactating women, calculate RDA based on age and then add the appropriate number of additional grams listed in the table.

[e]Retinol equivalents: 1 retinol equivalent = 1 μg retinol or 6 μg β-carotene.

SOURCE: Reprinted with permission from *Recommended Dietary Allowances*: 10th Edition. Copyright © 1989 by the National Academy of Sciences. Courtesy of the National Academy Press, Washington, D.C.

LAB 8-1   *Your Daily Diet Versus the Food Guide Pyramid*

Keep a record of everything you eat for 3 consecutive days. Record all foods and beverages you consume, breaking each food item into its component parts (for example, a turkey sandwich would be listed as 2 slices of bread, 3 oz of turkey, 1 tsp of mayonnaise, and so on). Complete the first two columns of the chart during the course of the day; fill in the remaining information at the end of the day using Figure 8-5 and pp. 207–208 in your text. For fats, oils, and sweets—foods from the tip of the Pyramid—put a star (*) in the Food Group column.

DAY 1

Food	Portion Size	Food Group	Number of Servings*

Daily Total

Food Group	Number of Servings
Milk, yogurt, cheese	
Meat, poultry, fish, dry beans, eggs, nuts	
Fruits	
Vegetables	
Breads, cereals, rice, pasta	

*Your portion sizes may be smaller or larger than the serving sizes given in the Food Guide Pyramid; list the actual number of Food Guide Pyramid servings contained in the foods you eat.

DAY 2

Food	Portion Size	Food Group	Number of Servings*

Daily Total

Food Group	Number of Servings
Milk, yogurt, cheese	
Meat, poultry, fish, dry beans, eggs, nuts	
Fruits	
Vegetables	
Breads, cereals, rice, pasta	

*Your portion sizes may be smaller or larger than the serving sizes given in the Food Guide Pyramid; list the actual number of Food Guide Pyramid servings contained in the foods you eat.

DAY 3

Food	Portion Size	Food Group	Number of Servings*

Daily Total

Food Group	Number of Servings
Milk, yogurt, cheese	
Meat, poultry, fish, dry beans, eggs, nuts	
Fruits	
Vegetables	
Breads, cereals, rice, pasta	

*Your portion sizes may be smaller or larger than the serving sizes given in the Food Guide Pyramid; list the actual number of Food Guide Pyramid servings contained in the foods you eat.

Next, average your serving totals for the 3 days, and enter them in the chart below. Fill in the recommended serving totals that apply to you from Figure 8-5 and Table 8-4.

Food Group	Recommended Number of Servings	Actual Number of Servings
Milk, yogurt, cheese		
Meat, poultry, fish, dry beans, eggs, nuts		
Fruits		
Vegetables		
Breads, cereals, rice, pasta		

Are there any groups for which you need to increase your consumption? Decrease your consumption? List any areas of concern below, along with ideas for changing them. If you see that you are falling short in one food group, such as fruits or vegetables, but have many starred items from the fats, oils, and sweets category, you might try decreasing those items in favor of an apple, a bunch of grapes, or some baby carrots. Think carefully about the reasons behind your food choices. For example, if you eat doughnuts for breakfast every morning because you feel rushed, make a list of ways to save time to allow for a more healthful breakfast.

Problem: _____

Possible solutions: _____

_____

_____

_____

_____

Problem: _____

Possible solutions: _____

_____

_____

_____

_____

Problem: _____

Possible solutions: _____

_____

_____

_____

_____

To monitor your progress toward your goal, enter the results of this lab in the Preprogram Assessment column of Appendix D. After several weeks of dietary changes, do this lab again and enter the results in the Postprogram Assessment column of Appendix D. How do the results compare?

LAB 8-2 *Dietary Analysis*

You can complete this activity using either a nutrition analysis software program or the food composition data in Appendix B and the charts printed below. Information about the nutrient content of foods is also available online; see the For More Information section for recommended Web sites.

Part I Analyze Your Diet for 3 Days

If you are using the software, follow the instructions to complete an analysis of your diet on 3 separate days; otherwise, complete the charts on the first three pages of this lab. Then go on to the second part of the lab.

Date _____ Day: M Tu W Th F Sa Su

Food	Amount	Calories	Protein (g)	Fat, total (g)	Saturated fat (g)	Carbohydrate[a] (g)	Dietary fiber (g)	Cholesterol (mg)	Sodium (mg)	Calcium (mg)	Iron (mg)
Recommended totals[b]			10–15%	≤30%	<10%	≥55%	20–35 g	≤300 mg	≤2400 mg	mg	mg
Actual totals[c]		cal	g / %	g / %	g / %	g / %	g	mg	mg	mg	mg

[a]To obtain a value for total grams of carbohydrate from Appendix B, add the values in the columns for carbohydrates ("Carb.") and added sugars ("Sug.").
[b]Fill in the appropriate RDA or DRI values for calcium and iron from Tables 1 and 2 in the Nutrition Resources section.
[c]Total the values in each column. To calculate the percentage of total calories from protein, carbohydrate, fat, and saturated fat, use the formulas on p. 197. Protein and carbohydrate provide 4 calories per gram; fat provides 9 calories per gram. For example, if you consume a total of 270 grams of carbohydrate and 2000 calories, your percentage of total calories from carbohydrate would be (270 g × 4 cal/g) ÷ 2000 cal = 54%. Do not include data for alcoholic beverages in your calculations. Percentages may not total 100% due to rounding.

LABORATORY ACTIVITIES

Date_____   Day: M   Tu   W   Th   F   Sa   Su

Food	Amount	Calories	Protein (g)	Fat, total (g)	Saturated fat (g)	Carbohydrate[a] (g)	Dietary fiber (g)	Cholesterol (mg)	Sodium (mg)	Calcium (mg)	Iron (mg)
Recommended totals[b]			10–15%	≤30%	<10%	≥55%	20–35 g	≤300 mg	≤2400 mg	mg	mg
Actual totals[c]		cal	g / %	g / %	g / %	g / %	g	mg	mg	mg	mg

Food	Amount	Calories	Protein (g)	Fat, total (g)	Saturated fat (g)	Carbohydrate[a] (g)	Dietary fiber (g)	Cholesterol (mg)	Sodium (mg)	Calcium (mg)	Iron (mg)
Recommended totals[b]			10–15%	≤30%	<10%	≥55%	20–35 g	≤300 mg	≤2400 mg	mg	mg
Actual totals[c]		cal	g / %	g / %	g / %	g / %	g	mg	mg	mg	mg

Date_____ Day: M Tu W Th F Sa Su

To monitor your progress toward your goal, enter the results of one day's dietary analysis in the Preprogram Assessment column of Appendix D. After several weeks of dietary changes, do this lab again and enter the results in the Postprogram Assessment column of Appendix D. How do the results compare?

Part II   Making Changes in Your Diet to Meet the Dietary Guidelines

(*Note:* If your daily diet follows all the recommended intakes, you don't need to complete this section.) Choose one of your daily diet records. Make changes, additions, and deletions until it conforms to all or most of the Dietary Guidelines. Or, if you prefer, start from scratch to create a day's diet that meets all guidelines. Use the chart below to experiment and record your final, healthy sample diet for one day.

Date_____									Day: M Tu W Th F Sa Su		
Food	Amount	Calories	Protein (g)	Fat, total (g)	Saturated fat (g)	Carbohydrate[a] (g)	Dietary fiber (g)	Cholesterol (mg)	Sodium (mg)	Calcium (mg)	Iron (mg)
Recommended totals[b]			10–15%	≤30%	<10%	≥55%	20–35 g	≤300 mg	≤2400 mg	mg	mg
Actual totals[c]		cal	g / %	g / %	g / %	g / %	%	mg	mg	mg	mg

LAB 8-3 *Informed Food Choices*

Part I   Using Food Labels

Choose three food items to evaluate. You might want to select three similar items, such as regular, low-fat, and non-fat salad dressing, or three very different items. Record the information from their food labels in the table below. How do the items you chose compare?

Food Items			
Serving size			
Total calories	cal	cal	cal
Total fat—grams	g	g	g
—% Daily Value	%	%	%
Saturated fat—grams	g	g	g
—% Daily Value	%	%	%
Cholesterol—milligrams	mg	mg	mg
—% Daily Value	%	%	%
Sodium—milligrams	mg	mg	mg
—% Daily Value	%	%	%
Carbohydrates (total)—grams	g	g	g
—% Daily Value	%	%	%
Dietary fiber—grams	g	g	g
—% Daily Value	%	%	%
Sugars—grams	g	g	g
Protein—grams	g	g	g
Vitamin A—% Daily Value	%	%	%
Vitamin C—% Daily Value	%	%	%
Calcium—% Daily Value	%	%	%
Iron—% Daily Value	%	%	%

Part II Evaluating Fast Food

Use the information from Appendix C, Nutritional Content of Popular Items from Fast-Food Restaurants, to complete the chart on the next page for the last fast-food meal you ate. Add up your totals for the meal. Compare the values for fat, protein, carbohydrate, cholesterol, and sodium content for each food item and for the meal as a whole with the levels suggested by the Dietary Guidelines for Americans. Calculate the percent of total calories derived from fat, saturated fat, protein, and carbohydrate using the formulas given.

If you haven't recently been to one of the restaurants included in the appendix, fill in the chart for any sample meal you might eat. If some of the food items you selected don't appear in Appendix C, ask for a nutrition information brochure when you visit the restaurant, or check out online fast-food information: Arby's (http://www.arbysrestaurant.com), Burger King (http://www.burgerking.com), Domino's Pizza (http://www.dominos.com), Jack in the Box (http://www.jackinthebox.com), KFC (http://www.kfc.com), McDonald's (http://www.mcdonalds.com), Taco Bell (http://www.tacobell.com), Wendy's (http://www.wendys.com).

	Dietary Guidelines							Total[b]
Serving size (g)		g	g	g	g	g	g	g
Calories		cal	cal	cal	cal	cal	cal	cal
Total fat—grams		g	g	g	g	g	g	g
—% calories[a]	≤30%	%	%	%	%	%	%	%
Saturated fat—grams		g	g	g	g	g	g	g
—% calories[a]	<10%	%	%	%	%	%	%	%
Protein—grams		g	g	g	g	g	g	g
—% calories[a]	10–15%	%	%	%	%	%	%	%
Carbohydrate—grams		g	g	g	g	g	g	g
—% calories[a]	≥55%	%	%	%	%	%	%	%
Cholesterol[c]	100 mg	mg	mg	mg	mg	mg	mg	mg
Sodium[c]	800 mg	mg	mg	mg	mg	mg	mg	mg

[a]To calculate the percent of total calories from each food energy source (fat, carbohydrate, protein), use the following formula:

$$\frac{(\text{number of grams of energy source}) \times (\text{number of calories per gram of energy source})}{(\text{total calories in serving of food item})}$$

(*Note:* Fat and saturated fat provide 9 calories per gram; protein and carbohydrate provide 4 calories per gram.) For example, the percent of total calories from protein in a 150-calorie dish containing 10 grams of protein is

$$\frac{(10 \text{ grams of protein}) \times (4 \text{ calories per gram})}{(150 \text{ calories})} = \frac{40}{150} = 0.27, \text{ or } 27\% \text{ of total calories from protein}$$

[b]For the Total column, add up the total grams of fat, carbohydrate, and protein contained in your sample meal and calculate the percentages based on the total calories in the meal. (Percentages may not total 100% due to rounding.) For cholesterol and sodium values, add up the total number of milligrams.
[c]Recommended daily limits of cholesterol and sodium are divided by 3 here to give an approximate recommended limit for a single meal.

SOURCE: Insel, P. M., and W. T. Roth. 2000. Wellness Worksheet 53. *Core Concepts in Health,* 8th ed., 2000 update. Mountain View, Calif.: Mayfield.

LABORATORY ACTIVITIES

Nutritional Content of Common Foods

This food composition table has been prepared for Mayfield Publishing Company and is copyrighted by DINE Systems, Inc., the developer and publisher of the DINE System family of nutrition software for personal computers. The values in this food composition table were derived from the USDA Nutrient Data Base for Standard Reference Release 10 and nutrient composition information from more than 300 food companies. Nutrient values used for each food were determined by collapsing similar foods into one food, using the median nutrient values. In the food composition table, foods are listed within the following eight groups: fruits, vegetables, beverages, alcoholic beverages, grains, dairy, fats/sweets/other, and protein foods. Further information can be obtained from DINE Systems, Inc., 586 N. French Road, Amherst, NY 14228, 800-688-1848, 716-688-2400, 716-688-2505 (fax), dine@aol.com (e-mail), or at www.dinesystems.com. SOURCE: © 1994 DINE Systems, Inc.

Order of fields: Name, Amount/Unit, Calories, Protein, Total Fat, Saturated Fat, Carbohydrates (minus added sugar), Added Sugar, Fiber, Cholesterol, Sodium, Calcium, Iron.

FRUITS

Name	Amount/Unit	Cal.	Pro. g	TFat g	SFat g	Carb. g	Sug. g	Fbr. g	Chol. mg	Sod. mg	Calc. mg	Iron mg
Apples, sweetened	½ cup	68	0	0.11	0	12.5	3.25	2	0	334	334	0.3
Apples, unsweetened	½ frt, ½ cup	41	0.25	0	0	9.5	0	2.1	0	0	4	0.2
Applesauce, sweetened	½ cup	97	0.25	0	0	12	11	1.8	0	4	4	0.4
Applesauce, unsweetened	½ cup	53	0.25	0	0	12.5	0	2.5	0	2	4	0.2
Apricots, sweetened	3 hlv, ¼ cup	65	0.5	0	0	3.75	10.75	1.1	0	3	8	0.4
Apricots, unsweetened	3 halves	27	0.5	0	0	5.5	0	1.1	0	3	8	0.3
Banana	1 fruit	105	1	0.33	0.22	24	0	2.3	0	1	7	0.4
Blueberries, sweetened	½ cup	103	0.5	0.11	0	8.5	16.25	2.3	0	3	7	0.4
Blueberries, unsweetened	½ cup	41	0.5	0.22	0	9	0	1.7	0	2	5	0.2
Cherries, sweetened	½ cup	106	0.75	0	0	12.25	13	0.9	0	4	13	0.4
Cherries, unsweetened	10 frt, ½ cup	44	0.75	0	0	10	0	0.9	0	2	12	0.4
Dates	5 frt, ¼ cup	118	0.75	0.22	0.11	28.5	0	3.7	0	1	14	0.5
Dried fruit	¼ cup	92	1	0	0	21.75	0	2.4	0	9	11	0.7
Figs, sweetened	2 fruit	45	0.25	0	0	7	3.75	1.3	0	1	15	0.2
Figs, unsweetened	2 frt, ¼ cup	74	0.75	0.33	0.11	17.5	0	4.2	0	3	39	0.6
Fruit cocktail, sweetened	½ cup	83	0.5	0	0	8.75	11	1.4	0	8	8	0.3
Fruit cocktail, unsweetened	½ cup	50	0.5	0	0	11.5	0	1.4	0	4	6	0.3
Grapefruit, sweetened	½ cup	76	0.5	0	0	10	8	0.5	0	2	18	0.5
Grapefruit, unsweetened	½ frt, ½ cup	39	0.5	0	0	9	0	0.7	0	0	14	0.2
Grapes, sweetened	½ cup	94	0.5	0	0	10.5	12	0.5	0	7	12	1.2
Grapes, unsweetened	20 frt, ½ cup	48	0.5	0	0	11.5	0	0.5	0	2	8	0.2
Guava	1 fruit	45	0.5	0.33	0.11	9.5	0	5	0	2	18	0.3
Juice, unsweetened	¾ cup	90	0.5	0	0	22.5	0	0.2	0	8	16	0.5
Kiwifruit	1 fruit	46	0.75	0.33	0.11	10	0	2.1	0	4	20	0.3
Mango	½ frt, ½ cup	61	0.5	0.11	0	14.25	0	1.8	0	2	9	0.2
Melon	½ cup	30	0.5	0	0	7	0	0.7	0	9	8	0.2
Nectarines	1 fruit	68	1	0.56	0	14.5	0	3.3	0	0	6	0.2
Orange	1 frt, ¾ cup	63	1	0	0	14	0	3.9	0	1	53	0.2
Papaya	½ frt, ½ cup	56	0.75	0	0	12.75	0	1.8	0	4	35	0.2

Name	Amount/Unit	Cal.	Pro. g	TFat g	SFat g	Carb. g	Sug. g	Fbr. g	Chol. mg	Sod. mg	Calc. mg	Iron mg
Peaches, sweetened	½ cup	94	0.5	0	0	5.25	17	1.2	0	8	3	0.4
Peaches, unsweetened	1 frt, ½ cup	44	0.5	0	0	10.75	0	1.3	0	3	5	0.1
Pears, sweetened	2 halves	103	0.5	0	0	6	18.5	3.2	0	8	8	0.4
Pears, unsweetened	2 hlv, ½ cup	60	0.5	0	0	15	0	3	0	4	10	0.2
Pineapple, sweetened	2 slices, ½ cup	93	0.5	0	0	7.5	15	0.9	0	2	15	0.4
Pineapple, unsweetened	2 slices, ½ cup	70	0.25	0	0	17.5	0	0.9	0	2	6	0.4
Plums, sweetened	2 fruit	67	0.5	0.11	0	8	7.75	0.7	0	17	9	0.7
Plums, unsweetened	1 raw, 2 canned	37	0.5	0	0	8.25	0	0.9	0	1	5	0.2
Prunes, cooked	½ cup	136	1.25	0.33	0	32	0	4.9	0	3	29	1.4
Prunes, dried	½ cup	209	2	0.44	0	49.25	0	6.8	0	4	45	2.1
Pumpkin, canned	½ cup	41	0.75	0.11	0.11	8.75	0	3.5	0	6	32	1.7
Raisins	¼ cup	109	1	0	0	26	0	2.5	0	5	19	0.8
Raspberries, sweetened	½ cup	117	0.75	0.11	0	12	18.25	4.2	0	0	19	0.5
Raspberries, unsweetened	½ cup	30	0.5	0.22	0	6.5	0	3	0	0	14	0.3
Strawberries, sweetened	½ cup	100	0.5	0.11	0	9	15	2	0	4	14	0.6
Strawberries, unsweetened	½ cup	24	0.5	0.22	0	5.5	0	1.6	0	2	11	0.5
Tangerines, sweetened	½ cup	76	0.5	0	0	10	8.5	0.9	0	8	9	0.4
Tangerines, unsweetened	1 frt, ½ cup	43	0.5	0	0	9.75	0	0.9	0	2	14	0.1
Watermelon	½ cup	25	0.5	0.22	0.22	5	0	0.3	0	2	6	0.2

VEGETABLES

Name	Amount/Unit	Cal.	Pro. g	TFat g	SFat g	Carb. g	Sug. g	Fbr. g	Chol. mg	Sod. mg	Calc. mg	Iron mg
Asparagus	6 spears, ½ cup	24	1.75	0.33	0.11	3.75	0	1.5	0	4	22	0.6
Asparagus, canned	½ cup	21	1.5	0.33	0.11	2.75	0	1.9	0	425	17	1.5
Avocados	½ frt, ½ cup	166	2	14.22	2.56	7.25	0	2.7	0	10	12	1
Bamboo shoots	¼ cup	4	0.25	0	0	0.5	0	0.3	0	1	4	0.1
Bamboo shoots, canned	¼ cup	6	0.5	0.11	0	1	0	0.6	0	2	1	0.1
Bean sprouts	½ cup	16	1.25	0	0	2.75	0	2.2	0	3	7	0.5
Bean sprouts, canned	½ cup	8	0.75	0	0	1.25	0	2.3	0	149	9	0.3
Beets, canned	½ cup	36	0.75	0	0	8	0	2.9	0	324	17	0.8
Beets, pickled	½ cup	82	0.75	0	0	8.5	11.25	2.8	0	250	13	0.5
Beets, raw, cooked	½ cup	31	0.75	0	0	6.75	0	2.5	0	49	11	0.6
Bok choy, chinese cabbage	½ cup	5	0.25	0	0	0.75	0	0.6	0	23	37	0.3
Broccoli, cooked	½ cup	24	1.75	0.11	0	4.25	0	2.5	0	15	68	0.8
Broccoli, raw	½ cup	12	0.75	0.11	0	2	0	1.5	0	12	21	0.4
Brussels sprouts	½ cup	32	1.5	0.33	0.11	5.75	0	2.4	0	18	24	0.8
Cabbage, raw or cooked	½ c rw, ¼ c ckd	9	0.25	0	0	1.75	0	1	0	7	13	0.2
Carrots, canned	½ cup	17	0.25	0.11	0	3.75	0	2.7	0	176	19	0.5
Carrots, raw or cooked	½ cup	26	0.5	0	0	5.75	0	2.2	0	43	21	0.4
Cauliflower, raw or cooked	½ cup	15	0.75	0.11	0	2.5	0	1.3	0	7	15	0.3
Celery, raw or cooked	½ cup	10	0.25	0	0	2.25	0	1.4	0	51	25	0.2
Coleslaw	½ cup	154	0.5	14.44	2.67	4.25	1	1.5	7	287	32	0.4
Corn	½ cup	80	1.75	0.33	0	17.5	0	4.6	0	4	2	0.5
Corn, canned	½ cup	83	1.5	0.44	0.11	13	5.5	4.7	0	324	5	0.4
Cucumber	½ cup	7	0.25	0	0	1.5	0	0.7	0	1	7	0.1
Eggplant	½ cup	13	0.25	0	0	3	0	1	0	2	3	0.2
French fries	½ cup	174	1.75	7.33	3.22	19	0	2.6	0	37	6	0.6
Fried vegetables/onions	½ cup, 6 rings	180	2	10.78	2.67	15.5	0	1	0	150	12	0.7
Green beans, canned	½ cup	13	0.75	0	0	2.5	0	1.5	0	170	18	0.6
Green beans, raw or cooked	½ cup	20	1	0	0	4	0	1.8	0	3	30	0.7

Name	Amount/Unit	Cal.	Pro. g	TFat g	SFat g	Carb. g	Sug. g	Fbr. g	Chol. mg	Sod. mg	Calc. mg	Iron mg
Greens, mustard, turnip, ckd	½ cup	15	1	0.11	0	2.5	0	1.4	0	16	87	0.7
Greens, mustard, turnip, raw	½ cup	7	0.5	0	0	1.5	0	0.9	0	9	41	0.4
Greens, turnip, canned	½ cup	17	1	0.22	0.11	2.5	0	2.2	0	325	138	1.8
Kale, raw or cooked	½ cup	20	0.75	0.11	0	3	0	1.7	0	15	47	0.6
Lettuce, endive	½ cup	4	0.25	0	0	0.75	0	0.7	0	6	13	0.2
Lettuce, iceberg	1 leaf	3	0	0	0	0.5	0	0.3	0	2	4	0.1
Miso	½ cup	284	14.25	7.33	1.11	39.25	0	7.4	0	5032	92	3.8
Mixed vegetables, canned	½ cup	39	1.25	0.11	0	8	0	3.5	0	122	22	0.9
Mixed vegetables, frozen	½ cup	22	0.75	0	0	4.5	0	2	0	22	27	0.6
Mushrooms, canned	½ cup	19	1	0.11	0	3.25	0	1.1	0	178	1	0.6
Mushrooms, fresh, cooked	½ cup	25	1.75	0.11	0	4.25	0	1.5	0	1	7	1.7
Mushrooms, raw	½ cup	9	0.5	0	0	1.5	0	0.6	0	1	2	0.4
Okra	½ cup	26	1	0.11	0	5.5	0	2.1	0	5	55	0.5
Onions	½ cup	29	0.5	0.11	0	6.25	0	1.4	0	8	20	0.3
Parsnips	½ cup	64	0.75	0.11	0	14.75	0	3.2	0	8	30	0.5
Peas, green	½ cup	63	3.75	0.11	0	11.5	0	3.5	0	70	19	1.2
Peas, green, canned	½ cup	59	3.25	0.11	0	8	2.75	5.3	0	186	17	0.8
Peas, snowpeas	½ cup	35	2.25	0.11	0	5.75	0	3.4	0	4	37	1.6
Peppers, hot	2 tablespoons	8	0.25	0	0	1.5	0	0.2	0	1	3	0.2
Peppers, sweet, green	½ cup	12	0.25	0.11	0	2.25	0	0.6	0	2	3	0.6
Peppers, sweet, red	½ cup	12	0.25	0.11	0	2.25	0	0.8	0	2	3	0.6
Potato, baked/boiled	½ bkd/1 bld	113	1.5	0	0	26.5	0	2.6	0	7	9	0.4
Potatoes, mashed	½ cup	118	1.5	4.56	1.44	17	0	1.8	4	340	40	0.3
Potato skins, cheese, bacon	2 halves	302	11	15.89	7.44	27.5	0	1.4	34	267	225	4.5
Rutabaga	½ cup	35	0.75	0.11	0	7.5	0	2.1	0	19	43	0.5
Salad, potato	½ cup	153	3	7.78	1.89	15	1.5	1.9	47	512	19	0.5
Salad, three bean	½ cup	80	2	0	0	16.25	1.75	5	0	540	20	3.6
Sauerkraut	½ cup	22	0.75	0.11	0	4.5	0	4.1	0	780	36	1.7
Soup, vegetable	1 cup	81	2	1.56	0.44	11.25	2.25	0.5	2	892	16	1
Spaghetti sauce	½ cup	118	2	5	0.89	12.75	1.5	3.3	0	589	20	1.1
Spaghetti sauce with meat	½ cup	80	2	3.11	0.67	12.5	2	3.3	2	630	20	1.1
Spinach, canned	½ cup	25	1.75	0.33	0.11	3.25	0	3.9	0	29	135	2.5
Spinach, fresh, cooked	½ cup	24	1.75	0.11	0	3.75	0	3	0	73	131	1.7
Spinach, raw	½ cup	6	0.5	0	0	0.75	0	1.1	0	22	28	0.8
Squash, summer	½ cup	18	0.5	0.11	0	3.75	0	1.5	0	3	22	0.4
Squash, winter	½ cup	41	0.75	0.11	0	9.5	0	3	0	4	23	0.6
Squash, zucchini, fresh, ckd	1 c rw, ½ c ckd	18	0.75	0	0	3.5	0	1.4	0	2	19	0.5
Sweet potato	½ cup	98	1.25	0	0	23	0	4	0	11	30	0.5
Sweet potato, candied	½ cup	190	1	0	0	26.5	20	4.4	0	60	20	0.7
Tomatoes, canned or stewed	½ cup	34	0.75	0.11	0	6.5	0.25	2.4	0	305	33	0.7
Tomatoes, raw	½ cup	17	0.5	0.11	0	3.5	0	1.3	0	8	6	0.5
Water chestnuts, canned	½ cup	34	0.25	0	0	8.25	0	1.5	0	3	3	0.3
Water chestnuts, raw	½ cup	66	0.75	0	0	15.75	0	1.4	0	9	7	0.4
Watercress, raw	½ cup	2	0.25	0	0	0.25	0	0.2	0	7	20	0

BEVERAGES

Name	Amount/Unit	Cal.	Pro. g	TFat g	SFat g	Carb. g	Sug. g	Fbr. g	Chol. mg	Sod. mg	Calc. mg	Iron mg
Beer, nonalcoholic	12 fluid ounces	55	0.75	0	0	11	0	0	0	19	25	0.1
Wine, nonalcoholic	5 fluid ounces	42	0.5	0	0	9.75	0	0	0	7	12	0.6
Cola	12 fluid ounces	150	0	0	0	0	37	0	0	70	0	0

(continued)

Beverages (continued)

Name	Amount/Unit	Cal.	Pro. g	TFat g	SFat g	Carb. g	Sug. g	Fbr. g	Chol. mg	Sod. mg	Calc. mg	Iron mg
Cola, diet	12 fluid ounces	2	0.25	0	0	0.25	0	0	0	70	0	0
Cola, diet, no caffeine	12 fluid ounces	2	0	0	0	0	0	0	0	70	0	0
Cola, no caffeine	12 fluid ounces	155	0	0	0	0	38.75	0	0	73	0	0
Mellow Yellow, Mountain Dew	12 fluid ounces	177	0	0	0	0	44	0	0	30	0	0
Noncola, diet, no caffeine	12 fluid ounces	4	0	0	0	0.5	0	0	0	42	0	0
Noncola, no caffeine	12 fluid ounces	157	0	0	0	0	37.75	0	0	46	2	0.1
Juice drink	¾ cup/1 box	106	0	0	0	6.5	19.5	0	0	7	1	1
Coffee	1 cup	5	0.25	0	0	1	0	0	0	7	6	0.6
Coffee, decaffeinated	1 cup	3	0.25	0	0	0.75	0	0	0	8	8	0.1
Postum	1 teaspoon	12	0	0	0	3	0	1.3	0	0	0	0
Tea, herbal, no caffeine	1 cup	4	0	0	0	0.75	0	0	0	3	5	0.2
Tea, plain	1 cup	3	0	0	0	0.5	0	0	0	0	0	0

ALCOHOLIC BEVERAGES

Name	Amount/Unit	Cal.	Pro. g	TFat g	SFat g	Carb. g	Sug. g	Fbr. g	Chol. mg	Sod. mg	Calc. mg	Iron mg
Beer	12 fluid ounces	145	1	0	0	13.25	0	0	0	8	12	0
Beer, light	12 fluid ounces	110	1	0	0	7	0	0	0	8	15	0
Chianti	5 fluid ounces	106	0.25	0	0	2.5	0	0	0	8	12	0.6
Cocktail, mixed drink	1 cocktail	139	0	0	0	1	1.5	0	0	6	4	0.1
Liqueur	1 glass, 1½ oz	167	0	0.11	0	8.5	9.5	0	0	4	1	0
Liquor	1 jigger	110	0	0	0	0	0	0	0	0	0	0
Vermouth	5 fluid ounces	100	0.25	0	0	1	0	0	0	8	12	0.4
Wine	5 fluid ounces	104	0.25	0	0	2.5	0	0	0	12	12	0.4
Wine, light	5 fluid ounces	73	0.5	0	0	1	0	0	0	10	13	0.6
Wine cooler	12 fluid ounces	173	0.75	0	0	7.75	9.75	0	0	25	32	1.4

GRAINS

Name	Amount/Unit	Cal.	Pro. g	TFat g	SFat g	Carb. g	Sug. g	Fbr. g	Chol. mg	Sod. mg	Calc. mg	Iron mg
Cereal, bran, fiber	⅓ cup	62	2	0.78	0.22	7.75	2.75	3.8	0	113	13	3
Cereal, frosted	1 cup	147	1.75	0.11	0	18.75	14.75	0.5	0	93	4	2.4
Cereal, fruit-flavored	1 cup	110	1.75	0.22	0.11	12	13	0.5	0	168	5	4.5
Cereal, granola	¼ cup	130	3	4.80	0.80	13.5	1.5	1.7	0	55	19	0.9
Cereal, oat flakes	1 cup	182	5	1.78	0.44	24.75	4.5	3.2	0	115	32	5.8
Cereal, other, cold	1 cup	110	2	0.22	0.11	19.5	3	0.6	0	226	4	1.8
Cereal, other, hot	⅔ cup	100	3	0	0	22	0	0.7	0	54	18	1.1
Cereal, whole-grain	¾ cup	105	3	0.78	0.22	19	0	2.3	0	160	8	1.4
Granola, fat-free	¼ cup	90	2	0	0	21	0.25	2.5	0	20	0	0.4
Oatmeal, flavored	1 packet	140	4	2.22	0.44	18	8.25	2.4	0	181	100	4.5
Oatmeal, plain	⅔ cup cooked	109	4	1.78	0.33	18.25	0	3.3	0	1	15	1.9
Pancakes, waffles	2 pnck/2 wfl	173	4.75	4	1.11	26	3.5	1	44	503	100	1.5
Bagel	1 bagel	175	7	1.22	0.22	32.5	2.25	1.5	0	325	20	1.8
Biscuit	1 biscuit	100	2	3.78	1.22	13.5	0	0.5	2	262	47	0.7
Bread or roll, wheat	1 slice, 1 roll	65	2	0.89	0.22	10	2	1.4	0	106	20	0.7
Bread or roll, white	1 slice, 1 roll	70	2.75	1.11	0.33	11	2	0.5	0	132	20	0.7
Bread, mixed-grain	1 slice	65	2	0.89	0.22	9.75	2.25	1.4	0	106	27	0.8
Bread, oatmeal	1 slice	90	4	1.78	0.33	10.5	4	1.5	0	140	40	1.1
Bread, pita, wheat	1 pita (6" diam)	145	5.5	0.89	0.22	28.5	0.5	4.1	0	360	50	1.4

Name	Amount/Unit	Cal.	Pro. g	TFat g	SFat g	Carb. g	Sug. g	Fbr. g	Chol. mg	Sod. mg	Calc. mg	Iron mg
Bread, pita, white	1 pita (6″ diam)	160	6	1	0.22	30	1	1.1	0	300	80	0.7
Bread, raisin	1 slice	70	2	1	0.33	8.25	3	0.9	0	85	20	0.7
Bread, rye, pumpernickel	1 slice	80	2.75	0.89	0.11	13	1	1.1	0	185	22	1.1
Bread, wheat, diet	1 slice	40	2.5	0.56	0.11	4.25	2	2	0	120	40	0.7
Bread, white, diet	1 slice	40	3	0	0	6	1	2	0	110	40	0.7
Bread, whole wheat	1 slice, 1 roll	70	2.75	1.11	0.22	10	1.25	1.9	0	160	20	1
Breadsticks	⅓ lrg/2 sm	36	1.25	0.78	0.22	6	0.5	0.6	0	72	0	0.2
Cornbread, hush puppies	2.5″ sq/3 hpup	166	3	5.33	1.78	25.75	0	1.6	42	421	87	0.8
Croissants	1 croissant	310	7	19	11.22	27	6	2	0	240	38	1.8
Danish, nonfat	1 piece	90	2	0	0	20	9.75	0.2	0	85	20	0
English muffin	1 muffin	130	5	0.89	0.33	25	1.5	1.6	0	280	96	1.7
Muffin	1 muffin	140	3	4.67	1.56	11.75	8	1.2	21	198	42	1.1
Muffins, fat free	1 muffin	155	3	0.11	0	35	11.5	0.9	0	140	50	0.5
Roll, hmbrgr, hot dog, wheat	1 roll	114	4	1.11	0.22	21.25	0.75	2.5	0	242	46	1
Roll, hmbrgr, hot dog, white	1 roll	138	3.25	2.44	0.67	22.5	2	1.4	0	271	67	1.3
Roll, hoagie, sub	½ roll	200	5.5	3.56	0.89	34.25	2	0.9	0	342	50	1.9
Stuffing	½ cup	210	4.5	12.67	3	17.5	2.5	0.5	22	578	40	1.1
Cake, nonfat	1 piece/slice	70	1.5	0	0	16	7.75	0.6	0	85	0	0
Cookies, nonfat	2 cookies	75	1	0	0	17.5	6.5	0.6	0	115	0	0.2
Cracker sandwiches	2 lrg, 5 sm	70	1.75	3.11	1.11	7.75	0.75	0.2	1	135	20	0.4
Crackers, butter type	5 lrg, 10 sm	70	1	3.56	1.11	8	0.25	0.2	1	193	4	0.4
Crackers, crispbread	1 lrg, 2 sm	40	1	0.89	0.33	8.5	0	1.6	0	112	0	0.5
Crackers, low-fat	2 lrg, 5 sm	60	2.25	2.33	0.33	10	0	0.6	0	100	0	0.4
Crackers, wheat	4 crackers	70	1	2.22	0.44	8	0.5	1.5	0	75	0	0.4
Matzo or melba toast	½ matzo, 5 melba	72	2.75	0.67	0.22	14	1.5	0.6	0	189	2	1
Barley, cooked	½ cup	84	2.25	0.11	0	18.5	0	2.5	0	3	11	0.5
Bulgur	½ cup	113	4.25	0.22	0	23.5	0	3	0	3	13	3.7
Couscous	⅔ cup	120	4	0	0	26	0	4.3	0	5	0	0.7
Grits	½ cup	73	1.5	0.11	0	16	0	0.3	0	136	0	0.8
Lasagna, meat	1 serving	350	27.5	23.11	6	31	1.5	2.6	73	1040	275	2.1
Lasagna, vegetable	1 serving	315	22	12	5.89	27	0.5	4.6	40	970	350	2.3
Macaroni and cheese	½ cup	191	6	8.56	2.67	22.75	0	1.4	18	434	71	1.2
Macaroni, whole-wheat	1 cup	202	8	1.11	0.22	39	0	7.4	0	10	20	4.5
Noodles, chow mein	½ cup	130	3	6.44	1.11	14.5	0	0.5	2	228	4	0.8
Noodles, egg, macaroni	1 cup	190	7	0.56	0.11	37	0	1.1	0	30	14	2.1
Pasta w/parmesan cheese	½ cup	252	6.5	14.67	6.33	22.5	0	1.1	38	479	78	1.5
Salad, pasta	½ cup	250	4	16	3.33	20.75	0	0.7	28	410	40	0.7
Spaghetti	1 cup	200	7.5	1	0.22	40.5	0	1.1	0	19	14	2
Spaghetti w/meatballs	1 cup	307	12	10.56	3.89	37	0	2.7	34	1220	53	3.3
Spaghetti, whole-wheat	1 cup	200	9	1.11	0.22	39.5	0	5.8	0	10	20	2.7
Rice cake	1 large cake	35	0.75	0	0	7.5	0	0.3	0	13	0	0
Rice, brown	½ cup	115	2.5	0.67	0.22	25	0	1.8	0	2	12	0.5
Rice, long-grain/wild, mix	½ cup	137	3	2	0.56	23	2	0.9	0	579	11	1.1
Rice, seasoned	½ cup	150	3.5	3.78	1.67	23	1	1	5	700	13	1.2
Rice, white	½ cup	92	2	0	0	20.5	0	0.5	0	225	10	0.7
Tabouli	½ cup	170	3	8.67	1.33	20	0	1.6	0	290	0	0.7
Taco shell	1 shell	50	0	2	1.11	8	0	0.2	0	5	0	0
Tortilla	1 tortilla	65	2	1	0.11	12	0	0.9	0	1	42	0.6

B

Name	Amount/Unit	Cal.	Pro. g	TFat g	SFat g	Carb. g	Sug. g	Fbr. g	Chol. mg	Sod. mg	Calc. mg	Iron mg
Buttermilk	1 cup	99	8.75	2	1.33	11.25	0	0	9	257	285	0.1
Hot cocoa prepared w/milk	1 cup	218	8	9	5.67	13.5	11.25	3	33	123	298	0.8
Meal replacement drinks	1 cup	200	14	1	0.44	36	17	4	5	230	500	6.3
Milk, chocolate	1 cup	179	8.5	4.67	3	10.5	14.5	1.1	17	150	284	0.6
Milk, low-fat	1 cup	112	8.75	3.56	2.22	11.25	0	0	14	123	299	0.1
Milk, skim	1 cup	86	9	0.44	0.33	11.5	0	0	4	126	302	0.1
Milk, whole	1 cup	150	8.5	7.67	5	11	0	0	33	120	291	0.1
Cheese spread	2 tablespoons	81	3.5	6.56	4.33	2	0	1	89	293	95	1
Cheese, American	1 ounce, 1 slice	106	6.75	8.22	5.44	0.5	0	0	27	406	174	0.1
Cheese, cheddar	1 ounce, 1 slice	113	7.5	8.67	5.89	0.5	0	0	30	177	203	0.2
Cheese, cottage	½ cup	113	14.5	4.78	3.11	3	0	0	17	440	65	0.2
Cheese, cottage, nonfat	½ cup	90	14	0	0	7	0	0	10	400	60	0
Cheese, cottage, low-fat	½ cup	96	15	1.22	0.78	4	0	0	5	440	74	0.2
Cheese, mozzarella	1 ounce, 1 slice	80	6	5.67	3.67	0.5	0	0	22	106	147	0.1
Cheese, mozzarella, light	1 ounce	72	7.25	4.11	2.78	0.75	0	0	16	150	183	0.1
Cheese, parmesan	1 tablespoon	23	2.25	1.44	0.89	0.25	0	0	4	93	69	0.1
Cheese, provolone	1 ounce, 1 slice	100	7.75	7	4.78	0.5	0	0	20	248	214	0.2
Cheese, reduced-fat	1 ounce	80	8	5	3	1	0	0	20	220	350	0
Cheese, ricotta	½ cup	216	15	14.89	10	3.75	0	0	63	104	257	0.5
Cheese, ricotta, part-skim	½ cup	166	14.5	8.67	5.67	6.25	0	0	37	143	369	0.3
Cheese, Swiss	1 ounce	101	8	6.89	4.67	0.75	0	0	25	231	246	0.1
Ice cream	½ cup	148	2.5	7.44	4.67	4.5	11.75	0.2	30	58	88	0.3
Ice milk	½ cup	110	3	2.78	1.89	10	8	0.3	8	75	100	1
Tofutti	½ cup	150	2.5	6.67	1.11	9	11	1.5	0	105	1	0.6
Yogurt, frozen	½ cup	100	3	1.78	1.11	8	10.25	0.1	7	59	100	1
Yogurt, low-fat w/fruit	1 container	240	9	3	2	27	16	0.3	10	120	330	1
Yogurt, nonfat w/fruit	1 container	95	3.5	0	0	8	12	0	0	70	150	1
Yogurt, plain, low-fat	1 container	142	11.25	3.67	2.44	15.75	0	0	15	160	422	0.6
Yogurt, plain, nonfat	1 container	110	11	0.22	0.22	16	0	0	4	160	430	1
Yogurt, plain, whole-milk	1 container	145	8.75	6.89	4.56	11.5	0	0	32	123	312	0.6
Yogurt, w/frt, art. swtner	1 container	90	7	0.67	0.44	14	0	0.5	5	110	250	1

Name	Amount/Unit	Cal.	Pro. g	TFat g	SFat g	Carb. g	Sug. g	Fbr. g	Chol. mg	Sod. mg	Calc. mg	Iron mg
Bacon	1 slice	36	5.25	1.78	0.67	0	0	0	12	360	2	0.2
Bacon bits	1 tablespoon	21	2.5	1.11	0.33	0	0	0	6	181	1	0.1
Butter	1 tablespoon	104	0	11.44	7.22	0	0	0	32	119	2	1
Gravy	¼ cup	30	1	1.44	0.56	2.25	0.5	0.1	1	260	3	0.4
Lard	1 tablespoon	115	0	12.22	5	0	0	0	12	0	0	0
Margarine, stick	1 tablespoon	101	0	10.56	2	0	0	0	0	133	4	0
Margarine, stick, light	1 tablespoon	60	0	6.67	1	0	0	0	0	110	1	1
Margarine, tub	1 tablespoon	101	0	8.89	2	0	0	0	0	152	4	0
Margarine, tub, light	1 tablespoon	50	0	5.89	1	0	0	0	0	110	1	1
Mayonnaise	1 tablespoon	100	0.25	11	1.89	0.25	0.25	0	8	74	1	1
Mayonnaise, light	1 tablespoon	48	0.25	4.56	1	0.75	1	0	5	95	1	1
Mayonnaise, nonfat	1 tablespoon	12	0	0	0	3	3	0	0	190	0	0
Miracle Whip	1 tablespoon	64	0	5.89	0.89	2.5	0.5	0	5	95	2	1
Miracle Whip, nonfat	1 tablespoon	20	0	0	0	5	5	0	0	210	0	0
Oil	1 tablespoon	120	0	12.78	1.89	0	0	0	0	0	0	0.1

Name	Amount/Unit	Cal.	Pro. g	TFat g	SFat g	Carb. g	Sug. g	Fbr. g	Chol. mg	Sod. mg	Calc. mg	Iron mg
Salad dressing	1 tablespoon	80	0	8.22	1.33	0.25	0.25	1	0	146	2	1
Salad dressing, light	1 tablespoon	16	0.25	0.33	0.11	0.75	0.5	0.3	0	137	1	1
Salad dressing, no oil	1 tablespoon	12	0	0	0	2.5	0	0.7	0	0	1	1
Salad dressing, nonfat	1 tablespoon	16	0	0	0	3	3	0	0	143	0	0
Brownie	1¾" square	150	2	6.22	1.67	6.5	15	0.9	10	105	1	0.7
Cake	1 piece/slice	280	4	11.33	3	15.25	22.25	0.5	56	285	57	1
Candy, choc/peanut butter	1 pkg, 1½ oz	237	6	13.78	5.89	4	22	2.5	3	90	34	0.7
Candy, chocolate	1-ounce piece	150	2	8.22	4.78	2.25	15	0.8	6	24	50	0.3
Candy, chocolate-covered	1 ounce	132	1.25	5.56	2.11	3	13.25	1.5	3	43	33	0.4
Candy, fudge	1" cube	88	0.75	3	0.78	1.25	13.25	0.3	2	40	20	0.2
Candy, hard	5 pieces	110	0	0	0	0	27.5	0	0	7	1	0.1
Cookies, fig bars	2 fig bars	100	1	1.78	0.44	10.5	10.5	1.2	1	90	20	0.7
Cookies, oatmeal raisin	3 cookies	195	2.25	8.11	1.89	13.5	13.5	1.4	1	150	0	0.8
Cookies, other	3 cookies	180	1.5	8.11	2.89	10	15	0.3	3	131	1	0.7
Danish	1 roll	252	4.5	11.67	3.67	10.25	19	0.7	14	249	36	1.1
Diet bar	1 bar	120	2	4	1.44	19	9.5	3	1	30	150	2.7
Doughnut or sweet roll	1 serving	201	3	8.11	2.89	12.5	13.25	0.6	19	145	21	0.8
Frozen desserts, nonfat	½ cup	100	2	0.22	0.11	23.5	9.5	0.4	1	48	100	0
Frzn yogurt cone, low-fat	1 serving	105	4	1	0.56	22	13	0.1	3	80	112	0.2
Frzn yogurt sundae, low-fat	1 serving	240	6	3	2.33	50.5	43	0.8	6	170	190	0.1
Gelatin	½ cup	105	2	1	1	23	22	0	0	57	0	0
Gelatin, sugar-free	½ cup	8	1.5	0	0	0	0	0	0	31	0	0
Granola bars	1 bar	133	2	6	2	18.25	13	0.6	0	70	20	0.5
Pie, custard or cream	⅙ of 9" pie	346	6.75	13.11	6.22	20.75	25.75	1	125	375	122	0.8
Pie, fruit	⅙ of 9" pie	405	4	16.22	5.33	34.75	25.25	4	6	423	17	1.6
Pie, pecan	⅙ of 9" pie	575	7	29.67	5.67	33	37.25	2.2	100	305	65	4.6
Pudding	½ cup	150	4.5	2.22	1.44	10	18	0	9	443	152	0
Pudding, diet	½ cup	90	4	2.44	1.56	13	0	0.4	9	423	152	0.1
Cream, whipped	1 tablespoon	15	0.25	1.33	1.11	0.25	0.25	0	2	4	3	1
Dessert topping, no sugar	1 tablespoon	5	0	0.56	0.44	0	0	1	4	5	2	1
Jam or jelly	2 teaspoons	35	0	0	0	1	7.5	0.1	0	1	1	1
Cream, coffee, half & half	1 tablespoon	25	0.5	2.22	1.44	0.5	0	0	8	6	15	0
Nutrasweet, Equal	1 packet	4	0.5	0	0	0	0.5	0	0	0	0	0
Saccharin	1 packet	2	0	0	0	0	0	0	0	2	0	0
Salt	4 shakes	0	0	0	0	0	0	0	0	64	0	0
Sugar	1 teaspoon	15	0	0	0	0	3.75	0	0	0	0	0
Syrup, pancake, table	2 tablespoons	110	0	0	0	0	27.5	0	0	21	1	1
Coffee whitener	1 tablespoon	22	0	2.11	1.33	0	1	0	0	12	1	1
Cream cheese	2 tablespoons	106	2.5	10.22	6.67	1	0	0	34	90	24	0.4
Cream cheese, light	2 tablespoons	80	3	7	4	1	0	0	25	115	20	1
Sour cream	1 tablespoon	26	0.25	2.56	1.56	0.5	0	0	5	17	14	0
Sour cream, imitation	1 tablespoon	25	0.75	2.33	2	0.75	0	0	1	10	7	0
Sour cream, nonfat	1 tablespoon	8	1	0	0	1	0	0	0	10	20	0
Catsup	1 tablespoon	17	0	0	0	2.75	1.5	0.2	0	168	3	0.1
Cheese sauce	¼ cup	71	3.5	3.56	1.89	6.5	0	0	10	412	139	0.1
Chili sauce	1 tablespoon	17	0.25	0	0	2.75	1.25	0.9	0	196	2	0.1
Hollandaise sauce	¼ cup	230	2.25	23.22	8.44	2.5	0	0	140	316	50	1
Mustard	1 teaspoon	6	0.25	0.33	0	0.25	0	0	0	60	0	0
Olives	3 olives	15	0.25	1.56	0.22	0.25	0	0.3	0	234	8	0.2
Pickles, dill	2 spears	7	0	0.11	0	1	0.75	0.9	0	584	9	0.4
Pickles, sweet	1 pickle, 3 sl.	18	0	0	0	0.5	4	0.3	0	107	2	0.2
Soy sauce	1 tablespoon	10	1.25	0	0	1.25	0	0	0	1015	3	0.4

(continued)

Fats, Sweets, Other (continued)

Name	Amount/Unit	Cal.	Pro. g	TFat g	SFat g	Carb. g	Sug. g	Fbr. g	Chol. mg	Sod. mg	Calc. mg	Iron mg
Steak, Worcestershire sauce	1 tablespoon	11	0	0	0	1	1.75	0	0	143	0	0
White sauce	¼ cup	99	2.5	5.67	2.22	6	0	0.1	8	222	73	0.2
Soup, beef or chicken	1 cup	74	4.25	2.22	0.67	8.5	0	1	7	910	17	0.9
Soup, bouillon, broth	1 cube/packet	9	0.75	0.22	0.11	0.25	1	0	1	965	1	0.1
Soup, broth-based, no-salt	1 cup	135	5.75	3.89	0.78	16.5	0	2.8	0	115	47	1.8
Soup, cream, chowder	1 cup	140	5.5	6.11	2.89	14	0	0.9	22	1010	150	0.6
Soup, low-salt	1 cup	110	4	3	1	12	0	0.5	2	100	17	1.3
Soup, miso	1 cup	152	4.5	6.44	0.89	19	0	3	0	490	20	1.3
Breakfast milk powder	1 packet	130	6	0	0	0	26.25	0.4	0	185	80	4.5
Hot chocolate mix	1 envelope	110	1.5	2.78	1.56	3.5	16	1.1	2	165	40	0.7
Meal replacement bar	1 serving	270	11	14	5	24	22.5	0	0	330	250	4.5
Milkshake	10 oz, 1¼ cup	368	10	12.78	8.22	26.5	19.25	0.5	54	243	375	0.5
Milkshake, low-fat	1 serving	320	10.75	1.33	0.56	66	44.75	0	10	170	327	0.1
Popcorn	1 cup	32	0.75	1.44	0.44	5.5	0	0.8	0	68	0	0.2
Potato chips, corn chips	1 cup	152	2	9.44	1.78	15	0	1.4	0	229	15	0.4
Pretzels	⅔ cup	110	2.75	0.89	0.22	21.75	1	0.9	0	610	9	1.4
Tortilla chips	1 cup	95	1.25	4.67	1.33	12	0	0.9	0	123	23	0.3

PROTEIN FOODS

Name	Amount/Unit	Cal.	Pro. g	TFat g	SFat g	Carb. g	Sug. g	Fbr. g	Chol. mg	Sod. mg	Calc. mg	Iron mg
Biscuit w/egg, meat, cheese	1 biscuit	489	18.75	31.22	9.67	29	4	0.8	347	1240	151	2.9
Egg salad	½ cup	267	11	22.89	5.78	1	3	0.3	418	513	43	1.8
Egg, boiled, poached	1 egg	79	6.5	5.56	2.11	0.5	0	0	274	69	28	1
Egg, fried, scrambled	1 egg	89	6.25	6.78	3	1	0	0	281	150	37	0.9
Egg, omelet	1 omelet	342	23.25	25.44	12.56	4	0	0	861	553	243	2.8
Egg, substitute	¼ cup	43	5.5	1.56	0.22	1.5	0	0	0	115	30	0.8
Chicken breast sandwich	1 sandwich	509	26	26.89	4.78	34.75	1.75	1.2	83	1082	80	2.7
Chicken salad	½ cup	179	14.75	12.22	2.89	0.75	0.75	0.3	118	329	21	0.9
Chicken wings	10 wings	1282	90	91.11	35.78	11.5	5	0.2	326	1750	62	4
Chicken, turkey, no skin	4 ounces	137	27.25	3.33	1.11	0	0	0	77	58	12	1.3
Chicken, turkey, w/skin	4 ounces	145	19.75	7.22	2.44	0	0	0	57	49	10	0.9
Chicken, fried, no skin	4 ounces	107	19.25	4.22	1.33	0.25	0	0	50	46	9	0.8
Chicken, fried, w/skin	4 ounces	206	21	11.22	3.22	6.25	0	0.2	69	199	14	1.1
Chicken, mixed dish	1 cup	365	15.25	17.78	5.56	13.5	0	1	103	600	30	2.2
Beef stew	1 cup	207	13.25	9	4.22	16.5	0.5	2.5	53	616	29	2.6
Beef, corned	4 ounces	242	24.25	16.11	7	0	0.25	0	87	1024	15	2
Beef, grnd, hmbrgr, not fried	4 ounces	200	21.25	13.67	6.11	0	0	0	70	60	8	1.9
Beef, grnd, hmbrgr, fried	4 ounces	207	21.25	13.56	5.89	0	0	0	68	62	8	1.9
Beef, mixed dish	1 cup	310	19.25	13.56	5.89	23.5	1.25	2.1	68	840	52	3.5
Beef, roast beef	4 ounces	198	21.25	11.11	4.89	0	0	0	59	47	6	2.1
Cheeseburger (large) w/roll	1 sandwich	711	32	43.33	16.78	33	4	1	113	1164	295	5
Cheeseburger (low-fat) w/roll	1 sandwich	370	24	14	5	35	3.5	1.6	75	890	200	3.6
Cheeseburger (small) w/roll	1 sandwich	461	29	27.56	13.67	25.25	3	0.8	95	906	245	3.3
Hamburger (large) w/roll	1 sandwich	594	27.5	33	12.67	33.25	2	0.9	101	688	87	4.8
Hamburger (low-fat) w/roll	1 sandwich	320	22	10	4	35	3.5	1.6	60	670	150	3.6
Hamburger (small) w/roll	1 sandwich	355	22	19.33	8.22	22.25	3	1.7	95	556	71	3.2
Liver	4 ounces	169	23.5	6	2.67	3.25	0	0	344	69	10	7.7
Pate	1 tablespoon	41	2	3.67	1.44	0	0	0	51	91	9	0.7
Roast beef sandwich	1 sandwich	353	27.25	14.89	7.33	30.25	2.25	0.7	49	766	87	4.1

Name	Amount/Unit	Cal.	Pro. g	TFat g	SFat g	Carb. g	Sug. g	Fbr. g	Chol. mg	Sod. mg	Calc. mg	Iron mg
Tripe	4 ounces	61	12.5	1.11	0.67	0	0	0	58	44	77	0.3
Veal	4 ounces	177	21.75	9.78	4.78	0	0	0	78	52	9	2.7
Veal, mixed dish	1 serving	327	28.25	17.78	9.78	9.5	0.75	1.7	137	634	138	3.7
Bacon substitute	1 strip	52	3	4.11	1.56	0	0	0	13	207	1	0.2
Ham	4 ounces	165	21	8.67	3.11	0	0	0	54	1419	8	1
Hot dog	1 hot dog	144	5.75	12.89	5.22	0.25	1.25	0	30	547	20	0.7
Hot dog and roll	1 sandwich	298	9.25	17.56	6.67	20	2.5	0.7	29	880	60	2.2
Pork feet	8 ounces	138	14.5	8.78	3.22	0	0	0	71	597	32	1.1
Pork rinds	4 ounces	610	69	34.67	13.33	0	0	0	106	3033	25	0.7
Pork spareribs	4 ounces	176	13.75	13.11	5.22	0	0	0	54	41	21	0.8
Pork, fresh, fried	4 ounces	192	14.5	14.89	5.67	0	0	0	55	33	5	0.5
Pork, fresh, roasted	4 ounces	164	15.75	10.22	3.89	0	0	0	54	37	4	0.6
Sausage	1 ounce	88	4	7.44	2.89	0	0.5	0	14	258	4	0.4
Lamb	4 ounces	225	26.25	14.78	7.11	0	0	0	91	65	10	2
Caviar	1 tablespoon	40	4.25	2.11	0.78	0.5	0	0	94	240	44	1.8
Clams, oysters, shrimp, fried	4 pieces	103	5.25	6.11	1.11	6	0	0.1	23	183	20	0.6
Clams, oysters, shrimp	½ cup	71	12.25	1.22	0.33	2.5	0	0	62	108	41	6
Crabmeat	3 ounces	86	12.5	1	0.22	4.5	0	0	26	713	25	0.4
Fish casserole	1 cup	407	18.5	23.78	7.56	26.25	0.75	1.8	70	1314	182	2.3
Fish sandwich	1 sandwich	488	19	26.56	5.89	39.25	3.75	1.5	70	928	46	2
Fish, fried	4 ounces	279	11.5	15.33	3.56	21.5	1.5	0.9	52	467	0	0.7
Fish, not fried	4 ounces	108	22.75	1.33	0.44	10	0	0	60	76	17	0.5
Fish, smoked, pickled	1 ounce	56	6.25	2.33	0.67	0	0	0	14	235	5	0.3
Seafood or fish salad	½ cup	160	13.5	9.78	2.33	1.75	0.25	0.4	142	250	31	0.9
Tuna in oil	½ cup	142	22	5.44	1.11	0	0	0	18	275	7	0.8
Tuna in water	½ cup	90	19.25	1.44	0.44	0	0	0	28	400	0	0.7
Chili con carne	1 cup	286	15.75	12.44	5.78	28.5	0	6.5	43	964	86	3
Chili, vegetarian	1 cup	240	18	12	1.78	13	2	16.4	0	860	6	3.2
Luncheon meat, beef, pork	1 ounce slice	76	4.25	6.11	2.56	0	0.5	0	18	348	3	0.4
Luncheon meat, chkn, trky	1 ounce slice	32	5.75	0.67	0.22	0	0	0	12	358	3	0.3
Pepperoni	1 slice	27	1.25	2.33	0.89	0.25	0	0	5	112	1	0.1
Pizza, cheese topping	2 slices	352	21.75	13.44	7.33	36.25	0.75	3	33	890	474	2.3
Pizza, French bread	1 slice	410	17.5	19.22	8	39	2	2	35	1030	200	2.7
Pizza, meat topping	2 slices	445	25	17	8	50	0.5	4.3	31	906	263	3
Pizza, vegetable topping	2 slices	419	24.75	10.33	5.56	64.25	1	10	19	685	285	5
Chop suey	1 cup	300	26	16	4.33	13	0	1.5	68	1053	60	4.8
Chow mein, beef or chicken	¾ cup	85	6.5	1.44	0.56	5.25	0.75	1.4	26	845	80	1.3
Eggroll	1 eggroll	173	6.75	4.56	0.89	25	3	0.8	7	471	20	1.1
Sweet & sour chicken, pork	1 cup	426	17.5	13.89	3.33	23.5	31.75	1.3	83	1209	27	1.9
Burrito	2 burritos	426	16	14.33	7.11	57.75	0	6.4	65	1116	105	4.5
Chimichanga	1 chimichanga	425	18.5	17.11	8.33	41.25	0	5.2	30	933	145	4
Enchilada	1 enchilada	322	10.5	16.89	9.67	30	0	5.8	42	1052	276	2.2
Taco	1 small	370	21	18.44	11.11	26.5	0	3.4	57	802	221	2.4
Taco salad	1½ cups	279	13.5	13.33	6.67	24	0	4.3	44	763	192	2.3
Tostada	1 tostada	325	13.75	13.89	9.67	28	0	7.5	40	834	214	2.2
Beans, baked	½ cup	140	6	1.67	0.67	15	7.5	6	8	423	60	2.1
Beans, black	½ cup	113	6.5	0.33	0.11	20.75	0	4.4	0	1	24	1.8
Beans, kidney, pinto	½ cup	115	6.5	0.33	0.11	22.25	0	4.5	0	2	33	2.4
Beans, kidney, pinto, canned	½ cup	104	5.75	0.22	0	19.5	0	6.1	0	445	35	1.6
Beans, lima	½ cup	94	5.5	0.22	0.11	17.5	0	4.6	0	26	25	1.8
Beans, lima, canned	½ cup	93	4.75	0.22	0.11	17.5	0	5.8	0	309	35	2

(continued)

Protein Foods (continued)

Name	Amount/Unit	Cal.	Pro. g	TFat g	SFat g	Carb. g	Sug. g	Fbr. g	Chol. mg	Sod. mg	Calc. mg	Iron mg
Beans, navy, chickpeas	½ cup	132	6.75	1	0.22	23.75	0	4.8	0	4	52	2.4
Beans, navy, chickpeas, cnd	½ cup	146	7	0.78	0.11	27.5	0	5	0	473	51	2
Beans, white, canned	½ cup	153	8.25	0.22	0.11	29.25	0	5	0	7	96	3.9
Beans, white, split peas	½ cup	125	7	0.22	0.11	23	0	5.3	0	2	66	2.6
Broadbeans, fava	½ cup	93	5.5	0.22	0	17	0	4.4	0	4	31	1.3
Broadbeans, fava, canned	½ cup	91	6	0.11	0	16.25	0	4.5	0	580	34	1.3
Chickpeas	½ cup	138	6.5	1.67	0.11	24.75	0	4.8	0	183	39	2
Lentils	½ cup	115	7.75	0.22	0	20.25	0	2.8	0	2	19	3.3
Peas, black-eyed	½ cup	100	5.75	0.33	0.11	18.25	0	8.3	0	3	21	2.2
Peas, black-eyed, canned	½ cup	92	5	0.33	0.11	16.5	0	8.2	0	359	24	1.2
Soybeans, roasted	¼ cup	205	14.25	10.22	1.56	13.5	0	1.9	0	1	89	2
Tahini	1 tablespoon	92	2.5	7.33	1.11	3.75	0	1.5	0	10	109	2.2
Nuts, mixed	3 tablespoons	170	4.25	13.56	2.22	6.25	0	1.6	0	170	20	1.1
Peanut butter	2 tablespoons	190	9	14.56	2.78	4.5	2	2.4	0	150	11	0.6
Peanuts	3 tablespoons	164	6.25	12.33	1.78	5.25	0	2.5	0	110	7	0.5

Nutritional Content of Popular Items from Fast-Food Restaurants

Arby's

	Serving size	Calories	Protein	Total fat	Saturated fat	Total carbohydrate	Sugars	Fiber	Cholesterol	Sodium	Vitamin A	Vitamin C	Calcium	Iron	% calories from fat
	g		g	g	g	g	g	g	mg	mg	\% Daily Value				
Regular roast beef	158	400	23	20	7	36	N/A	3	40	1030	N/A	0	5	25	43
Super roast beef	247	530	24	27	9	50	N/A	5	40	1190	N/A	15	8	30	44
Fish fillet	223	540	23	27	7	51	N/A	2	40	880	N/A	2	8	20	45
Big Montana®	313	720	50	40	17	44	N/A	7	110	2270	N/A	*	8	50	49
French dip	200	490	30	22	8	42	N/A	3	56	1440	N/A	*	12	35	41
Turkey sub	303	670	30	39	10	49	N/A	3	60	2130	N/A	15	35	25	53
Light roast turkey deluxe	196	230	19	5	1	33	N/A	4	33	870	N/A	15	6	15	18
Grilled chicken deluxe	247	420	30	16	4	42	N/A	3	60	930	N/A	20	8	15	33
Cheddar curly fries	170	450	7	25	6	52	N/A	0	5	1420	N/A	20	20	2	48
Potato cakes	85	220	2	14	3	21	N/A	0	0	460	N/A	*	*	6	59
Honey French dressing	71	390	0	27	4	24	N/A	0	0	530	N/A	0	0	*	72
French-toastix	124	370	7	17	10	48	N/A	4	0	440	N/A	0	7	10	41
Jamocha shake	292	380	8	9	6	66	N/A	0	10	300	N/A	7	25	5	22

N/A: not available.   *Contains less than 2% of the Daily Value of these nutrients.

SOURCE: Triare Restaurant Group, 1998–2000, http://www.arbysrestaurant.com. Permission pending.

Burger King

	Serving size	Calories	Protein	Total fat	Saturated fat	Total carbohydrate	Sugars	Fiber	Cholesterol	Sodium	Vitamin A	Vitamin C	Calcium	Iron	% calories from fat
	g		g	g	g	g	g	g	mg	mg	\% Daily Value				
Whopper®	270	660	29	40	12	47	8	3	85	900	10	15	10	25	55
Whopper Jr.®	158	400	19	24	8	28	3	2	55	530	4	8	8	15	55
Double Whopper® with cheese	374	1010	55	67	26	47	8	3	180	1460	15	15	30	40	59
BK Big Fish® sandwich	252	720	23	43	9	59	4	3	80	1180	2	0	8	20	54
BK Broiler® chicken sandwich	247	530	29	26	5	45	5	2	105	1060	6	10	6	15	43
Chicken Tenders® (8 piece)	123	350	22	22	7	17	0	1	65	940	0	0	2	4	57
Ranch dipping sauce	28	170	0	17	3	2	N/A	N/A	0	200	N/A	N/A	N/A	N/A	94
Barbecue dipping sauce	28	35	0	0	0	9	N/A	N/A	0	400	N/A	N/A	N/A	N/A	0
Chicken sandwich	229	710	26	43	9	54	4	2	60	1400	0	0	10	20	55
French fries (medium, salted)	116	400	3	21	8	50	0	4	0	820	0	0	0	4	48
Onion rings (king size)	151	600	8	30	7	74	7	6	4	880	0	0	15	8	45
Chocolate shake (medium)	397	440	12	10	6	75	67	4	30	330	8	0	30	15	20
Croissan'wich® w/sausage, egg, and cheese	152	530	18	41	13	23	4	1	185	1120	8	0	15	15	70
French toast sticks (5)	113	440	7	23	5	51	12	3	2	490	0	0	6	10	48
Dutch apple pie	113	300	3	15	3	39	22	2	0	230	0	10	0	8	47

N/A: not available.

SOURCE: Burger King Corporation, 1996–1999, http://www.burgerking.com. Burger King® trademarks, trade name, and Nutirtional Guide are reproduced with permission from Burger King Brands, Inc.

Appendix C   Nutritional Content of Popular Items from Fast-Food Restaurants   C-1

Domino's Pizza

(1 serving = ¼ of a 12-inch or 14-inch pizza; 1 6-inch pizza)

	Serving size g	Calories	Protein g	Total fat g	Saturated fat g	Total carbohydrate g	Sugars g	Fiber g	Cholesterol mg	Sodium mg	Vitamin A IU	Vitamin C mg	Calcium mg	Iron mg	% calories from fat
14-inch lg. hand-tossed cheese	219	516	21	15	7	75	6	4	32	1080	920	0	261	4	N/A
14-inch lg. thin crust cheese	148	382	17	17	7	43	6	2	32	1172	875	0	315	1	N/A
14-inch lg. deep dish cheese	256	677	26	30	11	80	9	5	41	1575	1050	.5	335	6	N/A
12-inch med. hand-tossed cheese	159	375	15	11	5	55	5	3	23	776	657	0	187	3	N/A
12-inch med. thin crust cheese	106	273	12	12	5	31	4	2	23	835	624	0	225	1	N/A
12-inch med. deep dish cheese	181	482	19	22	8	56	6	3	30	1123	754	.4	241	4	N/A
6-inch deep dish cheese	215	598	23	28	10	68	7	4	36	1341	870	.5	295	5	N/A
Toppings: pepperoni	*	99	4	9	4	<1	<1	<1	21	364	6	.1	7	.3	N/A
ham	*	32	4	1	<1	1	<1	0	13	292	.7	.1	3	.3	N/A
Italian sausage	*	110	5	9	3	3	<1	<1	23	342	54	.1	16	.6	N/A
bacon	*	153	8	13	5	<1	<1	0	23	424	0	9	3	.4	N/A
beef	*	111	5	10	4	<1	<1	<1	21	309	.2	0	3	.5	N/A
anchovies	*	45	8	2	<1	0	0	0	18	790	15	0	50	1	N/A
extra cheese	*	68	5	5	3	1	<1	<1	16	228	294	0	117	.1	N/A
cheddar cheese	*	71	4	6	4	<1	<1	0	19	110	188	0	128	.1	N/A
Barbecue wings (1 average piece)	25	50	6	2	<1	2	1	<1	26	175	42	.1	6	.3	N/A
Hot wings (1 average piece)	25	45	5	2	<1	<1	<1	<1	26	354	136	1	5	.3	N/A
Breadsticks (1 piece)	37	116	3	4	<1	18	<1	<1	0	152	20	.1	6	1	N/A
Cheesy bread (1 piece)	43	142	4	6	2	18	<1	<1	6	183	92	.1	47	1	N/A

* Topping information is based on minimal portioning requirements for one serving of a 14-inch large pizza; add the values for toppings to the values for a cheese pizza. The following toppings supply fewer than 30 calories per serving: green and yellow peppers, onion, olives, mushrooms, pineapple.
† Contains less than 2% of the Daily Value of these nutrients.

SOURCE: Domino's Pizza, 1999, http://www.dominos.com. Reproduced with permission from Domino's Pizza LLC.

Jack in the Box

	Serving size g	Calories	Protein g	Total fat g	Saturated fat g	Total carbohydrate g	Sugars g	Fiber g	Cholesterol mg	Sodium mg	Vitamin A	Vitamin C	Calcium	Iron	% calories from fat
											% Daily Value				
Breakfast Jack®	126	280	17	12	5	28	3	1	190	750	8	6	15	20	39
Supreme croissant	163	530	23	32	13	37	6	0	225	960	8	6	10	10	55
Hamburger	103	280	12	12	4	30	5	2	30	490	2	2	10	20	39
Jumbo Jack®	267	590	27	37	11	39	10	2	90	670	10	15	15	25	56
Sourdough Jack	233	690	34	45	15	37	3	2	105	1180	15	15	20	25	59
Chicken fajita pita	187	280	24	9	4	25	5	3	75	840	25	0	15	15	29
Grilled chicken fillet	242	480	27	24	6	39	6	4	65	1110	8	15	20	25	46
Chicken supreme	237	570	21	37	8	39	5	3	70	1440	15	15	20	15	60
Ultimate cheeseburger	288	950	52	66	26	37	7	1	195	1370	15	1	30	40	62
Garden chicken salad	253	200	23	9	4	8	4	3	65	420	70	20	20	4	40
Blue cheese dressing	57	210	1	15	2.5	11	4	0	25	750	0	0	2	0	62
Chicken teriyaki bowl	502	670	26	4	1	128	27	3	15	1730	130	40	10	25	6
Monster taco	125	270	12	17	6	19	2	4	30	670	8	2	20	8	56
Egg rolls (3 pieces)	170	440	15	24	6	40	5	4	35	1020	15	20	8	25	50
Chicken breast pieces (5)	150	360	27	17	3	24	0	1	80	970	4	2	2	10	42
Stuffed jalapeños (10 pieces)	240	750	20	44	17	65	7	5	80	2470	30	50	45	10	53
Barbeque dipping sauce	28	45	1	0	0	11	7	0	0	310	0	4	0	0	0
Seasoned curly fries	125	410	6	23	5	45	0	4	0	1010	6	0	4	10	51
Onion rings	125	410	6	23	5	45	0	4	0	1010	4	30	4	15	51
Cappuccino ice cream shake	16*	630	11	29	17	80	58	0	90	320	15	0	35	0	41

*Fluid ounces

SOURCE: Jack in the Box Inc., 1999, http://www.jackinthebox.com. Reproduced with permission from Jack in the Box Inc.

KFC

	Serving size (g)	Calories	Protein (g)	Total fat (g)	Saturated fat (g)	Total carbohydrate (g)	Sugars (g)	Fiber (g)	Cholesterol (mg)	Sodium (mg)	Vitamin A	Vitamin C	Calcium	Iron	% calories from fat
											% Daily Value				
Original Recipe®: breast	153	400	29	24	6	16	0	1	135	1116	*	*	4	6	55
thigh	91	250	16	18	4.5	6	0	1	95	747	*	*	2	4	64
Extra Tasty Crispy™: breast	168	470	31	28	7	25	0	1	80	930	*	*	4	6	53
thigh	118	370	19	25	6	18	0	2	70	540	*	*	2	4	59
Hot & Spicy: breast	180	505	38	29	8	23	0	1	162	1170	*	*	6	6	53
thigh	107	355	19	26	7	13	0	1	126	630	*	*	2	4	63
Popcorn chicken (large)	170	620	30	40	10	36	0	0	73	1046	0	0	2	4	57
Honey BBQ Wings Pieces (6)	189	607	33	38	10	33	18	1	193	1145	8	8	4	8	57
Hot Wings® Pieces (6)	135	471	27	33	8	18	0	2	150	1230	*	*	4	8	63
Colonel's Crispy Strips™ (3)	92	261	20	16	4	10	0	3	40	658	*	*	*	3	54
Chunky chicken pot pie	368	770	29	42	13	69	8	5	70	2160	80	2	10	10	49
Corn on the cob	162	150	5	1.5	0	35	8	2	0	20	2	6	*	*	10
Mashed potatoes w/gravy	136	120	1	6	1	17	0	2	<1	440	*	*	*	2	42
BBQ baked beans	156	190	6	3	1	33	13	6	5	760	8	*	8	10	13
Potato salad	160	230	4	14	2	23	9	23	15	540	10	*	2	15	57
Cole slaw	142	180	2	9	1.5	21	20	3	5	280	*	60	4	4	44
Biscuit (1)	56	180	4	10	2.5	20	2	<1	0	560	*	*	2	6	44
Double chocolate chip cake	76	320	4	16	4	41	28	1	55	230	0	0	4	10	44
Pecan pie (slice)	113	490	5	23	5	66	31	2	65	510	4	0	2	8	41

*Contains less than 2% of the Daily Value of these nutrients.

SOURCE: KFC Corporation, 2000, http://www.kfc.com. Reproduced with permission from Kentucky Fried Chicken Corporation.

Taco Bell

	Serving size (oz)	Calories	Protein (g)	Total fat (g)	Saturated fat (g)	Total carbohydrate (g)	Sugars (g)	Fiber (g)	Cholesterol (mg)	Sodium (mg)	Vitamin A	Vitamin C	Calcium	Iron	% calories from fat
											% Daily Value				
Taco	2.75	170	9	10	4	12	<1	3	30	340	8	0	8	4	53
Taco Supreme®	4	210	9	14	6	14	2	3	40	350	8	6	10	6	57
Double Decker Taco Supreme®	7	380	15	18	7	39	3	9	40	760	8	6	15	10	45
Soft taco	3.5	210	11	10	4	20	1	3	30	570	8	0	8	6	43
Burrito Supreme®	9	430	17	18	7	50	4	9	40	1210	50	8	15	15	40
Big Beef Burrito Supreme®	10.5	510	23	23	9	52	4	11	60	1500	50	8	15	15	41
7-layer burrito	10	520	16	22	7	65	4	13	25	1270	30	10	20	20	38
Beef Gordita Supreme®	5.5	300	17	14	5	27	4	3	35	550	2	6	15	10	40
Chicken Gordita Santa Fe™	5.5	370	17	20	4	30	3	3	40	610	4	6	15	10	49
Big Beef MexiMelt®	4.75	290	15	15	7	22	2	4	45	830	10	0	20	6	48
Taco salad with salsa	19	850	30	52	14	69	12	16	70	2250	290	50	30	35	55
Taco salad w/o shell	16.5	430	25	22	10	36	12	15	70	1990	150	50	30	25	47
Beef Chalupa Baja™	5.5	420	14	27	7	30	3	3	35	760	6	8	15	15	57
Chicken Chalupa Santa Fe™	5.5	440	17	26	6	30	2	2	40	560	4	8	10	10	57
Steak Chalupa Supreme™	5.5	360	17	20	7	27	3	2	35	500	2	6	15	15	50
Big Beef Nachos Supreme	7	440	14	24	7	44	3	9	35	800	8	6	15	15	48
Nachos BellGrande®	11	760	20	39	11	83	4	17	35	1300	10	8	20	20	46
Pintos 'n cheese	4.5	180	9	8	4	18	1	10	15	640	45	0	15	10	44
Mexican rice	4.75	190	5	9	3.5	23	<1	<1	15	750	100	2	15	8	42

SOURCE: Taco Bell Corporation, 1999, http://www.tacobell.com. Reproduced with permission from the Taco Bell Corporation.

Wendy's

	Serving size	Calories	Protein	Total fat	Saturated fat	Total carbohydrate	Sugars	Fiber	Cholesterol	Sodium	Vitamin A	Vitamin C	Calcium	Iron	% calories from fat
	g		g	g	g	g	g	g	mg	mg		% Daily Value			
Single w/everything	219	420	25	20	7	37	8	3	70	930	6	10	15	25	43
Big Bacon Classic	282	580	33	31	12	45	11	3	95	1500	15	20	25	30	48
Jr. hamburger	118	280	15	10	3.5	34	7	2	30	610	2	2	10	20	32
Jr. bacon cheeseburger	166	390	20	20	8	34	7	2	55	870	8	10	15	20	46
Grilled chicken sandwich	189	300	24	8	1.5	36	8	2	55	730	4	10	10	15	23
Garden veggie pita	257	400	11	17	3.5	52	8	6	15	780	60	90	15	20	38
Caesar vinaigrette pita dressing	17	70	0	7	1	1	0	0	0	170	0	0	2	0	86
Caesar side salad (no dressing)	92	110	9	6	2.5	6	1	1	15	600	35	25	15	6	45
Grilled chicken salad (no dressing)	338	190	22	8	1.5	10	5	4	45	680	120	60	20	10	42
Taco salad (no dressing)	468	380	26	19	10	28	8	8	65	1040	45	45	35	25	45
Blue cheese dressing (2T)	28	180	1	19	3.5	0	0	0	15	170	0	0	2	0	94
Ranch dressing, reduced fat (2T)	28	60	1	5	1	2	1	0	10	240	0	0	2	0	83
Soft breadstick	44	130	4	3	0.5	23	N/A	1	5	250	0	0	4	9	23
French fries (Biggie®)	159	470	7	23	3.5	61	0	6	0	150	0	15	3	7	43
Baked potato w/broccoli & cheese	411	470	9	14	2.5	80	6	9	5	470	35	120	20	25	28
Baked potato w/chili & cheese	439	630	20	24	9	83	7	9	40	780	20	60	35	30	35
Chili, small, plain	227	210	15	7	2.5	21	5	5	30	800	8	6	8	16	29
Chili, large w/cheese & crackers	363	405	31	16.5	7	37	8	7	60	1380	14	10	22	26	36
Chicken nuggets (5)	75	230	11	16	3	11	0	0	30	470	0	2	2	2	61
Frosty™ dairy dessert, medium	298	440	11	11	7	73	56	0	50	260	20	0	41	8	23

N/A: not available.

SOURCE: Wendy's International, Inf., 2000, http://www.wendys.com. Reproduced with permission from Wendy's International, Inc.

Monitoring Your Progress

Name _____ **Section** _____ **Date** _____

As you completed the 11 labs listed below, you entered the results in the Preprogram Assessment column of this lab. Now that you have been involved in a fitness and wellness program for some time, do the labs again and enter your new results in the Postprogram Assessment column. You will probably notice improvement in several areas. Congratulations! If you are not satisfied with your progress thus far, refer to the tips for successful behavior change in Chapter 1 and throughout this book. Remember—fitness and wellness are forever. The time you invest now in developing a comprehensive, individualized program will pay off in a richer, more vital life in the years to come.

	Preprogram Assessment	Postprogram Assessment
LAB 2-1 Activity Profile	Light activity: _____ hours Moderate activity: _____ hours Vigorous activity: _____ hours Stairs climbed: _____ flights _ Exercise index: _____ Classification: _____	Light activity: _____ hours Moderate activity: _____ hours Vigorous activity: _____ hours Stairs climbed: _____ flights Exercise index: _____ Classification: _____
LAB 3-1 Cardiorespiratory Endurance 1-mile walk test 3-minute step test 1.5-mile run-walk test Åstrand-Rhyming test	$\dot{V}O_{2max}$: _____ Rating: _____ $\dot{V}O_{2max}$: _____ Rating: _____ $\dot{V}O_{2max}$: _____ Rating: _____ $\dot{V}O_{2max}$: _____ Rating: _____	$\dot{V}O_{2max}$: _____ Rating: _____ $\dot{V}O_{2max}$: _____ Rating: _____ $\dot{V}O_{2max}$: _____ Rating: _____ $\dot{V}O_{2max}$: _____ Rating: _____
LAB 4-1 Muscular Strength Maximum bench press test Maximum leg press test Hand grip strength test	Weight: _____ lb Rating: _____ Weight: _____ lb Rating: _____ Weight: _____ kg Rating: _____	Weight: _____ lb Rating: _____ Weight: _____ lb Rating: _____ Weight: _____ kg Rating: _____
LAB 4-2 Muscular Endurance 60-second sit-up test Curl-up test Push-up test	Number: _____ Rating: _____ Number: _____ Rating: _____ Number: _____ Rating: _____	Number: _____ Rating: _____ Number: _____ Rating: _____ Number: _____ Rating: _____

	Preprogram Assessment	Postprogram Assessment
LAB 5-1 Flexibility Sit-and-reach test	Score: ____ in. Rating: _____	Score: ____ in. Rating: _____
LAB 6-1 Body Composition Body mass index Skinfold measurements (or other method for determining percent body fat) Waist circumference Waist-to-hip-circumference ratio	BMI: _____ kg/m² Rating: _____ Sum of 3 skinfolds: _____ mm Percent body fat: _____% Rating: _____ Circumference: _____ Rating (√ high risk): _____ Ratio: _____ Rating (√ high risk): _____	BMI: _____ kg/m² Rating: _____ Sum of 3 skinfolds: _____ mm Percent body fat: _____% Rating: _____ Circumference: _____ Rating (√ high risk): _____ Ratio: _____ Rating (√ high risk): _____
LAB 8-1 Daily Diet Number of servings Number of servings Number of servings Number of servings Number of servings	Milk, cheese, etc.: ____ Meat, poultry, fish, etc.: ____ Fruits: ____ Vegetables: ____ Breads, cereals, rice, etc.: ____	Milk, cheese, etc.: ____ Meat, poultry, fish, etc.: ____ Fruits: ____ Vegetables: ____ Breads, cereals, rice, etc.: ____
LAB 8-2 Dietary Analysis Percentage of calories Percentage of calories Percentage of calories Percentage of calories	From protein: _____% From fat: _____% From saturated fat: _____% From carbohydrate: _____%	From protein: _____% From fat: _____% From saturated fat: _____% From carbohydrate: _____%
LAB 9-1 Daily Energy Balance	Approximate daily energy expenditure: ____ cal/day	Approximate daily energy expenditure: ____ cal/day
LAB 10-1 Identifying Stressors	Average weekly stress score: ___	Average weekly stress score: ___
LAB 11-1 Cardiovascular Health CVD risk assessment Hostility assessment	Score: ____ Estimated risk: ____ Score: _____ Rating: _____	Score: ____ Estimated risk: ____ Score: _____ Rating: _____

Index

Boldface numbers indicate pages on which glossary definitions appear. A "*t*" indicates that the information is in a table.

abdominal belts and back injuries, 133
abdominal curl, 98
ACE (American Council on Exercise), 31
across-the-body stretch, 121
ACSM. *See* American College of Sports Medicine (ACSM)
active stretching, **118**, 119–120
additives in food, 217
adenosine triphosphate (ATP), **42**–43
    immediate energy system and, 43
    oxidative energy system and, 44
adipose tissue, 146, **147**
adolescents, exercise program design and, 176–177
aerobic, **42**, 43–44
aging and older adults
    diet planning for, 214
    exercise for, 46
    exercise program design and, 176–177
agonist muscle groups, **75**–76
alcohol use
    nutritional content of alcoholic beverages, B-4
    wellness and, 6
alternate leg stretcher, 124
altitude and exercise, 57
alveoli, **42**
amenorrhea, 150, **151**
    female athlete triad condition, **149**
American College of Sports Medicine (ACSM), 27–28, 29, 31, 77, 120
American Council on Exercise (ACE), 31
American Heart Association, on obesity, 147
amino acids, 194, **195**
amino acid supplements, 81*t*, 82
amphetamines, athletes and, 83
anabolic steroids, 80, 81*t*, 82
anaerobic, **42**, 43
anemia, **202**
anorectic drugs, 83–84
anorexia nervosa, female athlete triad condition, **149**
antagonist muscle groups, **75**–76
antioxidants, **200**, 201, 205
aorta, 40, **41**
appetite suppressants, 83–84
Arby's, nutritional content of popular items, C-1
arteries, **41**
arthritis, exercise program design and, 175
assessments
    body composition, 157–162
    cardiorespiratory endurance level, 61–66
    desirable body weight, 163–164
    dietary analysis, 235–238
    fitness facility, 113–114
    flexibility, 137–142
    Food Guide Pyramid versus your daily diet, 231–234
    lifestyle evaluation, 17–18
    muscular endurance, 107–110
    muscular strength, 103–106
    physical activity profile, 35–36
    postprogram assessments, D-1 to D-2
    safety of exercise (PAR-Q), 37–38
asthma, exercise program design and, 175–176
Åstrand-Rhyming cycle ergometer test, 49, 63–65

athletes
    amphetamine use by, 83
    diet planning for, 214–215
    female athlete triad condition, **149**
    See also sports
ATP. *See* adenosine triphosphate (ATP)
atrium, 40, **41**

BAC. *See* blood alcohol concentration
back bridge, 130
back extensions, 98
back injuries
    abdominal belts and, 133
    See also low-back pain
ballistic stretching, **118**, 119
behavior change
    developing a plan, 10–12
    health journal sample, 11
    personal contracts for, 12, 13
behaviors, wellness and, 3–6
bench press, 88, 93
beverages, nutritional content, B-3 to B-4
BIA (bioelectrical impedance analysis), 153
biceps curl, 90
bicycles, bicycling program, 183–184, 185*t*
bioelectrical impedance analysis (BIA), 153
blood alcohol concentration (BAC), 3
blood pressure, 44
    cardiorespiratory endurance exercise and, 45
    See also hypertension
blood vessels, 41–42
BMI. *See* body mass index
Bod Pod, 153
body composition, 24, **25**, 145–164
    assessing, 150–154
    assessment calculations, 157–162
    distribution of body fat, 147, 149, 153–154
    exercise and, 154, 155
    importance of, 146–150
    ratings table, 161
    resistance exercises and, 99
    sports and fitness activities for, 168*t*–169*t*
    strength training and, 70
body mass index (BMI), **151**–152
    calculating, 157
body weight
    determining desirable weight, 163–164
    determining target weight, 154
    wellness and, 6
    See also obesity
Borg scale, 52
breads, cereals, rice, and pasta group, 207
    nutritional content of, B-4 to B-5
    recommendations versus average American diet, 210*t*
    whole-grain types of, 209
bulimia nervosa, female athlete triad condition, **149**
Burger King, nutritional content of popular items, C-1
butter, 223–224

caffeine, athletes and, 83
calculations, body composition, 157–162
caliper, **152**–153
calorie costs, 170–**171**
    bicycling, 185*t*
    in-line skating, 188*t*
    sports and fitness activities, 168*t*–169*t*
    swimming, 186*t*
    walking/jogging/running program, 181*t*
calories, expended per day in physical activity, 21–22, 23

cancer, cardiorespiratory endurance exercise and, 46
capillaries, 41–42
carbohydrates, 198–**199**
    daily intake goals, 197
    recommended intake, 199
cardiorespiratory endurance, **23**–24, 39–68
    assessing, 47–50
    assessing level of, 61–66
    benefits of exercise for, 44–47
    cautions and fitness prerequisites for assessments, 50
    exercise effects on, 49
    exercise program design, 51–53
    exercise program worksheet, 67–68
    physical activity pyramid and, 28
    physiology of exercise for, 40–44
    sports and fitness activities for, 168*t*–169*t*
cardiorespiratory system, 40–42
cardiovascular disease (CVD), **47**
    cardiorespiratory endurance exercise and, 46
cellular metabolism, cardiorespiratory endurance exercise and, 45
cellulite, 155
certified organic, **220**
cheese. *See* milk, yogurt, and cheese group
children
    DRIs for, 228*t*–229*t*
    exercise program design and, 176–177
    RDAs for, 230*t*
cholesterol, **195**
    butter and margarine compared, 223–224
    cardiorespiratory endurance exercise and, 46
chromium picolinate, 81*t*, 83
chronic disease, **2**
    cardiorespiratory endurance exercise and, 46–47
    death from, 4*t*
    quality of life and, 3
cigarette smoking, 6
clenbuterol, 83
clonidine, 82
cocaine, athletes and, 83
collagen, **117**
collars for weights, 79
college students, diet planning for, 213–214
commitment. *See* motivation and commitment
concentric muscle contraction, 74, **75**
consumer issues
    dietary supplement labels, 216
    exercise equipment, 58
    food labels, 216
    footwear for exercise, 172–173
    health clubs, choosing, 33
contracts. *See* personal contracts
cooking tips for food safety, 219
coronary heart disease (CHD), **47**
    cardiorespiratory endurance exercise and, 46
    See also cardiovascular disease
creatine monohydrate, 81*t*, 83
cross-training, 56, **168**–169
cruciferous vegetables, **205**
crunch, 91
curl-up, 91
Cybex. *See* exercise machines
cycle ergometer test, 49, 63–65

daily log
    for personal fitness plan, 171
    See also food journal
Daily Values, **206**
dairy group. *See* milk, yogurt, and cheese group
death
    causes of in the U.S., 4*t*